ASHTANGA YOGA

Yoga in the Tradition of Śrī K. Pattabhi Jois

Petri Räisänen

IN MEMORIAM

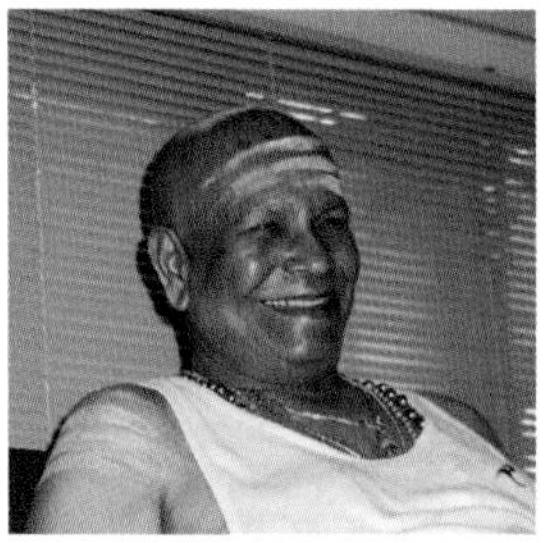

Yogāsana-viśārada Vedānta-vidvān
Śrī Krishna Pattabhi Jois

FULL MOON DAY JULY 1915 – MAY 18, 2009

My deepest gratitude for Gurujī;
for his knowledge, love and work
in making this world a better place.
You made our lives a miracle.
Let your light always shine.

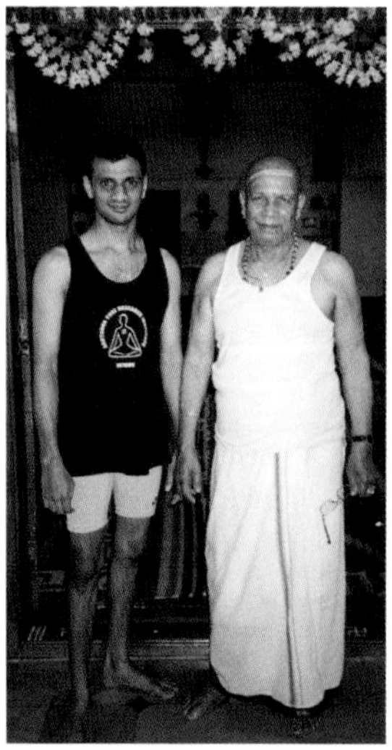

ASHTANGA YOGA

Yoga in the Tradition of Śrī K. Pattabhi Jois

THE DEFINITIVE PRIMARY SERIES PRACTICE MANUAL

Hence an aspirant, by the grace of his guru and constant practice of yoga,
can someday realize, before casting off his mortal coil,
the Indweller that is of the nature of supreme peace and eternal bliss.

Śrī K. Pattabhi Jois, *Yoga Mala*

Petri Räisänen AUTHOR AND MODEL

Alexander Berg PHOTOGRAPHER

Nicole Rassmuson GRAPHIC DESIGNER AND ILLUSTRATOR

Erica Berg TRANSLATOR

Magnus Nygren PRODUCER

YOGAWORDS

Ashtanga Yoga
Yoga in the Tradition of Śrī K. Pattabhi Jois
The definitive primary series practice manual

First published in 2005 by Bokförlaget Prisma in Swedish translation as *Kraften bakom yoga, Ashtangayogans åtta delar enligt Śrī K. Pattabhi Jois*

This revised and updated English language edition first published by YogaWords Ltd 2013

Published in the English language by arrangement with Otava Group Agency, Helsinki, Finland

Based on Śrī K. Pattabhi Jois' interviews (R. Sharath Jois, translator; recorded by Petri Räisänen) in Mysore, 2003–2004. Edited in 2013.

ISBN 978-1-906756-05-5

British Library Cataloguing-in-Publication Data
A catalogue record for this book is available from the British Library

Printed and bound in the EU by Graficas 94, Spain

This book has been printed on paper that is sourced and harvested from sustainable forests and is FSC accredited

YogaWords Ltd
32 Clarendon Road
London N8 0DJ

www.yogawords.com

I dedicate this book

ASHTANGA YOGA

Yoga in the Tradition of Śrī K. Pattabhi Jois

to my teacher, my guru

Yogāsana-viśārada Vedānta-vidvān

Śrī Krishna Pattabhi Jois

with deep gratitude

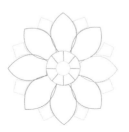

contents

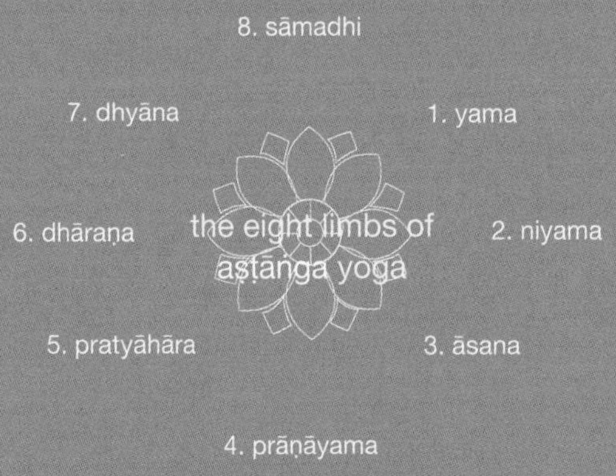
8. sāmadhi
7. dhyāna
1. yama
6. dhāraṇa
the eight limbs of aṣṭāṅga yoga
2. niyama
5. pratyāhāra
3. āsana
4. prāṇāyama

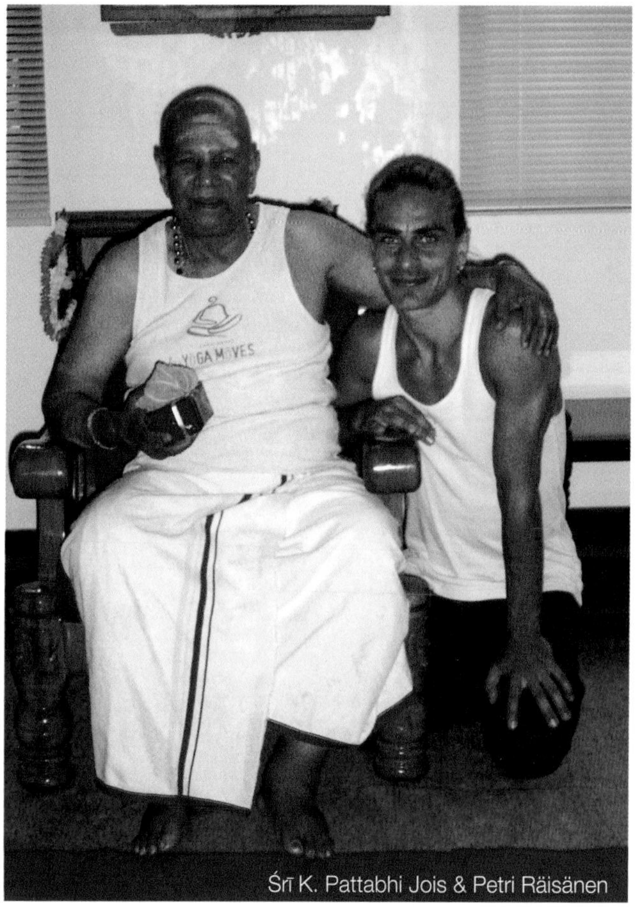

Śrī K. Pattabhi Jois & Petri Räisänen

translator's note

When translating this in-depth and layered text from Swedish, I was already working from a translation of the original Finnish version. Having known Petri over the years, and through discussing together his intentions with this book, I hope to have honored the original tone of Petri's writing.

foreword

Aṣṭāṅga yoga has become popular worldwide, and teachings from ancient yogic texts are now accessible to people everywhere. These texts tell us that with regular practice it is possible to attain a healthy body and mind and to realize the Self, our innermost soul, which in its nature is eternal peace, limitless freedom and happiness.

It is important for students to practice āsana (yoga postures) in the correct order and to follow the exact vinyāsa method. It is in this way that the body, mind and spirit can develop intelligence and harmony.

Petri Räisänen's fine book honors the tradition of Aṣṭāṅga yoga. I have gone through the vinyāsa techniques in all of the āsanas with him, and discussed philosophical questions that affect the practice, and I give my blessing to Petri and to this book. I hope that this book reaches a wide audience of readers, so that the teachings and beauty of yoga continue to spread.

Lokāḥ samastāḥ sukhino bhavantu (May all beings be happy and prosperous).

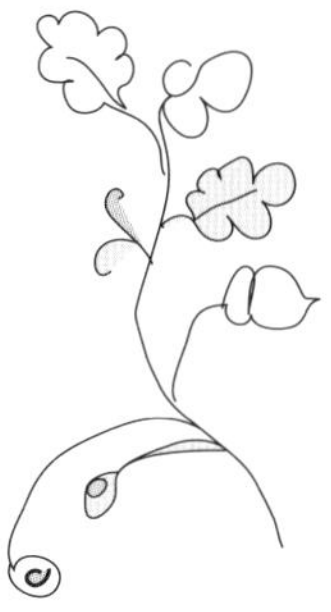

ŚRĪ K. PATTABHI JOIS

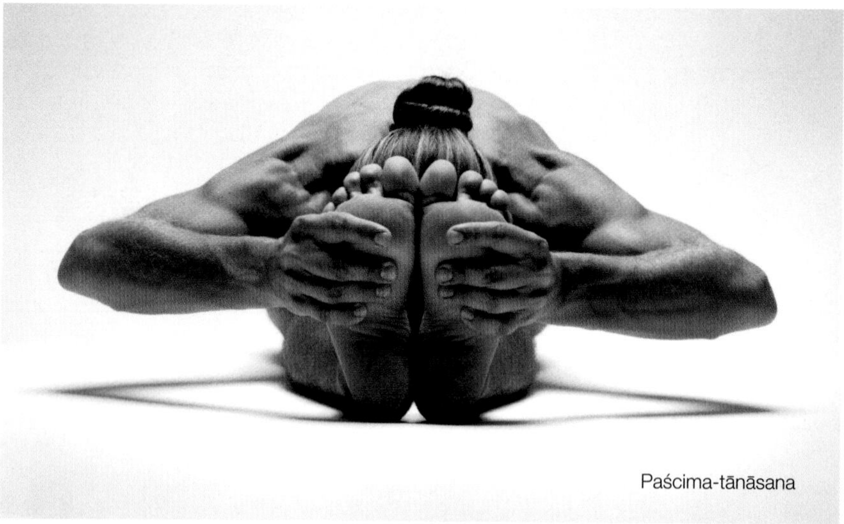
Paścima-tānāsana

introduction

The living tradition of Aṣṭāṅga yoga

Aṣṭāṅga yoga is a practice and philosophy that develops one's psychological and spiritual health. It has been kept alive for thousands of years from one generation to the next by being passed on through a lineage of gurus. It has not endured by staying fixed in the past, rather it is a living tradition that has maintained its integrity while adjusting to people's needs and the demands of the time. Aṣṭāṅga Yoga is not bound to one particular religion, political lineage or any other association. What this yoga tradition does do is connect us to the life-force that flows through all beings, and most importantly, remains grounded in a deep sense of respect for the gurus, for it is they who uphold and form the knowledge made accessible to us through practice.

Śrī K. Pattabhi Jois studied for over two decades with his guru, T. Krishnamacharya. From this period of intense study, complemented with the study of holy texts, through his own practice and teaching efforts to thousands of students, his knowledge of Aṣṭāṅga Yoga has been spread worldwide.

I have had the great blessing and fortune of studying with Śrī K. Pattabhi Jois and came to see that he deeply honored the traditional relationship of guru and student in that he was always willing to answer questions with endless generosity. It is through the generous sharing of this knowledge that has made this book possible. I have noticed over the years that many variations of Pattabhi Jois's Aṣṭāṅga yoga system have cropped up. It is my intention and hope that with this book I can clarify and pass on, as best I can, the traditional form of Aṣṭāṅga yoga, and how it is practiced in Mysore today.

My own path within Aṣṭāṅga yoga began on September 21,1989. I was twenty-two years old, interested in different cultures, religions and philosophies, and friends recommended that I should try Aṣṭāṅga yoga. I had played ice hockey for many years and stretched a bit after hockey practice, but nothing could compare to what I felt in that first yoga class. In my first class, led by Tove Palmgren, we were taken through the entire Primary series. I felt like I had stretched my body for the first time in my life. I felt I had truly encountered my body in an entirely new way. After class, my entire body shook with fatigue and I nearly choked with laughter from deep within. I was so sore I could barely walk for a week, yet I was full of excitement, as if I had just met my first love. I went to class again the following week, and the next. Later on that year, Derek Ireland and Radha Warrell, who were health and beauty personified, gave a workshop in Helsinki. I was further inspired by Derek and Radha and traveled to their school in Crete, deepening my connection and love for the practice. Over the span of the next five years, my visits to the yoga shala went from weekly to bi-weekly, and soon after extended to four and five times a week. Eventually I took on the traditional six-day-a-week practice. From the years of ice hockey and soccer training in my youth, I was accustomed to intense physical activity and training, and though my body was quite strong, it was also stiff and heavy. It took nearly seven years of dedicated practice for me to feel my body transform into lightness and softness, which in turn carried my mind along for the ride . . . likewise softening and lightening it up.

In 1994 Lino Miele's book *Aṣṭāṅga Yoga under the guidance of Śrī K. Pattabhi Jois* was published. Lino came to Finland that same year, heralding the beginning of a new era of Aṣṭāṅga yoga in Finland. The practice became slower, deeper and more meditative. Lino taught my dear friend, Juha Javanainen, and me the vinyāsa-count system (p. 61), the āsana names in Sanskrit, and the opening and closing mantras (pp. 67-69). It was with Lino's help that I first traveled to India in 1996. I went to study with him at Kovalam Beach, along the Malabar coast in the south-western state of Kerala. I met the guru of Aṣṭāṅga yoga, Śrī K. Pattabhi Jois in Mysore, India in January 1997. Later on, in the same year, I changed my work as a massage therapist, bone-setter and folk-healer to become an Aṣṭāṅga yoga teacher. Juha and I also co-founded Astanga Yoga Helsinki in 1997. Our school has become what is now one of the world's largest schools that specializes in the pure and traditional form of Aṣṭāṅga yoga, with often more than 400 students per day. Juha went on to translate *Yoga Mala* from English into Finnish in 2002.

In 2000, I traveled to Boulder, Colorado, where Aṣṭāṅga yoga teacher Richard Freeman had organized a two-week workshop with Pattabhi Jois. I remember sitting at his feet during the evening discourses and wondering, "How could he have answered all of my questions without even hearing them?" His depth of knowledge and gentle presence burrowed themselves into my heart and I felt that I had found my guru without even having searched for him. Shortly after, I traveled to New York City, where I met my fifth yoga teacher, Eddie Stern, who first translated Pattabhi Jois's *Yoga Mala* into English from its original language of Kannada in 1999. In addition to following religious Hindu traditions and running a South Indian Hindu temple in NYC, Stern's style of teaching and knowledge of yoga made a deep impression on me, and I felt as though I was walking along the rich path towards yoga's noble yet humble goal.

Back in Helsinki, in 2001, Pattabhi Jois and his family honored us greatly by coming to visit our school. During that visit, Pattabhi Jois and his grandson Sharath authorized Juha and me to continue teaching the traditional Aṣṭāṅga yoga method. For one unforgettable week, alongside Jois' daughter Saraswati, and Sharath, his grandson, Pattabhi Jois taught, shared and met over a hundred students at our school in Helsinki. This encounter was documented in the video "Meeting with Gurujī." They returned to Helsinki in 2006 and Sharath came on his own in 2009 and 2011.

It was never my intention to write a book on Aṣṭāṅga yoga. My own knowledge and understanding of yoga, Indian culture and Sanskrit has felt small and insignificant, and it seemed impossible to accept the offer to write this book. Upon recalling Pattabhi Jois's words in *Yoga Mala*, "This is because they get their information from books on the practice of yoga written by the people who want to spread word of the science of yoga out of a love and respect for it, but without knowing it properly themselves," I thought of all the yoga books, ranging widely in quality and accuracy, that have come out in this time of yoga's booming popularity. Well aware of the risks in choosing to write a book on the science of yoga and its background, I still felt called to share this practice that had transformed my life. I have seen too many modifications of the āsanas, inexperienced teachers and books that don't capture Aṣṭāṅga yoga's multi-faceted beauty, and I have done my best to offer this book as both an accurate documentation of the practice, as it presently stands in Mysore, and as a tool to open up the spirit of the practice.

The āsana technique described in this book may differ from how students learned in Mysore in the '60s or how it was practiced in the '80s, as Aṣṭāṅga yoga has significantly grown and shifted since Pattabhi Jois's first journey to North America in 1975. At that time, for example, āsanas were given out much more quickly; some students learned three series in just three months. Today, it would take about three years for a highly flexible and stable-minded student to accomplish the same. Some āsanas were practised in a different order than they are today, and prāṇāyama (breathing) practice was introduced after a few months of practice. Some readers will recognize other changes, such as Jānu-śīrṣāsana A, which used to be practised with the head to the knee whereas now practitioners bend forwards into a "chin-to-shin" position; or in Prasārita-pādottānāsana C, where the palms are often turned outwards instead of inwards. A further example can be found in Utthita-hasta-pādāṅguṣṭhāsana, when the leg was lifted up only to a

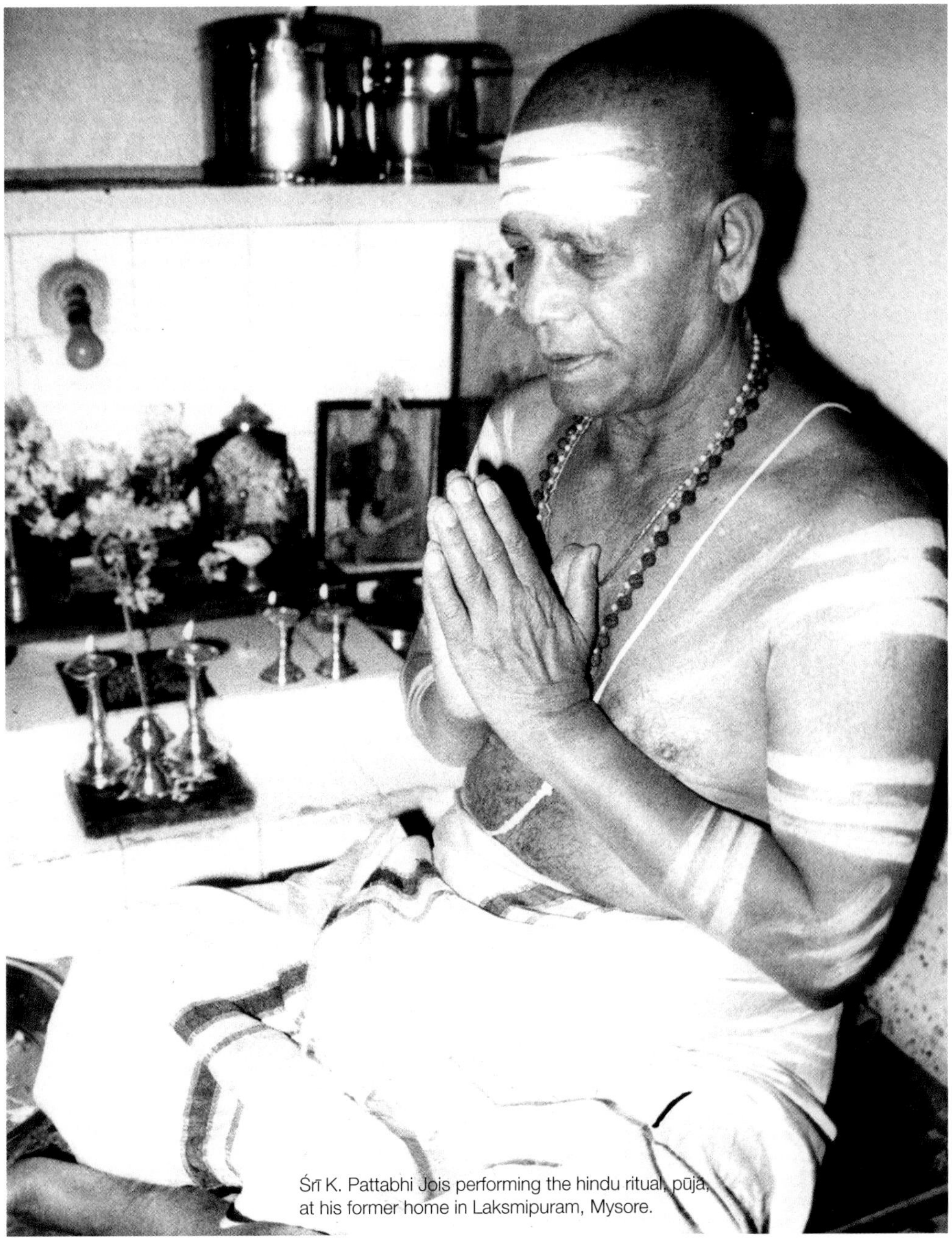
Śrī K. Pattabhi Jois performing the hindu ritual, pūjā, at his former home in Laksmipuram, Mysore.

horizontal level and the head placed down onto the knee. The dṛṣṭi (gazing points) have changed in many āsanas from the nose-tip to the big toe or from between the eyebrows to the nose-tip. While gathering the research for this book, I discovered many details that were new to me, such as the position of the back foot in the standing poses, which should be at a 85–90 degree angle, as well as a different breathing pattern in Utkaṭāsana and Vīrabhadrāsana. I also became aware of variations in the spelling and translation of the following āsana names: Tiryaṅ-mukhaikapāda-paścima-tānāsana is usually spelled Triang-, which means three parts (*tri-aṅga*); Ūrdhva-mukha-paścimottānāsana is often spelled Paścima-tānāsana. Gurujī used the letter "o" when describing

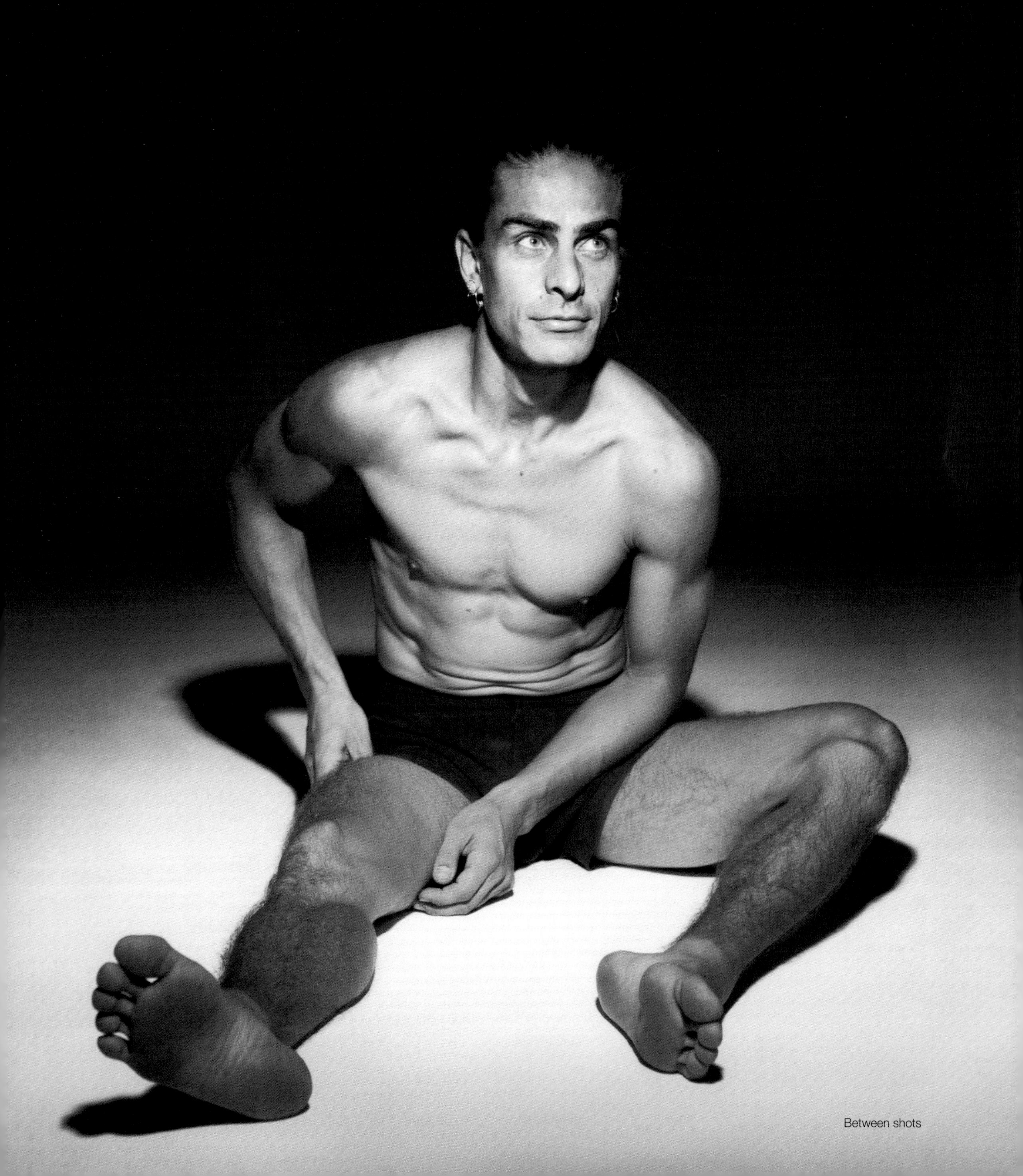

Between shots

an upright position like Ūrdhva-mukha-paścimottānāsana and the letter "a" in a horizontal position such as Paścima-tānāsana. The same goes for Pārśvottānāsana (upright) and Pūrva-tānāsana (horizontal).

In terms of pronunciation, Pattabhi Jois used the words samasthiti, utpluti and śānti in the nominative case, that is, ending with a *visarga* (samasthitiḥ, utplutiḥ and śāntiḥ, pronounced samasthitihi, utplutihi and śāntihi). This book follows Pattabhi Jois's usage of the terms.

Over time, a distinction has also developed between Western and Indian styles of āsana practice. The Western style often focuses excessively on "exact" outer alignment and incorporates an overly intense form of breathing, whereas in the Indian style one focuses more on conserving the body's energy and breath, while finding an internal alignment through sensing one's inner flow of energy. The practice has also been affected by varying trends developed primarily by Western yogis. At one point, students practised handstands as foundational āsanas, or would do Hanumānāsana and Sama-koṇāsana (front and side splits) after Prasārita-pādottānāsana D. Up until the end of the '80s, some people would practise both in the morning and evening. Towards the end of the '90s, Pattabhi Jois and Sharath Jois started to clear away extra vinyāsas and superfluous positions from the vinyāsa system. In 2006, Gurujī announced that his research had been completed and that the practice was ready to be taught in its essential form.

To verify that the information in the book is correct, follows the Indian tradition in its entirety, and is in accordance with Pattabhi Jois and his grandson, Sharath Jois (formerly known as Sharath Rangaswamy), I was fortunate enough to meet with them both every afternoon for two months in 2003 and 2004 at the office of the Aṣṭāṅga Yoga Institute in Mysore. I asked an endless number of questions and wrote fervently as they gave their time so generously. I would present the more detailed questions in English to Sharath, who would then translate them into Kannada (the Southern Indian language of Karnataka state) for Pattabhi Jois, whom I sat beside. Pattabhi Jois would think for a moment, and then reply by citing entire passages in Sanskrit and Kannada to Sharath, who then translated them back into English. We went through the vinyāsa technique and alignment for each posture extremely carefully; so carefully, indeed, that Pattabhi and Sharath laughed at my pedantic "Western" nature. They actually didn't want to give strict rules such as the alignment of the fingers, toes, or shoulders in various āsanas. Such details have to be learned straight from a teacher on an individual basis, keeping different body types and capabilities in mind. We spoke only briefly about the physical benefits of the postures since this information is covered so well in *Yoga Mala* and *Aṣṭāṅga Yoga*, and Pattabhi Jois recommended that I use these books to list the effects of each āsana. Pattabhi Jois and Sharath were also not terribly keen to give advice specifically for beginners, as the practice is meant to be learned directly through an experienced teacher or guru and only then can students receive the specific attention they need. I have, however, written some words of advice for beginners, so that they can understand as closely as possible the technique for the foundational āsanas, since practising these incorrectly not only reduces the efficiency of the benefits and effects of the āsana, but can be harmful as well.

The opening and closing mantras in this book are Pattabhi Jois's own English translations from my book on the intermediate series (2006–2007) which have been transliterated and edited by Sanskrit scholar, Måns Broo, and myself.

As a former Finnish folk-healer, I have been particularly interested in the parts of Aṣṭāṅga yoga which operate on the level of the body's energy flow, and I was able to receive advice from Pattabhi Jois and Sharath on these topics. This information appears in short chapters (Prāṇa, nāḍīs, vāyu and cakras p. 41–42) in this book. According to Pattabhi Jois and Sharath, comprehension of the latter limbs of Aṣṭāṅga is only necessary for a devoted practitioner, and to speak of these parts in a book about the Primary series is not essential. I have included them in this text as a way to further entice the new practitioner into the quieter and more subtle realms of this practice. This section is also of interest for those students who are already quite established in their practice and ready to explore other aspects of the yogic journey.

Writing this book did not come without a certain degree of sacrifice and difficulty, as my own teaching and workshop schedule continued throughout the entire writing process. It was written over a two-year period in seven different countries. I completed the first draft in 2003, written simply from my own experience and with a few widely known and well-reputed source materials for assistance, before making my yearly trip to India. When Pattabhi Jois, Sharath and I discussed the book, I saw that my knowledge and understanding had been faulty in many areas, and I understood that the references I had been using were often incorrect or no longer current. For example, I rewrote the section on āsana alone nine times while continuing to revise other sections of the book.

A shift in āsana practice has taken place since *Yoga Mala* was translated into English in 1999, which has caused some confusion. I myself had to change what I had learned and read in *Yoga Mala* as to how one did the postures in Mysore in 2004. With Sharath's permission, I decided to leave the dṛṣṭi (gazing points) for the sun salutations and yoga-mudrā as they are in Gurujī's book, but to mention which dṛṣṭi were being used in Mysore at the time. I also had to add one vinyāsa, with Gurujī's permission, to Ūrdva-mukha-paścimottānāsana.

Throughout the entire process, I witnessed my guru's wisdom in action, as he would spontaneously cite entire textual passages and speak on this science of yoga and how Aṣṭāṅga distinguishes itself from other styles of yoga. At first, I found myself confused by my guru's knowledge and noticed that if I asked the same question on a different day, using another choice of words, he would often respond with contradictory answers. At first this puzzled me, but then I began to see that he was answering according to my ability to listen on those days, or according to what I really needed to hear. It became necessary to ask the same questions on different days in order to get a broader answer. As a result of these interactions, I realized not only how fundamental a guru is for a student's development but also how the guru is essential in keeping the yogic tradition alive.

In meeting with Gurujī, I was most struck by his unbelievably warm and positive attitude towards me as a student, working to collect this knowledge and share it in a new book. It made an enormous impression on me that he had such a sense of responsibility for the knowledge of prāṇāyama practice and samantrika-mantras. He felt one can only learn these practices directly from him, or from students who have truly mastered these particular practices, and that it was not appropriate to include them in a book.

I would like to offer my greatest respects to Śrī K. Pattabhi Jois and R. Sharath Jois for their patience and love, for teaching from their deep source of knowledge and for giving their energy tirelessly, which continues to guide students along the path of yoga. I thank them from the bottom of my heart for all the support and knowledge they have given in the writing of this book, without which it would not have been possible or at the very least, meaningless.

how to use this book

Aṣṭāṅga Yoga: Yoga in the Tradition of Śrī K. Pattabhi Jois paints a broad but detailed picture of Aṣṭāṅga yoga. It discusses āsana practice, energy flow, yoga philosophy and spiritual development, and is written for both beginners and advanced practitioners alike. Ideally, the text should first be read through in its entirety, and after you have established a regular practice, the book will serve as a useful reference guide for such points as the vinyāsa counting system (p. 61) and the correct use of dṛṣṭi and bandhas (see symbols on pp. 56–57). Though the main focus of the book is to describe with clarity and in great detail how the āsana practice is done, much attention is given to other aspects of Aṣṭāṅga yoga, including its history and background. In the practice-manual part of the book, each āsana (posture, pose, or stance) is described in two ways:

1. In the main text, in addition to the āsana, I explain the breathing, gazing points (dṛṣṭi), energetic locks (bandhas), as well as the proper vinyāsa count, as it has been taught in Mysore, India. For each āsana, I describe where it begins, how it is done, and how to transition from one āsana into the next. Almost all the āsanas are depicted in a photograph, with a few illustrated in line drawings. In some cases, depending on the student's ability, there are a number of acceptable variations, such as ways to get into and out of the pose. These alternatives have been explained in further detail.
2. To supplement the main text, there is a chart on every āsana page that outlines the counting system of each vinyāsa. As Aṣṭāṅga yoga is built upon continuous movement, getting into and out of each pose is considered to be an essential part of the series and is counted in a systematic manner. In an effort to clarify this part of the practice and to document it in a clear manner, this information has been outlined in a chart on the side of the page. It can stand alone as a quick guide to help double check details, like dṛṣṭi, breathing and bandhas. Do note, however, that these charts are written in the traditional full-vinyāsa style, in which to count out the full system, one would return to Samasthitiḥ after each āsana. This is not how the practice is currently being done by most practitioners. To find the āsana as it is done today, follow the sequence in the area of the chart shaded in grey.

After describing how each āsana is performed, I have also included information regarding the physical, psychological and energetic benefits of the āsana, as well as tips for beginners. For the most part, these benefits have been described in *Yoga Mala*, and have been documented through practical observation and research, both over the thousands of years yoga has existed and through current, ongoing investigation. At times, the benefits described may not always have an immediate connection to modern allopathic medicine, and those with serious illnesses should consult a doctor before starting a yoga practice.

Beginners should keep in mind that the body's initial stiffness, level of strength and balance and overall ability will generally affect how one starts this practice. I have included "How To" information for beginners in each āsana that may differ from how one practises at a more proficient level. When the body and mind are ready for the original position, the student can follow the description of the āsana and vinyāsa without need for modification.

For all practitioners, regardless of any advice from the book, be sure always to listen to your own body and the signals it gives you, and keep its limitations, as well as capabilities, in mind. Remember that studying with an experienced teacher will be your best support in moving forwards safely and effectively in the practice. Take in each āsana and let it work on you. The practice aims to clean and strengthen both the body and mind, encouraging the practitioner towards a positive lifestyle. Coming to the practice with the right intention, one can find peace, happiness and self-acceptance even in the first session.

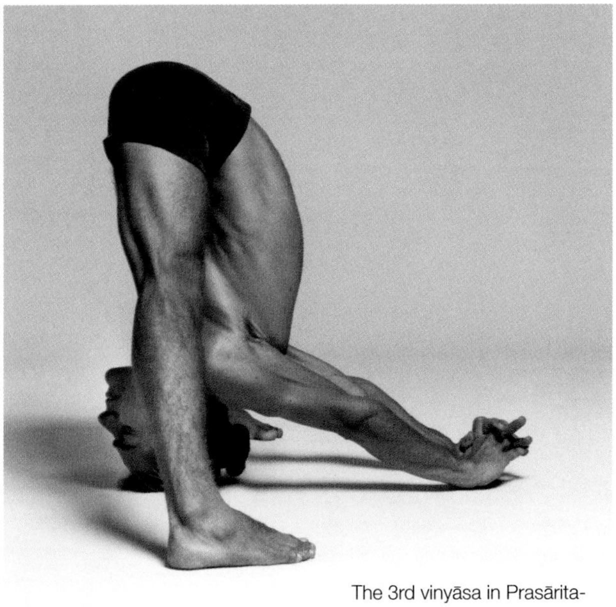

The 3rd vinyāsa in Prasārita-pādottānāsana C.

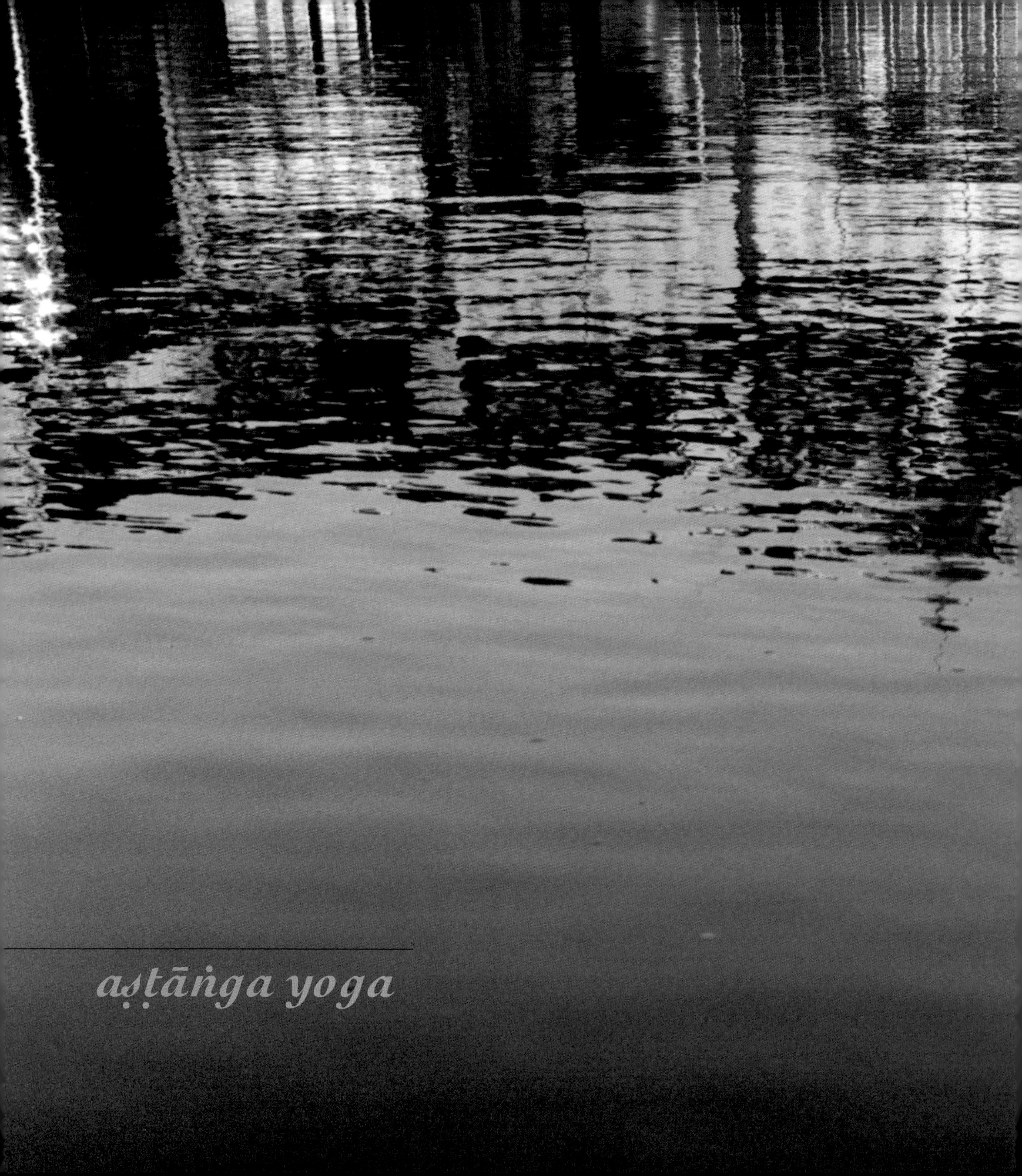

aṣṭāṅga yoga

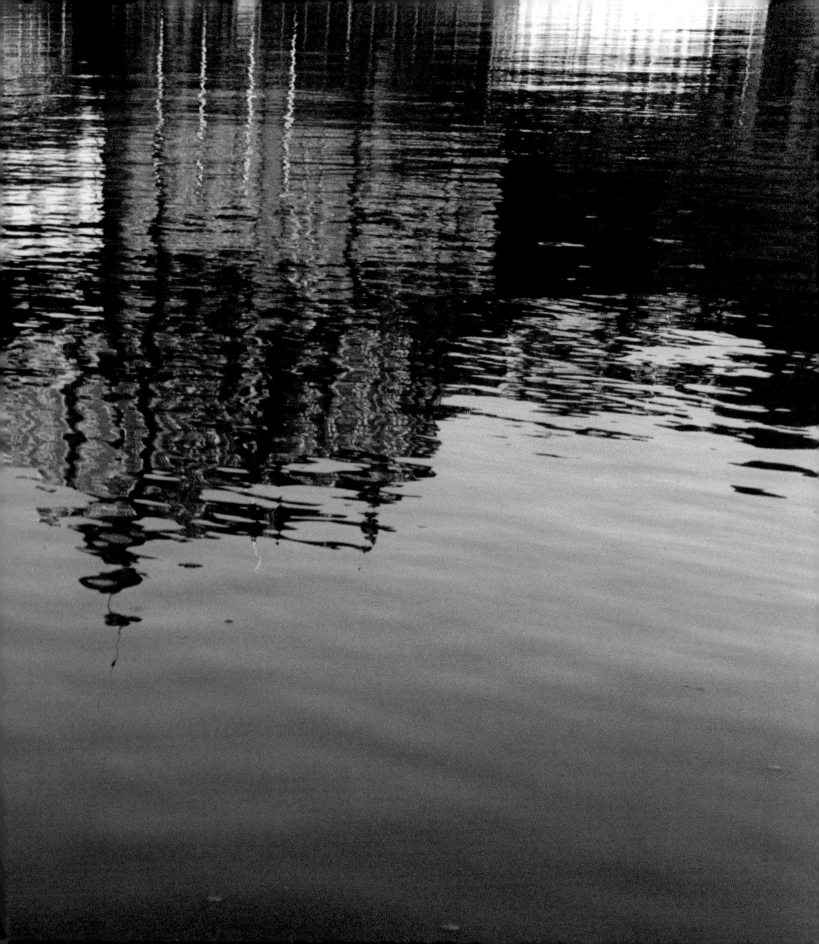

aṣṭāṅga yoga

Aṣṭāṅga yoga is often defined as an intense, athletic, and dynamic form of yoga. In many ways this is true, although Aṣṭāṅga does much more than just strengthen and stretch the body. By practising with awareness of breath, correct use of the dṛṣṭi (gazing points) and the bandhas (energetic locks), one can develop a sense of consciousness in both the body and the mind. According to Śrī K. Pattabhi Jois, Aṣṭāṅga yoga is a path that leads us to our own spirit, to our very nature.

Aṣṭāṅga yoga literally means eight limbs (*aṣṭau aṅga*), which Ṛṣi Patanjali defined in the *Yoga-sūtra* approximately 2000 years ago. The *Yoga-sūtra* are based on the teachings of early texts such as the Vedas, this knowledge having been passed down orally from guru to student. This authentic process of giving and receiving the teachings of the yoga tradition is known as parampara or lineage, which Pattabhi Jois describes in Yoga Mala as, ". . . a noble, desireless action (the practice of yoga) . . . which has been passed down, in an unbroken tradition, since time immemorial."

Aṣṭāṅga yoga seems to encapsulate a wide-range of yoga forms, which are commonly referred to within the teachings of the subject. When Pattabhi Jois was asked what Aṣṭāṅga yoga is and is not, he couldn't limit it. For him Aṣṭāṅga yoga was karma, jñāna, bhakti, kriyā, japa, haṭha, tantra, rāja... all in one limitless, ancient form. It is a complete yoga, which includes the whole yogic view.

Reading and studying the philosophy of yoga found in ancient, holy texts is only a fraction of the practice. Books can describe the path of yoga for us, but they cannot provide us with the direct experience of yoga. As Pattabhi Jois was fond of quoting, "Aṣṭāṅga Yoga is 99% practice and 1% theory." He firmly believed that practical training is the only way to cleanse the body and mind of blockages and obstacles, and to activate the physical, mental and spiritual renewal processes which lead to freedom and happiness.

In Aṣṭāṅga practice, the breath, āsana, vinyāsa krama (vinyāsa technique), bandhas and dṛṣṭi are all used in conjunction with one another, serving to warm up the body, providing a safe and wonderfully intense release in order for the body to practice asana. This inner heat generates a cleansing process which affects everything from the muscles, organs and nervous system, to the mind, intelligence and spirit; all that is found in the physical and energetic kośas (sheaths of being) as well as in the more refined layers.

"Do your practice and all is coming." – *Śrī K. Pattabhi Jois*

Instructions

To really benefit from your practice, try to create the best possible environment, one that supports the proper conditions for the practice to take place in. This pertains to both the external and internal factors that could affect your concentration and general attitude or mood.

If you are just starting out, it is strongly recommended that you find a place to study with a professional teacher, preferably in a yoga shala (yoga center or room) that teaches traditional Pattabhi Jois Aṣṭāṅga yoga. It is always best to begin under the supervision of an experienced teacher or guru, as he or she can best observe your progress and understanding of the practice. Books can introduce one to āsana yet they can in no way replace a teacher and the chance to get personal feedback, nor can they provide for one's specific issues or needs.

The yoga shala (or practice room) should be kept clean, warm and draft-free. The air should be fresh and the atmosphere in the shala should give you a sense of composure. It is also recommended that the yoga shala be built of natural materials which breathe and bring positive energy to the āsana practice. In older shalas in India, the floor was made of dried cow dung, which was considered to be a pure and hygienic building material. It is not recommended that you practice on an uneven floor, outside, in a damp cellar, or in a place without proper air circulation.

Yoga is, for the most part, inexpensive. It doesn't require much: only light-weight clothing that allows for free movement and perspiration. It is helpful to use a yoga mat, both to soften contact with the floor and to provide proper grip or traction. If you sweat excessively, bring a small hand towel to dry the mat and your surrounding area as you practise. In some āsanas, a mat alone may not provide enough cushioning, in which case a blanket designed for yoga practice or a cotton mat may be useful. These can also help the teacher when adjusting the student, as in the forward-bending postures.

Since yoga focuses so much on the breath, taking in the pranic energy found in fresh air, which occurs during respiration, it is highly recommended that you practise with a clean body and fresh, odor-free clothes. This is not only considerate for your own practice, but also for the other people in the shala. It's best to shower before yoga class, or at the very least wash your feet and armpits. After every practice, your clothes and hand towels should be washed. Everyone has a different constitution, and some people will naturally sweat more than others. Be mindful of your mat and cotton blankets and wash them as often as necessary to keep them clean and neutral in smell.

It is crucial to practise on an empty stomach. Do not eat for at least two hours, or drink for at least fifteen minutes, prior to doing āsana practice. You should not eat or drink anything, including water, during the practice. It is much easier to get into some of the more intense stretches, particularly the forward-bending or twisting poses, when the stomach is empty. It is also much more effective to access the bandhas (muscle and energy locks) on an empty stomach, while practising with a full stomach can cause cramping and, at times, nausea.

Before, during and after practice, it is important that everyone contributes to a pleasant and focused environment, free from interruption or disturbance. This means that the shala should remain as silent as possible, in respect for the teacher, other students and your own internal process. If you find you have philosophical questions that arise or any questions related to the āsanas that are not urgent, I suggest waiting until you have finished your practice and discussing them with your teacher at that time. You may find that some questions are unavoidable, and sometimes a teacher may speak or give verbal instructions during a Mysore class. For the most part, however, the less conversation there is in the shala, the better.

Set aside plenty of time afterwards for your body and mind to settle and recover. You may drink fluids after you have taken rest, although one should wait at least half an hour before eating, as the body needs time before it is ready to digest and benefit from the nutrients.

The best time to practise is in the morning, when the air is richest in prāṇa (life-giving energy), the mind has not yet become activated with excessive thought, the body is rested and the stomach is empty. Doing āsana in the morning will open and energize the body and mind for the rest of the day. On the other hand, be aware that it can take time to get accustomed to this routine, and the body is often stiffer in the morning than in the evening. Evening practice is also acceptable if it suits your rhythm or schedule better, or if it simply feels better, although traditionally there is no practice after sunset.

It is not a goal within Aṣṭāṅga yoga to you forget the outside world and develop an obsessive focus on the inner world of your own body and mind. Avoid the appeal of fanaticism. Yoga should be a source of support and strength for your everyday life, and should improve the quality of your life on all levels. Regarding how many poses you should do and how frequently, listen truthfully to your inner thoughts and feelings, and keep to the reality of your body's capabilities as well as your situation and phase in life. This should help you decide how much to do and when to stop. If you are going to a yoga shala, your teacher will be your best guide and partner in this developmental process.

Traditionally, the practice is done six mornings a week, with Saturday as the day of rest. Rest days are also taken on full and new moon days and on holidays. For women, it is not advised to do āsana during the first three days of menstruation, nor during the first trimester of pregnancy and the first three months postpartum (see p. 185).

Aṣṭāṅga yoga is beneficial for anyone interested, stiff or flexible, fit or unfit. You progress at your own level and in your own time, listening to your body, breath and mind. To stay motivated, it is important that you establish the right pace for yourself, moving forwards at a calm and steady pace. Resist the urge to compare yourself to others, as everyone benefits from this system of yoga in his or her own way.

This method is not intended for children under the age of twelve, as their bones have not yet fully grown, although it is perfectly safe and quite beneficial for them to learn about yoga āsana playfully, keeping a focus on the breath. There is no limit as to how old one can be and still maintain a practice. Āsana can be adjusted to the individual at the various stages of life. However, when pregnant or when experiencing serious illness, undergoing surgery or other acute ailments, you should speak with a doctor prior to engaging in any form of physical activity. The practice should never be done while sick with a fever or flu, or under the influence of alcohol, drugs or strong medicine. After an illness has passed, it is recommended to take at least one day of rest before beginning again gently. For example, if you already do Intermediate or Advanced series, start again with the Primary series for some time. After a long period of serious illness, discuss with your yoga teacher and doctor as to the best way to begin again, how quickly you should proceed, and which postures may be particularly beneficial for your recovery. It is more helpful, of course, if your medical doctor has some knowledge and understanding of yoga in general, and Aṣṭāṅga yoga in particular.

Aṣṭāṅga yoga opens the body up in a safe and natural way. Ujjayī breathing (pp. 52–53), the rhythm of the movements within the vinyāsa system, the drawing-in of the bandhas, and the heat generated in the body all lower the risk of injury. Despite this, one should avoid using too much strength or force in the postures, otherwise it may actually be detrimental to take on more strenuous āsana sequences. One should not be overly zealous in the practice either, as this can lead to injury. Always listen to your body, which will tell you where your limits are as well as when it feels beneficial to go deeper into a posture. For example, you can stretch forwards even if you feel tight and try to release the tension through deep, relaxed breathing. If you feel pain, ease up a bit. It will come when it is ready. We are not meant to perform āsana in exactly the same way everyday; some days the body will release deeply into the postures, and other days one will feel heavy and tight.

In addition to the healthy development of the body, Aṣṭāṅga yoga will purify and calm the mind. This system works on deep and subtle levels and, at times, certain memories or experiences from the past will arise. This is a healthy and natural part of the process. Each negative experience we have gone through lodges itself inside us as a blockage. In order for us to be freed from these experiences, we must let them resurface again and go through them once more, in a final farewell. Keep breathing and remember that as each experience is brought up and passes through us, we create more peace and clarity for the mind.

Study the order of the poses, the breathing and movement system (vinyāsa), and the names of the postures. This will clarify the practice, improve your concentration, and make it easier for you to communicate with your teacher and ask questions specific to any particular poses.

It is perfectly fine to continue with other kinds of physical activity while incorporating Aṣṭāṅga yoga into your life. In fact, the flexibility and inner strength gained through Aṣṭāṅga yoga can help improve other activities and reduce the risk of injury, as most injuries come from the body being too tight or stiff. If one continues with other physical forms of activity, it is highly advisable to adjust the yoga practice and make it useful and energizing, as opposed to working too intensely and draining both the body and mind.

Over time, yoga will bring about a positive change in a student's body and mind, including lifestyle choices such as diet as well as an overall approach to health. The practice develops naturally as the student's trust in it grows. Students often find that the biggest obstacle along the way is not, for example, inflexibility in the body or weakness in their muscles, but rather an inflexibility of the mind.

Often, the more you advance, the less you obsess with the need to achieve. Patience is cultivated. Small steps forwards, both physical and psychological, erase doubt and give you the energy to continue on along the path. Try to take note of your progress while giving yourself permission to regress once in a while, since progress doesn't always necessarily travel in an upwards, linear direction. At certain times, it may be useful to stay in an āsana longer than five breaths – one can stay anywhere from ten breaths up to three hours. It can be necessary sometimes to go "backwards" in order to restore the body's energy balance. With the right attitude, yoga is a genuine path towards meeting your true self, where you are happy and already content with the present moment, as it is.

There are three different ways to perform the vinyāsa between, and within, the postures:

1. Advanced practitioners who have the strength and flexibility to follow the vinyāsa count will keep working in the way described in the book.
2. The second option is for students who take a bit more time and effort to get into the āsanas and require a lighter option. Change sides from right to left without jumping back. You can jump back when you finish both sides of the āsana, to transition into the next one.
3. This is for people with pain or weakness, where jumping back would cause more pain, as opposed to bringing positive benefits. Do the āsanas in the same order as described in the āsana section, but skip the jumping-back section. Try to avoid pain. Breathe deeply and slowly, making it enjoyable. When you feel better and stronger, start to follow option two, and eventually the first vinyāsa technique.

Styles of practice

There are two traditional ways in which Aṣṭāṅga is taught: in a led class, where the vinyāsa system is counted out loud, or in a Mysore-style class, with everyone going through the āsana series individually, at his or her own pace, under the supervision of the teacher. When you cannot get to a class, you can do self-practice at home.

In a led class, the teacher counts out the vinyāsa and says the name of each āsana in Sanskrit, stating each inhalation and exhalation that comes with the āsana. The teacher establishes an even rhythm that the students follow together and gives verbal instructions for the alignment of the posture, the holding of the bandhas and which dṛṣṭi to use. In this way, one learns Aṣṭāṅga's exact vinyāsa technique to be followed in both a Mysore class and during self-practice. After learning the vinyāsa technique and sequence of the positions in a led class, it is easier to continue in a Mysore-style class.

In Aṣṭāṅga yoga, the word vinyāsa refers to the system in which each movement is linked either to an inhalation or an exhalation. In between each sthiti (state) of an āsana, there are a series of movements that link one āsana to the next. It is worth mentioning here that the new, trendy yoga styles like vinyāsa or vinyāsa-flow are not the same as Aṣṭāṅga yoga's vinyāsa krama (vinyāsa technique).

In Mysore-style, students move through the series independently, following their own rhythm and breath. The teacher gives mostly physical, hands-on adjustments, although he or she may also give verbal adjustments or instructions when necessary. The teacher may also count out the āsana or vinyāsa movements, or the rhythm of the breathing, if a student has forgotten the order or if some correction is needed. In a Mysore class, the teacher comes to know each student's process and can observe his or her individual development. The teacher also determines when a student is ready for new āsanas or poses. This readiness is a very individual thing, and often comes when a student can perform the preceding āsana with ease and fluidity. However, it may also come when the student needs the next challenge for their progress to continue. "Mysore- style" is named after the town in which Pattabhi Jois lived and taught for several decades. At his yoga shala, the teachings are primarily done in this manner, although over the years, led classes have been taught on Fridays and Sundays.

"Self-practice" is done at home, when traveling or when it is not possible to get to a class or shala. If and when you are alone, try to create a space that will best serve your needs, remembering that you should practise indoors, in a calm, clear space, with clean, warm air. You should also do your best to limit any interruptions that may arise, for example by turning off the telephone or keeping pets in another room.

In keeping with tradition, it is most favorable to have a teacher or a guru to guide you, as this is the fastest, safest and most rewarding way to learn, and ensures that you get the full benefits from the practice. If you find that you must do self-practice for many months of the year, I highly recommend that you take workshops or travel to Mysore to make sure you are still progressing correctly, not only in your physical form but with your breath, energy and intention.

Treatments

Yoga āsana and the traditional system of Indian medicine, āyurveda (āyur- life, veda- knowledge) go hand in hand. Treatments can include oil massage, oil baths, herbal medicine, exercise and analysis of one's body/mind constitution or doṣa: kapha: earth/oil, pitta: fire/water, vāta: air/ether. These treatments aid in creating better diet and lifestyle choices and habits. When needed, they can also assist in the purification process and are recommended for the yoga practitioner.

Food

Eating healthy, nutritious, vegetarian food is an essential part of yoga. Our food is broken down into vitamins, minerals, trace elements and bindu, or life-power (Amṛta-bindu, pp. 46–47), and is incorporated by the seven dhātus (p. 46) throughout the body. The quality of our food directly affects the body's ability to absorb the nutrients it needs in order to feel well. If possible, eating ecologically grown, biodynamic or organic food is recommended. Take into consideration the manner in which the food was grown, how it was treated, packaged and shipped, as every aspect affects the overall compound energy of the food.

Yoga practice will make you more sensitive and capable of sensing the relationship between the food we eat and our overall sense of well-being. Take things in small steps, just like in the development of āsana. The same diet does not work for everyone, and if you make sudden, radical changes in your diet, it may cause too much stress on the body. On the other hand, if you make dietary changes slowly and consciously, your body and mind will feel a natural urge to give up heavy, unhealthy, low-quality foods, and even other toxins found in cigarettes, alcohol or drugs. You will notice over time that your body will effortlessly turn towards lighter food and your mind will make healthier lifestyle choices in an attempt to maintain the sattvic (pure, clean) feeling one receives from consistent practice and through leading a simple yogic life.

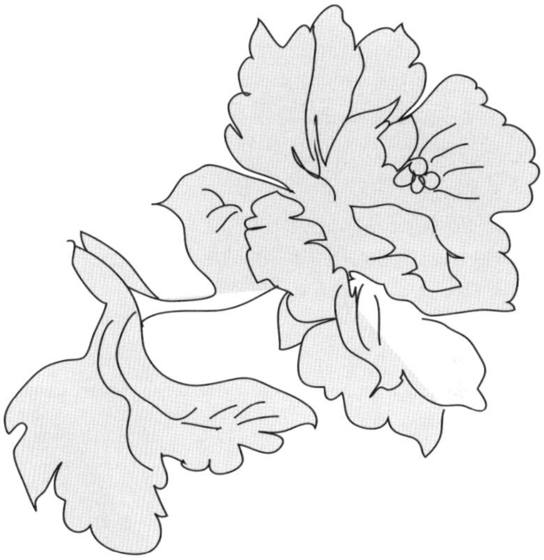

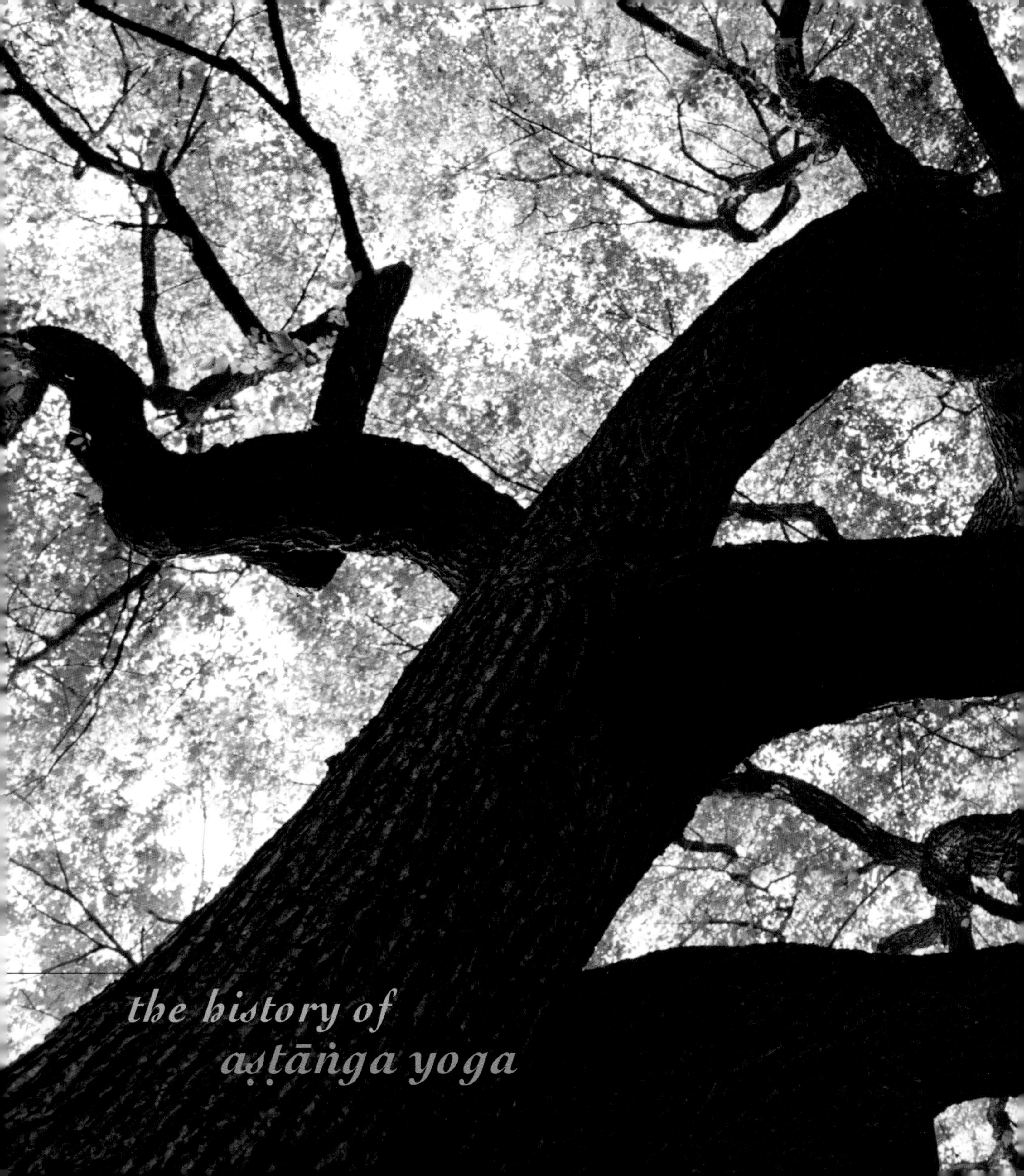

the history of aṣṭāṅga yoga

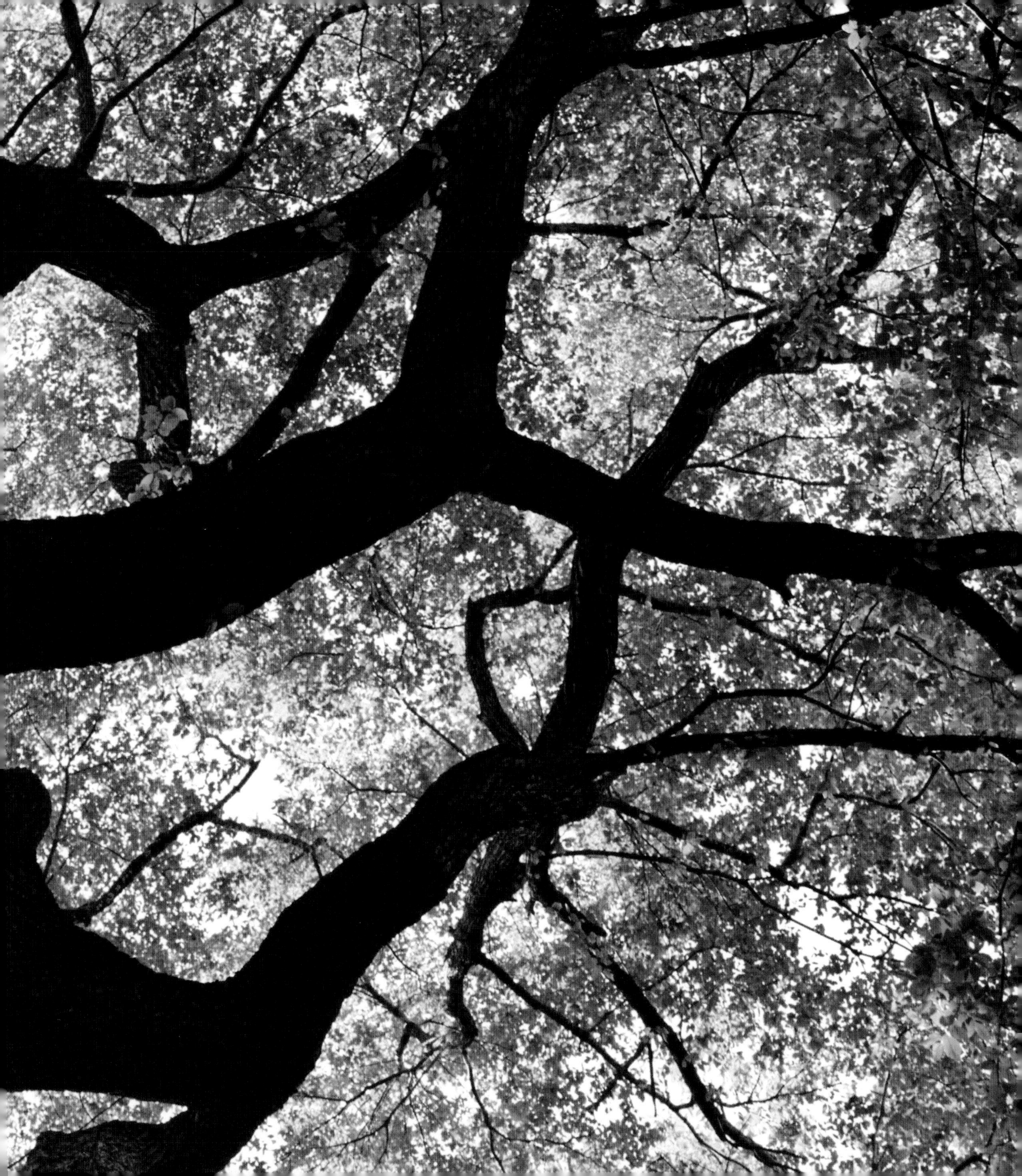

the history of aṣṭāṅga yoga

According to ancient holy texts, the history of yoga is as long as the history of mankind. In Indian mythology there are 330 million gods and goddesses, heroes and heroines, most with supernatural strength and mental and physical powers (siddhis) which are said to be the result of sustained yogic discipline.

More recent research and sources claim that yoga began more than 5,000 years ago. During that time, Aryan high culture reached the Indus Valley in the north of India. There they formed the four-part categorization system known as varṇa (class or color), more commonly referred to as the caste system. Later on, these Aryans came to be known as the Indo-Aryans, and knowledge of their spiritual traditions and yogic philosophy began to spread throughout the region and beyond. These teachings spread via oral tradition and through texts written on palm leaves. In this way, yoga became one of India's well-known systems of philosophy.

Six main philosophical schools developed, of which sāṃkhya and yoga are two. Sāṃkhya is considered to contain yogic theory while yoga contains the practical aspect of yoga. The four remaining schools are Nyāya, Vaiśeṣika, Mīmāṃsa, and Vedānta. These six philosophies explain various ways in which one can develop the body, mind, intellect and spirit. They have something to offer everyone from the religious and spiritual to the non-religious and atheist.

The first Indo-Aryan texts are the basis of all yoga and Indian spiritual texts. These include the four Vedas: *Ṛg-veda*, *Sāmaveda*, *Yajuveda* and *Atharvaveda*. The *Ṛg-veda*, written circa 1500 BCE is among the world's oldest spiritual texts. Often referred to as Vedānta, or the end of the Vedas, the *Upaniṣads* followed the Vedas. Next came the *Purāṇa* texts, Patanjali's *Yoga-sūtra*, and the epic poems, the *Mahābhārata*, which includes the *Bhagavad-gītā* and the *Rāmāyaṇa*, where Āditya-hṛdayam (prayer to Āditya, the sun deity) can be found. All of these texts expound on yogic philosophy to varying degrees of emphasis. Texts more directly related to the practices of yoga were written much later; these include the *Yoga-vaśiṣtha*, *Śiva-saṃhitā*, *Gheranda-saṃhitā*, *Haṭha-yoga-pradīpikā*, *Yoga-yajñavalkya-saṁhitā* and *Yoga-tārāvalī*.

These texts document and preserve an ancient oral tradition which has been passed on from guru to student. "Gu" means darkness, "ru" means lightness; and the "Guru" leads the student out of the dark and into the light, from ignorance into awakening. The wisdom within yoga had been kept secret among the brahmin families before the appropriate time came to spread the teachings out in order to serve and benefit humanity.

Ṛṣi Patanjali

The wise Bhagavan Patanjali is referred to as the pioneer and father of Aṣṭāṅga yoga. His work, the *Yoga-sūtra* or *Patanjala Yoga Darśana* (darśana - philosophical sight) defines Aṣṭāṅga yoga's eight limbs (disciplines or parts), from the practice of āsana to descriptions of yoga's ability to refine the body and mind, and, ultimately, lead to fundamental freedom (kaivalya). His way of illustrating the sūtras (lit. thread; aphorism, verse) has provided the blueprint for yoga masters throughout the ages to interpret and provide commentary on the sūtras.

There is very little historical knowledge of Patanjali's life and existence. It is claimed that Patanjali was also the author of the Mahābhāsya, the commentary for Pāṇinī's Sanskrit grammar as well as for the Caraka's classic āyurveda text. Some resources claim his birth place to be Gonarda, Trinkomale, India. Based on recent research, it is generally accepted that he lived somewhere between 200 BCE and 300 CE.

In Indian mythology, it is said that Patanjali is connected to the god Viṣṇu, and that Patanjali is, in fact, an incarnation of Ādiśeṣa, Lord Viṣṇu's living divan and 1,000-headed serpent. In whichever form he actually manifested, we can be thankful for the teachings he left behind. They define the practice of yoga today, which continues to spread and remain vital for the lives of so many, throughout India and the world.

Patanjali's sūtras reveal his enormous sensitivity and knowledge of the effects of yogic practices as well as his contact with non-rational states of mind and supernatural forces.

The *Yoga-sūtra* are organized in four chapters (pādas) and describe the yogic practices, their effects, and the possibilities of reaching the highest possible state (sāṃkhya view) – to revert human nature, prakṛti, to the original, pure consciousness, puruṣa.

1. *Samādhi-pāda* (absorption), means the path of samādhi (one-pointed contemplation, absorption). The first part of the text defines yoga and its goal, the human condition (chitta vritti), the obstacles in the mind to reach the goal of yoga, and the solutions to these afflictions.
2. *Sadhana-pāda* (practice), contains the definitions of kriyā-yoga (sūtra 2:1), as well as the eight limbs of yoga (sūtra 2:29), and the descriptions of the first five limbs, as well as the qualities needed to develop sensitivity in the mind and perception of the higher self. The first five limbs open the path to spiritual development by purifying the body and mind and accessing the spirit.
3. *Vibhūti-pāda* (powers) describes the power and possibility of the mind when distraction has been removed. This chapter also describes the sixth, seventh and eighth limbs.
4. *Kaivalya-pāda* (detachment, liberation) speaks of the mind's final insight: detachment of the mind (manas) and intellect (buddhi) from nature (prakṛti) and absorption with pure consciousness (puruṣa).

Ṛṣi Vāmana

What we know of Ṛṣi Vamana's life can be found in shlokas (verses) or śāstras (scriptural texts), teachings and legends passed on by oral tradition. Facts about the sages' personal lives were not passed down orally in the same way as their teachings were. According to Pattabhi Jois, the *Yoga Korunta* is considered to be Ṛṣi Vāmana's greatest work. It was written on palm leaves bound together to create a book, as was commonly done at the time, and contained most of the Aṣṭāṅga yoga series that T. Krishnamacharya taught Śrī K. Pattabhi Jois from 1927–1953.

One of the most well-known sentences in the *Yoga Korunta* is a key phrase regarding the approach we should keep in mind when practisng, "Vinā vinyāsa-yogena āsanādāīn na kārayet." ("Oh, yogi, do not do āsana without vinyāsa"). According to Ṛṣi Vāmana, it is the vinyāsa, the linking of breath and āsana in a continuous rhythm, that creates the tapas (heat) which initiates the purification process in the organs and nervous system, and provides the meditative quality, without which, āsana practice could be dangerous or ineffectual, at the very least. To our disappointment, for those of us used to accessing knowledge through books, the *Yoga Korunta* is completely lost. It is widely believe that this was due to the appetites of termites. Pattabhi Jois's book, *Yoga Mala*, was about to suffer the same fate, until his students rescued the original text from the attic above the shala. It is comforting to know that, while we don't have direct access to his book, Ṛṣi Vāmana's teachings survive to this day, through the efforts of T. Krishnamacharya and Pattabhi Jois, which continue to bear fruit through the teachings and work of their students in turn.

Śrī Tirumali Krishnamacharya

(title: Mīmāṃsa-tīrtha Vedānta-vāgīśa Sāṃkhya-yoga-śiromaṇi Śrī) According a number of biographies, Śrī T. Krishnamacharya (1888–1989) was given the best possible start in life. He was born in 1888, on 18th November to a well-respected yogic family in Muchukundapuram (Karnataka, Southern India). His father was Srinivasa Tatacharya and his mother was Ranganayakiamma, and it was his family tree (which can be found in the text, *Yoga-rahasya*) that led him to the sage Nāthamuni (born 823 CE). Nāthamuni fathered the Vaiṣṇava religious lineage, which honors Viṣṇu as the head god. When Krishnamacharya was five years old, he started learning Sanskrit and was initiated into the practice of yoga by his father, in the Yamunacharya tradition, named after Nāthamuni's grandchild (917–1042 CE). In order to carry on the teachings, his father also prepared him for his duties as the eldest son and educated him in the family's history.

Krishnamacharya began his studies under his father's gurukula (an place for study over a prescribed period of time). He woke up at two o'clock every morning and studied Vedānta, yoga āsana, Sanskrit, and religious rituals including pūjā, a daily offering made to the ishta devata (family god) Hayagriva, Lord Viṣṇu's horse-headed form. When Krishnamacharya was ten years old, his father died quite suddenly. His mother and her six children, of whom Krishnamacharya was the eldest, moved to Mysore, where his grandfather was the spiritual leader of one of India's most renowned spiritual schools, Brahmatantra Parakala Math. He took the boy under his wing and Krishnamacharya studied Vyakarana (Sanskrit grammar), Vedānta (Vedānta philosophy), Tarka (logic), and Sāṃkhya, the theoretical aspect within yoga.

As a 15-year old, he fulfilled one of his dreams and traveled on his own to his relatives' temple, Sathakopa in Alvar Tirunagar, Tamil Nadu, India. It is said that there, outside the temple, under a tamarind tree, he met his master, Nāthamuni, who gave him the holy text, *Yoga-rahasya*. Krishnamacharya was not satisfied with merely reading about the wisdom held within yoga, so in 1911 with the encouragement of his Banarasian (also called Varanasi) teacher and yoga charya (yoga master) Ganganath Jhan, he walked more than 120 miles to reach an area near Lake Manasarovar and Mt. Kailash. In this region of the Himalayan mountains, he was to meet his intended guru: the yoga master Yogisvara Śrī Ramamohan Brahmachari of Mukti Narayana Kshetra, Nepal.

There began what would become a seven-and-a-half year long relationship (gurukula) between guru and student. During this period, Ramamohan Brahmachari taught him more than 700 yoga poses (āsana) and the most essential breathing exercises (prāṇāyama). He also taught Krishnamacharya the health benefits of each āsana, and which ailments can be healed from practising them. Krishnamacharya also became well-versed in mantra recitation, and familiar with the most important yogic texts, such as the *Yoga-sūtra* of Patanjali (*Patanjala Yoga Darśana*) and *Haṭha-yoga-pradīpikā* (his recommended book list is mentioned at the beginning of the first part of the Yoga Makaranda).

After this period of intense study, instead of asking for any kind of monetary payment for the teachings, Ramamohan Brahmachari gave his blessings to Krishnamacharya and advised that he go back to Mysore, start a family and teach yoga. This was to be Krishnamacharya's form of repayment to his guru. Krishnamacharya was also given his guru's sandals, symbolizing the journey along the path of holy learning. Before returning to Mysore, Krishnamacharya visited universities in Calcutta, Allahabad, Patna, Barodas and Varanasi to complete his studies in philosophy and religion, while simultaenously embarking on his calling to teach yoga.

He completed his studies in record time, and earned the highest grade possible in Mīmāṁsa (Mīmāṃsa-tirtha-Mīmāṃsan, Master in Yogic Theory), in Nyāya (Nyāyacharya-Nyāyan, Professor in Philosophical Logic), in Vedānta (Master in Vedāntic Philosophy) and in Sāṃkhya (Master in Sāṃkhya Philosophy). Besides his university qualifications, he studied Ayurvedic medicine, Vedic astrology and music, not to mention 16 of the languages spoken in India and Tibet.

Upon his return to Mysore, he described his travels and studies to his family, and explained that he was asked and chosen to be a teacher of yogic studies. Krishnamacharya established himself as a yoga teacher and Ayurvedic healer (*ayur*- life, *veda*- knowledge) at the palace of the Maharaja, Krishnarajendra Wodeyar IV. Krishnamacharya met the Maharaja in Varanasi in 1926, cured him of various illnesses and they became close friends. In the previous year (1925), Krishnamacharya married Srimati Namagiriamma, and the first of their six children was born in 1931. Their fourth child, T.K.V. Desikachar, who went on to become a prominent yoga teacher and author, was born in 1938.

Krishnamacharya also taught small groups in the surrounding area of Mysore, including Hassan (about a two-hour drive from Mysore) where Patthabi Jois studied with him from 1927–1929. In 1931, at the request of the Maharaja, Krishnamacharya founded a yoga shala (school), located in a wing of the Jaganmohan Palace in central Mysore and taught there for twenty-two years until it closed down in 1952. At the yoga school, Krishnamacharya made a name for himself through his demonstrations of āsana, his way of speaking, and his wide range of knowledge as a yoga teacher. However, as the Maharaja's influence waned once India gained independence in 1947, the school could no longer support itself and had to close, much to the dismay of Krishnamacharya's students and the school. Krishnamacharya taught for a few more years in Mysore, although he felt that his time in the Maharaja's city had come to an end.

As this was his life's calling and his promise to his guru, Krishnamacharya felt driven to spread yoga to other parts of India, so he started traveling and presenting yoga throughout many cities and villages. In 1953, he moved with his wife and children to Madras (Chennai) and continued his work with the healing practices of yoga and Āyurveda, working in smaller groups and on an individual basis. In 1975, his son T.K.V. Desikachar co-founded the Krishnamacharya Yoga Mandiram (KYM), a school that continues to spread his father's teachings. Krishnamacharya continued teaching in Chennai until his passing on February 28th, 1989.

In addition to his immense knowledge of yoga, Krishnamacharya was also highly regarded for his ability to heal and for his psychic powers. He was known for being able to adapt yoga practice to the individual body and for the student's specific needs. He often knew his patients' symptoms or complaints before they would tell him and he had an uncanny ability to determine whether or not his students had done their homework before they said a word. He also authored books on his several areas of expertise: *Yoga-makaranda* in 1934 (*The Nectar of Yoga*, published in English in 2011), *Dhyāna-mālikā (Preparations for Meditation), Yogāñjali-sāra (The Heart of Yoga)* and *Yoga-rahasya (Yoga's Mystery)*. He gained world-wide visibility through the efforts of his son T.K.V. Desikachar, who wrote *The Heart of Yoga* (1995) and *Health, Healing and Beyond* (1998), as well as through his grandson, Desikachar's son, Kausthub Desikachar, who wrote Krishnamacharya's biography, *The Yoga Of The Yogi* (2005). One of Krishnamacharya's later students, A.G. Mohan, wrote another biography, *Krishnamacharya* (published in 2010) which provides an insightful perspective on the yoga master's life and teachings.

To prove the effects of āsana practice on the breath, mind and inner organs, Krishnamacharya demonstrated the results of his exercises to a French doctor in 1939. To the doctor's amazement, he was able to stop his breath and his pulse slowed down until his heart stopped beating completely. This technique, known as khecarī-mudrā (not recommend without proper guidance) has been described in texts like *Haṭha-yoga-pradīpikā* and *Gheranda-saṃhitā*.

Krishnamacharya is often considered to be the father of this modern era of yoga and a life's worth of commitment towards the subject continues to inform yoga teacers and students to this day. Krishnamacharya's teachings have been passed on through five prominent students who taught, or still teach, what they learned from their guru: Śrī K. Pattabhi Jois (began practising in 1927), B.K.S. Iyengar (began in 1934), Indra Devi (Krishnamacharya's first female and Western student, began in 1937), his son T.K.V. Desikachar (began in 1960) and A.G. Mohan (began in 1971). Due to the efforts of these individuals, not to mention Krishnamacharya's less well-known children and family members, this particular system towards the understanding of the self, which had all but died out during Krishnamacarya's time, continues to provide benefit for its practitioners and devotees of yoga.

Śrī K. Pattabhi Jois

(title: Yogāsana-viśārada Vedānta-vidvān)

Śrī Krishna Pattabhi Jois was born into a brahmin family (Hoysala Karnatakans caste) under a full moon (Guru Pūrṇimā day) in July 1915, in Kausika, near Hassan, Mysore district. The family followed the Smarta Sampradaya religious view and worshipped its founder Ādi-Śaṅkarācārya (788–820 CE) as their family guru. Jois' father was an astrologer, priest and landowner, and his mother cared for the home and their nine children. K. Pattabhi Jois was the fifth child, and when he was five years old, his father began to teach him Sanskrit, astrology, mantras (religious chants from the Vedas), slokas (verses), and brahmin rituals. He also began school that same year (1920) in Hassan.

Pattabhi Jois began practising Aṣṭāṅga yoga at the age of 12. He had seen a demonstration and heard a speech given by T. Krishnamacharya in Hassan's community hall in March, 1927, both of which affected him greatly. Two days later, after intense questioning by T. Krishnamacharya, Pattabhi Jois stood on a mat as a student (sasthaka) of Krishnamacharya and received his first lesson under his soon-to-be guru. He practisāed with him daily for a period of two years.

The path of yoga was not considered a suitable pursuit for a child from a regular brahmin family. At that time, yoga was thought of as preparation for the aspirant to lead the life of a sannyāsī or sannyāsīn (male or female ascetic), which meant living on the margins of society and certainly not being a family member and participating in householder duties. In an effort to avoid confrontation with his parents, Pattabhi Jois chose to keep secret, for a time, his deep interest in yoga. As a result, young Pattabhi Jois woke up two hours before his schoolmates, walked five kilometers along a path to Hassan, where T. Krishnamacharya's shala was located, did his practice while Krishnamacharya counted the vinyāsa and then headed off to regular school.

In 1930, after he was officially initiated as a brahmin by his father and was given the characteristic thread (upavīta) to be worn around his body, he moved to Mysore and enrolled himself in the Sanskrit University, Parkala Math.

In Mysore, Pattabhi Jois was reacquainted with his guru, T. Krishnamacharya, as the latter had been invited in 1931, by his student and friend, Krishnarajendra Wodeyar IV (1894–1940), the Maharaja of Mysore, to open a yoga shala at the Jaganmohan Palace. The guru-student relationship between T. Krishnamacharya and Pattabhi Jois was reestablished and continued in Mysore until 1953, at which point T. Krishnamacharya moved with his family to Madras, present-day Chennai.

T. Krishnamacharya's teaching followed the vinyāsa krama (vinyāsa technique) that he learned from his guru, Ramamohan Brahmacarya, in the Himalayas. Pattabhi Jois belonged to a group of about a hundred students who performed āsana according to the exact technique described therein. They learned all the āsana numbers, transitions from one āsana to the next, proper breathing and deep concentration. Their guru did not tolerate even the slightest sign of fatigue or forgetfulness. Pattabhi Jois progressed rapidly under his guru's watchful eyes and their guru-student relationship deepened, with T. Krishnamacharya instructing Pattabhi Jois daily on yogic theory, according to ancient texts and philosophical schools, and on the therapeutic and healing effects of the practice.

The Maharaja of Mysore, who was a famous student of T. Krishnamacharya, became convinced of Pattabhi Jois's capabilities and assigned him to be a headmaster of the yoga department at the Sanskrit University in 1937. This year was very memorable in Pattabhi Jois's life, as he began both his long teaching career and his more than sixty-year marriage to Savitramma (1923–1997).

Pattabhi Jois continued to study Sanskrit, teach Aṣṭāṅga yoga, and began to study advaita-vedānta (a school of philosophy based on Ādi-Śaṅkarācārya's 8th-century non-dualistic viewpoint where "everything is Brahman"). He earned the title, Professor of Vedānta (Vidvān) from Parakala Math in 1956. The title Yogāsana Visharada had already been presented to him in 1945 by Jagadguru Śaṅkarācārya from Puri. His students respectfully called him Gurujī. After 1956, in addition to teaching Aṣṭāṅga yoga, he became a teacher of Sanskrit and of the philosophical view of Advaita-vedānta. Pattabhi Jois continued teaching at the Sanskrit University until his retirement in 1973. After retirement he taught yoga for three years, from 1976–1978, at the Ayurvedic college (Government College of Indian Medicine) in Mysore and then devoted himself fully to teaching Aṣṭāṅga yoga at his home in Lakshmipuram, Mysore.

In 1948, Pattabhi Jois's students helped him buy a house in Lakshmipuram for himself and his family: his wife, Savitri "Ammaji," and their three children, Saraswati, Manju and Ramesh. He founded the Aṣṭāṅga Yoga Research Institute (Aṣṭāṅga Yoga Nilayam) and taught out of his home, with the purpose of researching the method of Aṣṭāṅga yoga in accordance with the holy texts.

Pattabhi Jois wrote *Yoga Mala* between 1958 and 1961, and it was published in his native language of Kannada in 1962. It is probable that the model for his book came from the *Yoga Korunta* and from Krishnamacharya's text *Yoga-makaranda*. In *Yoga Mala* he describes the Primary series of Aṣṭāṅga yoga (yoga-cikitsā), yogic philosophy, and how to integrate yoga with modern life. The book is a testimony to his immense knowledge, compiled from twenty-five years of study with Krishnamacharya, his complete dedication to the yogic path, and his belief in yoga's healing and spiritual powers.

The first Western students to study with Pattabhi Jois were the British diplomat John Bowers and his wife. Mr. Bowers was Director of the UNESCO Group Training Scheme for Fundamental Education and he conducted research on a project entitled "An Experiment in Mysore, India" for the Forestry and Fundamental Education department in Mysore. Bowers and his wife studied Aṣṭāṅga yoga for two weeks in 1947.

The third Western student was a Belgian man named Andre van Lysebeth, who came to Mysore as Gurujī's student in 1964. In the two months that he studied with Pattabhi Jois, van Lysebeth went through both the primary and intermediate series. In 1971, he documented the teachings he received from Gurujī, highlighting the breathing practices, in particular, in his book titled *Prāṇāyama*. First published in French, the book sparked an interest among Europeans to seek out Gurujī and make the pilgrimage to Mysore. In 1974, Pattabhi Jois was invited to speak at a yoga conference in Sao Paolo, Brazil, where he presented a paper he had written on yoga (written mostly in Kannada and some Sanskrit), and his presentation was translated into several languages. Among the first Americans to travel to Mysore in 1973 were Norman Allen, David Williams and Nancy Gilgoff. Deeply moved by their studies with him, David and Nancy invited Gurujī and his son Manju to Encinitas, California in 1975. After his second international invitation, Pattabhi Jois continued to teach workshops for thousands of students around the world, contributing tremendously to yoga's widespread accessibility in the Western world.

In May 2002, Pattabhi Jois opened a new shala in Gokulam, a quiet neighborhood in Mysore. Until then, the Aṣṭāṅga Yoga Research Institute had been located in Lakshmipuram, on the other side of the city, in what is commonly known among Aṣṭāṅga yoga students as the legendary "old shala". In this shala, there was space for about twelve yoga mats, placed right beside each other. At its busiest, 150 students would practice in the shala, the first group beginning at 4:30am and continuing on throughout the morning. There would be a long line on the stairs to the main room, and through a small window those waiting their turn could listen to Gurujī's teachings and catch a glimpse of him. He would be counting the vinyāsa and correcting āsanas, always equipped with his wonderful sense of humor. These students can remember Gurujī's wife, Savitri Jois, whom the family called Sathu and students called either Savitramma or Ammaji. She spoke happily with the students after practice and gave consolation after Gurujī's often hard, though heart-felt, teachings. Ammaji passed away quite suddenly and unexpectedly in 1997. Gurujī saw to the renovation of two temples of particular significance to him, located in his home village of Kaushika, which he dedicated to the memory of his wife.

Pattabhi Jois died in his home in Gokulam on May 18, 2009. The funeral was held on 31st May and hundreds of Gurujī's students, friends and relatives visited Mysore to pay respects to Gurujī, to his life and for his work. From 1937 until his passing in 2009, Gurujī followed his inner voice without tiring, and for 72 years was a devoted, respected and well-regarded yoga master.

Pattabhi Jois was a living example of the traditional guru-student teaching method: complete devotion (bhakti) to the guru and God. His teaching style was strict and clear while at the same time heart-felt and therapeutic. His verbal instructions and physical adjustments pointed out exactly where one needed to improve. Even though his way was considered brusque at times, or seemed to lack warmth or sympathy, there was always deep compassion behind his words. His powerful and often ringing laughter passed through practitioners' minds and brought with it an almost transcendental energy. Well into his senior years, Gurujī maintained as much vigor as when he was a younger man.
T. Krishnamacharya warned Jois' young wife, "If you ask your husband to bring Chamundi Hill to you (the temple mountain south of Mysore, named after the goddess, Śrī Cāmuṇḍeśvarī or Chamundi), he will do it."

The shala in Gokulam is now known as the Śrī Śrī K. Pattabhi Jois Aṣṭāṅga Yoga Institute (KPJAYI). His daughter, Saraswati Jois, and his grandson, Sharath Jois, current director of the shala (who began to assist Gurujī in 1990 at the age of 19) carry on the lineage and continue to pass on Gurujī's teachings.

aṣṭāṅga yoga's eight-limbed path

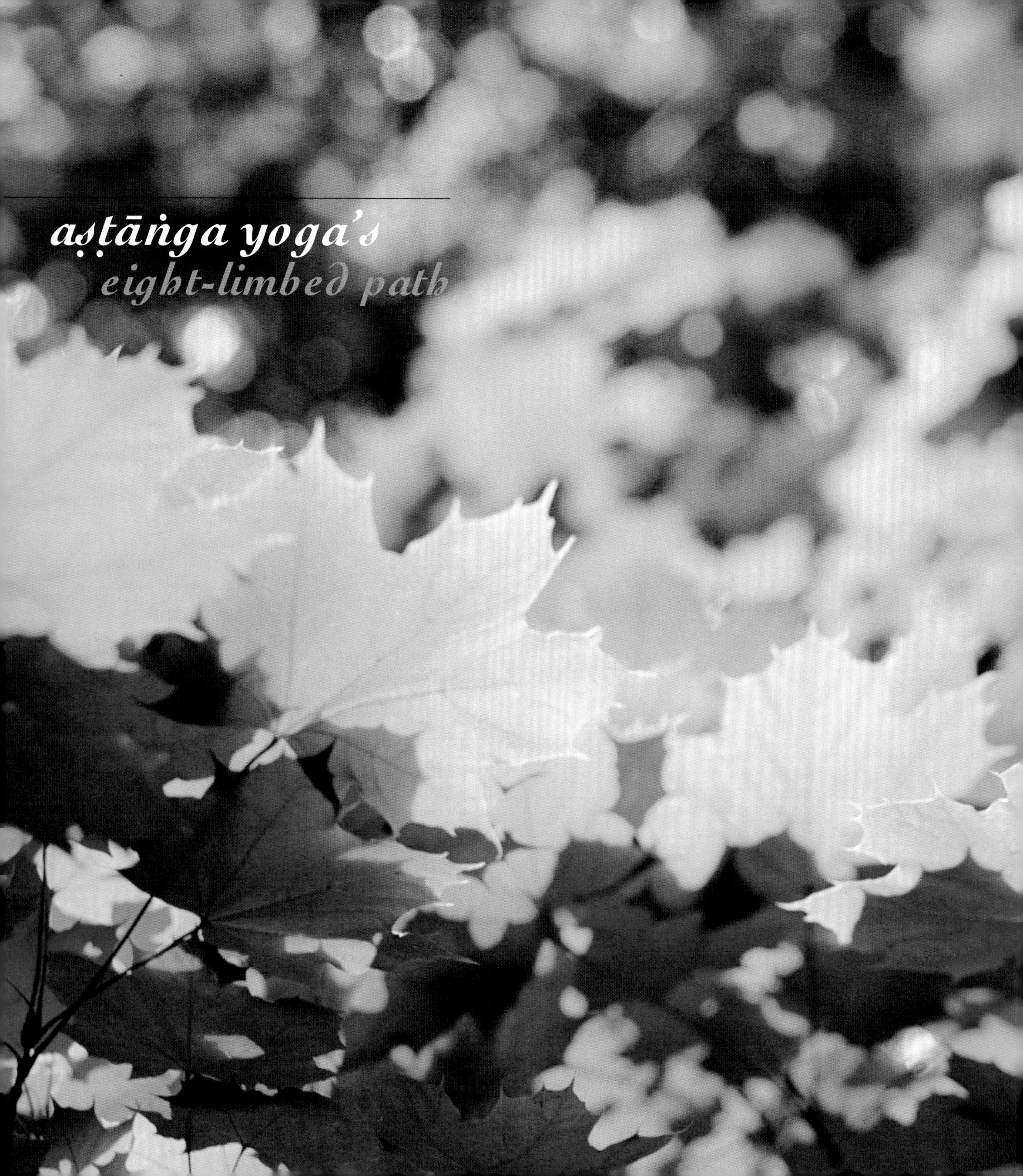

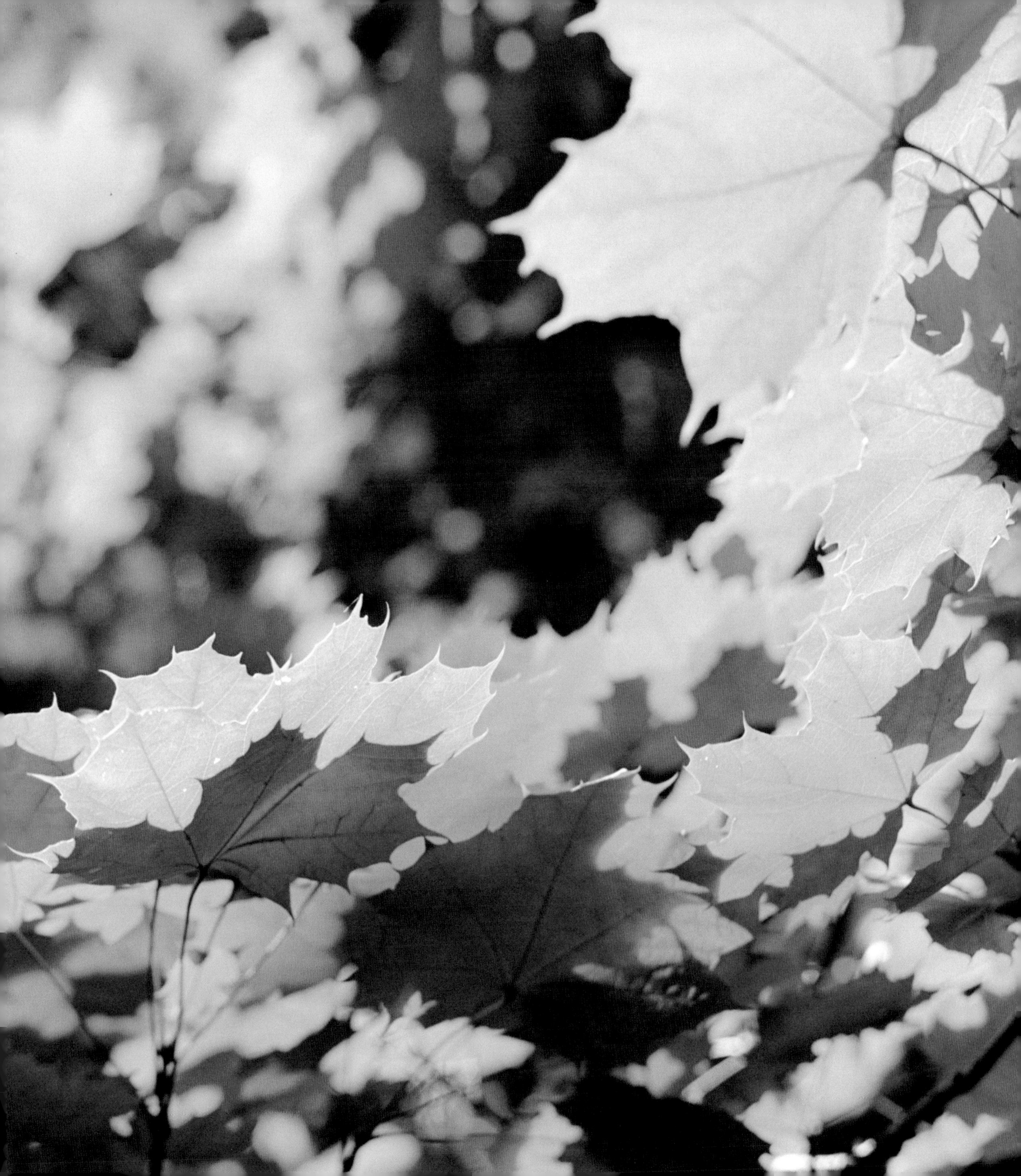

aṣṭāṅga yoga's eight-limbed path

Aṣṭau aṅga (eight limbs) are the eight foundational and philosophical principles of yoga that Ṛṣi Patanjali laid out in a clear order in the *Yoga-sūtra*. According to Patanjali, by following these principles, human beings can walk the path of spiritual development and liberate their bodies and minds from destructive habitual patterns which weaken life-force and cause us to remain in a state of ignorance from our true selves. Once freed from that which inhibits the flow of prāṇa (omnipresent life-energy), this prāṇa can then move freely through the energy channels, purifying the body and mind and preparing the aspirant for the highest goal of yoga which, according to the *Yoga-sūtra*, is the state of kaivalya (detachment from identification with the intellect; liberation from the cycle of death and rebirth). Pattabhi Jois outlined in *Yoga Mala* the six obstacles which inhibit this goal of self-realization: kāma (desire), krodha (hatred), moha (delusion), lobha (greed), mada (envy) and mātsarya (laziness, sloth).

According to the Aṣṭāṅga yoga tradition of Śrī K. Pattabhi Jois, one begins Patanjali's eight limbs with āsana, the third limb. Once firmly established in this limb, one can then pursue the fourth limb, prāṇāyama. Through the efforts of these third and fourth aṅgas, understanding of the first two limbs, yama and niyama will naturally arise. The *Maitri Upaniṣad* also suggests a similar order (sadaṅga – six limbs), confirming that one's body and mind must be strong, clean, and balanced before one is mindful enough to truly begin following yama and niyama.

Aṣṭāṅga yoga's first four limbs are called the external practices, for these take place mainly on the physical level and influence our interactions with other people and with the world around us. The last four limbs are the internal practices that govern our relationship mostly with our inner self. As with all other aspects of yoga, it is important to learn these limbs under the guidance of a guru or an experienced teacher. When studying āsana, learning from a teacher is the best way to prevent injury; likewise, when studying yogic theory, philosophy or meditative practices, a trusted teacher is the best way to prevent mental harm from occuring and to ensure a spiritual development that is safe, proper and balanced.

Once the first four limbs have been integrated within the individual, the body and mind will be ready for the final four limbs. These latter limbs affect the being on a subtle, refined level, and activate the most sensitive nāḍīs (energy channels). According to Pattabhi Jois, these four inner limbs foster the ability to sense Brahman, that which is infinite. In order to integrate and be open to the inner working of our daily lives, a healthy body, quiet mind and an awakened sensitivity is required. If one attempts to understand these limbs under the guidance of books alone, or with a teacher who is not deeply experienced, one can encounter problems. This is not to be taken lightly, as it is possible, through inappropriately practiced meditation, to create lasting psychological problems that can be nearly impossible or extremely challenging to recover from later on.

Yama: the first aṅga

Yama is concerned with self-control and ethical thinking and behavior. It teaches the student to cultivate an atmosphere of peace and respect within oneself, extending this towards other people and all beings. An individualistic mindset can often lead to indifference for others, whereas yama teaches us that we are all an equal part of this universe, which we all share. When we follow the universal laws of yama, we not only improve our own lives, but we bring about positivity in our interpersonal relationships with friends and family members, through our communities on the societal level and on a global level as well, due to the interconnected nature of the world in which we live.

The aṅga of yama requests or, frankly speaking, challenges us to follow five observances pertaining to moral conduct with other beings: ahiṃsā (non-violence), satya (truth and honesty), asteya (non-stealing), brahmacarya (associated with brahman, harnessing and wise use of life-power), and aparigraha (non-possessiveness, moderation).

Śrī K. Pattabhi Jois mentioned that it is very difficult to follow yama and niyama completely and without straying. Over time, yoga helps bring people closer to understanding and, eventually, applying these first two limbs.

1 Ahiṃsā

To practice and follow ahiṃsā is to respect all life through observance of non-violence. It means acceptance and tolerance of all of life's differences: religion, skin color, appearance, social status or class, and more. Ahiṃsā's teachings encompass forgiveness and humility, urging us to create peaceful energy both within ourselves and around the environments in which we interact and are engaged with. Ahiṃsā also includes practising kindness: ensuring that one does not injure others (or be the cause of injury) with words, thoughts or actions. "Others" includes all people, animals and elements in nature. Mohandas (Mahatma) Karamchand Gandhi brought the concept of ahiṃsā to global attention when he used non-violent civil disobedience and led India to gain its independence in 1947.

Āsana is an effective way to observe your own relationship with ahiṃsā. Moving forward in the physical postures without violence but rather with humility, ease and forgiveness towards both yourself and others is of utmost importance, making your practice a continually meaningful and safe journey.

2 Satya

Satya means being truthful in thought, word and action. It requires that one speak the truth, albeit with discriminative kindness (maitrī) and non-violence (ahiṃsā). It seems that sometimes a small lie, or not speaking one's thoughts, may save hurting another person's feelings. To observe and put satya into action legitimizes your words, thoughts and actions. In the end, all lies harm us and others, and a well-timed truth is always kinder in the long run.

In āsana practice, it behooves the student to accept the truth with regards to his or her body and how one can, or cannot, advance in the practice. The principle in Aṣṭāṅga yoga is that one should not move forward to the next āsana if one cannot perform the preceding āsana fluidly, with deep, calm breathing. Be truthful to yourself and others about where you realistically are in the āsana series, and about what you are ready to do or not. By following this, one can avoid unnecessary pain, savoring the process and making it enjoyable.

3 Asteya

Asteya means not stealing, which can sound quite obvious. However, this principle includes a broader definition of the term "stealing". In addition to the moral behavior of not stealing things which don't belong to you, such as another's property or physical belongings, on a more psychological level it means that one must not take advantage of other people, in effect stealing their energy or generosity, thoughts and feelings. For example, to win over another's trust and then break that trust is not in accordance with asteya, which teaches us to behave kindly, honestly and unselfishly. Envy is another example of straying from asteya, for it comes from a sense of lack and the desire to get what one does not have.

When one feels envious of another student who is more proficient in the āsanas and seems to be further along the journey, one should try to appreciate that student's effort and be inspired by his or her concentration and dedication. Bring your focus back to your breathing and enjoy the meditative movements. Experience the joy that comes from cultivating a more positive attitude and extend gratitude for both your own, and all the other students' small steps forwards in the practice.

4 Brahmacarya

Brahmacarya is often defined as celibacy, or refrainment from indiscriminate use of our sexual energy. According to yogic philosophy, sexual fluids are one of the seven dhātus (p. 46), and we must be respectful of these energies. By losing one's sexual fluids, which contain vital life-energy, the energy of the body and mind can be weakened; whereas retaining these fluids and the life-energies contained in them causes the body to grow stronger and the mind to function clearly.

If one were to follow this line of thinking completely, with the sole wish of increasing one's life-force or gaining insight into life's deepest truths, it would be impossible to have a family, or to engage in any sexual activity. Further examination of Aṣṭāṅga yoga's history shows that many gurus were, in fact, householders who lived according to the principles of brahmacarya, without adhering to a strictly celibate lifestyle reserved for renunciates. By carefully studying yogic texts, we see that brahmacarya does not only mean retention of sexual fluids. The *Yoga-sūtra* define the five great vows (mahāvratam), which include the prohibition of sexual activity of any kind (even in thoughts) and are to be observed by monks and renunciates. However, a small vow (anuvrata) also exists. This provides more flexibility, and offers rules on how to follow brahmacarya as a householder.

According to Indian philosophy, there are four stages in life (āśrama). Brahmacarya is the first of these four, meaning the stage of study, and is accompanied by a celibate lifestyle. One undertakes this stage before marriage, as a youth. The second stage is that of the householder (gṛhastha), which is the time of marriage and family, work and involving oneself in the material world. The next stage comes with old age, and is that of the hermit (vānaprastha), wherein one withdraws from worldly life and turns one's attention within. The final stage of life is that of renunciation (sannyāsa), wherein one fully gives oneself over to a life with very few possessions, turning towards spiritual contemplation, with complete devotion to the Divine. However, if one has a natural inclination towards brahmacarya, he or she can continue to live as a brahamchari or brahmacharini, without continuing onto the subsequent stages.

In *Yoga Mala*, Pattabhi Jois gives some advice to couples in a committed, monogamous relationship who would like to adhere to the principles of brahmacarya in this specific context:

1. The best time for sexual intercourse is between sunset and sunrise. Engaging in intercourse during the day can weaken the life-force.
2. According to Indian tradition, only those who are married should have intercourse, though one may extend this concept in the Western world to include life-partners and those in a committed relationship. It is said that even thinking sexual thoughts about a person other than your partner weakens your life-force, or bindu.
3. The most appropriate time for intercourse are between days four and sixteen of a woman's menstrual cycle, when her level of estrogen is at its peak and she is at her most fertile. (In this context, the main reason to engage in intercourse is for procreation.)
4. It is not recommended to have intercourse on new-moon or

full-moon days, as any activity which requires concentration, focus, and strong feelings should be abstained from on those days. This includes such activities as a strong āsana practice, air travel or important business meetings.

5. Righteousness or fairness (dharma), prosperity or purpose (artha), and physical or emotional pleasure or desire (kāma) should all be in balance.
6. To constantly think of the higher self, even during intercourse, unavoidably leads us to the state of brahmacarya, increasing our life-force and connection with the Divine.

In order to bring an awareness of bramhacharya into your āsana practice, continue to turn your attention inwards, becoming aware of the various sensations of life-force coursing through your body. In keeping with the intention as to why you and others come to the shala, dress in a practical and decent manner. If you happen to find yourself unwittingly drawn towards someone, return to that inner awareness, focus on your dṛṣṭi, and concentrate on the breath and meditative quality of the movements.

5 Aparigraha

Aparigraha literally means non-grabbing or non-holding, but in certain situations it can also mean release and letting go.

The less time we spend engaged with the delusions of the outer world, the more time we have to encounter our inner self and develop physically and spiritually. When we incorporate aparigraha into our lives, we develop moderation in thought, word and action. We openly and without regret relinquish the desire to own, letting go of all that is unnecessary in our lives. We should long for nothing, and only receive rewards and accept thanks for that which we truly deserve. We also aim to avoid pleasures that are clearly destructive.

Incorporating the ancient wisdom of aparigraha within our āsana practice is quite simple. We advance forwards by cultivating patience and moderation. One of the biggest obstacles in moving forwards is that one wishes to advance too quickly, yearning for more āsana, or starting intense prāṇāyama or meditation before the mind and nervous system are ready. One can also overestimate one's own levelof practice and perform āsana incorrectly. When engaged in a particular āsana or prāṇāyama practice, one should continually experience a deep letting go, rather than an urgent sense of acquisition. The more the body or mind holds onto an āsana, the less space there is available for the āsana to do its work by opening up and deepening within the body.

Niyama: the second aṅga

Niyama outlines five observances to follow in order to develop one's inner power and insight: śauca (purity), santoṣa (contentment), tapas (self-discipline/austerity), svādhyāya (self-study of sacred texts), īśvara-praṇidhāna (surrender to God).

1 Śauca

Śauca means purity and applies to both inner and outer purity. Bahiḥ-śauca means outer purity, and refers to the literal cleansing of the physical body. The importance of cleanliness and āsana practice have already been mentioned in the Instructions sections (p. 21). That said, it is useful to examine the way we think of the sweat released during practice. It is actually recommended that we massage our sweat back into our bodies, so that the minerals in our sweat can be incorporated back into our blood stream. Furthermore, in order to benefit fully from these essential minerals, one should refrain from bathing or showering immediately after practice. Instead, wait for fifteen minutes after practising and before bathing, to ensure that the minerals have been recirculated into your system and at which point, warm water and soap will cleanse away any remaining sweat. Antaḥ-śauca means inner purity, which is the cleansing of the deeply rooted mental impurities (chitta mala) and pollution (dukḥa) from the mind.

2 Santoṣa

Santoṣa is a state of deep, sustained contentment, accompanied by an acceptance of what is, regardless of one's particular circumstances. This comes when one can truly direct the mind inwards and towards the higher self. Santoṣa is present when one can experience mistakes, disappointment or despair as teachers, and find fulfillment in the continual learning process.

> "Every day is a good day, and every moment is a good moment." – *Śrī K. Pattabhi Jois*

3 Tapas

Tapas challenges us to exercise greater self-restraint. *Tap* means heat and through the practice of Aṣṭāṅga yoga's eight limbs (Patanjali's view), heat is generated to burn away the impurities of the body and mind, as well as the karmic imprints from our consciousness. Through such methods, one disciplines the body, mind and consciousness to be able to function as fully as possible. To put tapas into action is first of all to show up for your āsana and/or prāṇāyama practice consistently, and secondly to eat simple, clean vegetarian food in accordance with ahiṃsā, non-violence.

4 Svādhyāya

Svādhyāya means the studies towards realizing the Self through reading sacred texts, gaining awareness of speech and chanting mantras (japa-yoga). For the mantras to really take effect, and in order for their gifts to bear fruit, it is advised that the student should make the effort to learn proper pronunciation directly from a master.

5 Īśvara-praṇidhāna

Īśvara-praṇidhāna means full surrender of oneself to a higher power, in both thought and deed, without any expectation of a particular personal result, reward or benefit. By following the niyama of Īśvara-praṇidhāna, the student cleanses the subtler, more sensitive nāḍīs (energy channels) in the heart's energy center. Only then can prāṇa can then flow freely all the way up to the center of the head, brahma-randhra (p.46).

Āsana: the third aṅga

Aṣṭāṅga yoga is often described as an intense and powerful practice, requiring great body and mind control. Practising āsana daily develops a light, strong and pure body, which is required for spiritual development since it is much more difficult for a sick or weak body to create a stable mind or to live a long and vital life. Āsana also removes ailments that distract the mind as well as the body, while detoxifying the inner organs and nervous system. Positive growth on all levels is possible through consistent practice approached with the right intention. For some people āsana is another type of physical exercise, however, when performed with an understanding of the yogic texts and with awareness in breathing and concentration, āsana can take on a much deeper spiritual nature. By practising āsana with the proper vinyāsa technique and meditative focus, the mind becomes clear, strong and peaceful.

Prāṇa (life-force) balances itself out via the īḍā- and piṅgalā-nāḍīs (the left and right energy channels). The īḍā-nāḍī (ṭha or candra) is related to the moon, whereas piṅgalā-nāḍī (ha or sūrya) relates to the sun. From these two words ha and ṭha, the word "haṭha" is formed. From this we can understand the deeper layers of the word, and the goal of haṭha-yoga, which is to balance out these two nāḍīs, and pave the path for a meditative practice, or rāja-yoga. It is only through the process of āsana that we can transform the body into a temple for the soul.

Aṣṭāṅga yoga is comprised of six series, or collections of āsana, each of which have a specific function in the cleansing and strengthening of the mind and body. In addition to āsana, there are ongoing techniques that support and develop the practitioner's understanding of postures on a physical, mental and spiritual level. These are: sound breath (p. 52) – deep, energy-generating breathing for each inhalation and exhalation (pūraka and recaka); vinyāsa (p. 61) – the breath and movement, linking these two in order to create mental clarity as well as a meditative quality to the postures; bandhas (p. 53) – muscular and energy locks, operating within both the physical and energetic kośas (layers of the body); bandhas lighten and strengthen the body while directing the movement of the energy throughout the body; dṛṣṭi (p. 58) – gazing points that increase one's concentration and ability to focus; and meditation (dhyāna), which directs the mind inwards. These will be discussed in greater detail in the practice section of the book.

The first collection of āsana, which is featured in this book, is commonly known as the Primary series. It is known in Sanskrit as yoga-cikitsā, or roga-cikitsā (roga: illness or sickness; cikitsā: therapy). Yoga-cikitsā contains the sequence of āsanas that removes existing illness and ailments from the body, prevents new illnesses from arising and creates a strong and healthy body. In other words, the body is restored to its natural state of strength, flexibility, balance and relaxation. The primary series also alleviates chronic pain, removes excess fat from the body, improves blood circulation, and cleanses the inner organs, while developing one's ability to focus the mind.

The second collection of āsanas, the Intermediate series, is called Nāḍī-śodhana. Nāḍīs, which have previously been mentioned, are the channels that transport energy throughout the entire body, both on the physical and energetic plane. Śodhana means purification, so the intermediate series is the sequence of āsana which purifies the energy channels. It works on both the nervous system as well as on the subtler energy channels that exist in our energy body.

The third collection of āsanas contains four series; the Advanced A, B, C and D series. As a whole, this series is defined as sthira-bhāga, inner and outer strength, peace and beauty (sthira - stable, complete, entire; bhāga - grace, fortune, opulence; part or portion). These series trains the body and mind to stay consistently stable while remaining relaxed, light and present at the same time. The Advanced series demand a great deal of flexibility, strength, control of the breath and bandhas, and absolute concentration.

One should be able to perform each movement, each āsana, and each series with a full calm breath and without pain before moving onto the next āsana, or series of āsana. If one moves forwards before the body and mind are ready, this can deplete the energy reserves one has built up and leave one devoid of the resilience needed to perform more challenging āsanas. The benefits of the practice can also be negated if one skips over difficult āsanas or underestimates the importance of the method and does not follow the order of the āsanas, or the system of breathing with the proper vinyāsa count. This can cause even greater difficulties in progressing, as the series are already challenging enough. If done incorrectly, āsana can simply cause pain and add more strain to the muscles, nerves and mind.

"When the mind is quiet, the āsana is correct."
– *Śrī K. Pattabhi Jois*

Prāṇāyama: the fourth aṅga

The process of purification and stilling of the body and mind that starts with the āsana continues with prāṇāyama. Prāṇa is the life-force found in all elements; in yoga, however, emphasis is given to the breath, so air is considered the most valuable element in which prāṇa can be accessed. The throat cakra (viśuddha cakra) filters this prāṇa, or pure air, from the air we breathe. Ayama means long and refers to methods through which this life-power enters into and is extended within the body. Prāṇāyama is a practice in which one establishes various rhythms of inhalation (pūraka), exhalation (recaka), and retention (kumbhaka) while engaging the throat lock (jalandhara-bandha), root lock (mūla-bandha) and abdominal lock (uddīyana-bandha), and in some techniques, breathing through alternate nostrils using the hand mudrā (fingers blocking the nostrils). Note that jalandhara-bandha is only used during prāṇāyama while holding the breath (kumbhaka). It is not used while doing āsana.

Aṣṭāṅga yoga's prāṇāyama practice is made up of eight different exercises (mentioned in *Haṭha-yoga-pradīpikā*) that aid the body, mind and spirit in a number of ways. They have a similar effect on the body and mind as āsana practice has, such as curing illnesses, strengthening the body, purifying the nāḍīs and calming the mind. The purification process in prāṇāyama, however, targets the mind, nāḍīs, and movement of energy throughout the body, accessing the energetic and mental levels of our being.

When the mind is quiet and free from blockages, and prāṇa has been gathered successfully in the body, this prāṇa can then be guided towards the suṣumnā-nāḍī – the central channel in the network system of nāḍīs, energy channels that originate in the kāṇḍa (located just above the perineum). Located in the sacrum and next to the suṣumnā-nāḍī are three energy knots (granthi-traya). When these three knots are released, the entrance to the suṣumnā-nāḍī opens up and prāṇa can flow freely, purifying and cleansing the nāḍīs. Prāṇa can then naturally circulate through to the heart cakra (anāhata-cakra), and reach the crown of the head (sahasrāra-cakra), which is our connection to the higher self. Prāṇāyama prepares one, through deep purification and well-established inner balance, for this process to occur.

According to the tradition of Aṣṭāṅga yoga, it is considered safe to start with prāṇāyama only once strength, flexibility, and an understanding of the bandhas – not to mention the purification of the organs and nervous system – are evident in the body. Some students (and teachers) read about various kinds of breathing techniques in books, and start practising, or in some cases, teaching them to others. These self-taught techniques cannot officially be called prāṇāyama since, in the Aṣṭāṅga yoga tradition, prāṇāyama must be learned directly from a guru or a competent teacher. It is for this reason that I cannot present or explain prāṇāyama in this book, as it is crucial that students learn correctly and under safe guidance.

Prāṇāyama requires that one must be able to keep the body still and sit calmly in Padmāsana (lotus pose) with the hands in jñāna-mudrā (see description of Padmāsana, p. 173) for the duration of the practice. The inner organs, bandhas, flexibility, breath, nāḍīs and concentration should have been purified enough and developed through steady practice of at least the Primary and Intermediate series (yoga-cikitsā and nāḍī-śodhana). The āsana series prepare the body to take in prāṇa without causing dangerous side effects such as dizziness, stomach pain, cramping or joint pain, loss of concentration or confusion. The main thing is that the body should not be an issue while doing prāṇāyama. There are enough obstacles and challenges to overcome, so the body must be ready to act in full compliance with this subtle yet powerful purification process.

After one has understood and benefited from prāṇāyama, one is prepared for the following four limbs: pratyāhāra, dhāraṇa, dhyāna and samādhi.

Pratyāhāra: the fifth aṅga

Pratyāhāra, sense withdrawal, is the first of the remaining four limbs considered to be the internal practices (antahkarana). It occurs naturally from observing and incorporating the first four limbs (yama, niyama, āsana, prāṇāyama) which purify, strengthen and bring sensitivity to the body, nervous system and mind. Pratyāhāra is concerned with enhancing a more profound level of control over the mind. By practising or maintaining the state of pratyāhāra, obstacles of the mind such as distraction associated with the five senses drop away as the aspirant becomes more and more aligned with a pure, inner awareness. Once established, this inner focus results in the aspirant's ability to overcome and distance oneself from often unconscious and automatic reactions, triggered by the senses and habitual conditioning in relation to the external, material world.

At this point, awareness of the ultimate goal of yoga has started to become apparent as pratyāhāra shows us the Divine in everything and in everyone. Following this line of thought, Pattabhi Jois often stated that pratyāhāra is the internal essence found in every aṅga. In this way, it is not only the fifth aṅga, but one of the foremost goals of yoga practice.

"If you are looking at a wall and constantly focusing on God (state of pratyāhāra), the wall also transforms into God. Everything becomes God." – *Śrī K. Pattabhi Jois*

Dhāraṇa: the sixth aṅga

Dhāraṇa continues to refine our mind control, working towards maintaining a steady, stable and reliable mind. It occurs when the aspirant is able not only to establish concentration in the mind, but to sustain this unwavering focus while remaining connected with the Divine.

Dhyāna: the seventh aṅga

According to Pattabhi Jois, dhyāna (meditation) is not a technique or something to formally engage in. Rather, it is a process that eliminates identification with the ego, thus deepening and stabilizing the presence of God in our hearts. Working with āsana can raise awareness of a meditative state, a type of moving meditation, brought about by rhythmic breathing and the use of dṛṣṭi and bandhas. In order to enter a deep state of meditation, however, one should be able to hold Padmāsana comfortably for up to three hours, without feeling pain or any other distracting sensations in the body. This requires a strong, supple, calm body, which is the result of a dedicated āsana practice.

"A quiet mind is a strong body." – *Śrī K. Pattabhi Jois*

Samādhi: the eighth aṅga

Samādhi is described as a state in which the mind is deeply focused on one point and all thoughts cease to exist and disappear from consciousness. The mind is absorbed fully with the object of contemplation. This can be called the same (sama) state, or the highest level of meditation. This is the result of a long and dedicated commitment to the practice of all eight limbs of Aṣṭāṅga yoga. People who have experienced samādhi express it as happiness, bliss, or a sense of utter wholeness that is beyond description. It is a quiet understanding that exists deep within us, patiently waiting to be felt. Pattabhi Jois's often-quoted phrase, "Do your practice and all is coming" speaks of the path towards this final aṅga. Step by step, in this expansive awakening state of samādhi, we uncover what has been there all along and peel away the layers to experience our true nature.

According to Pattabhi Jois, there are two main kinds of samādhi: savikalpa-samādhi and nirvikalpa-samādhi. Savikalpa-samādhi means association with God, but not yet having acquired complete control of the mind. The moment the mind becomes attached to the distractions of the outer world, one leaves this state of samādhi and must enter into it again. Nirvikalpa samādhi is experienced when full control of the mind has been achieved, and the six distractions or obstacles of the mind (p. 32) have been dissolved entirely. In this type of samādhi, prāṇa courses energetically and freely through the suṣumnā-nāḍī and one has achieved what the legendary sage Vyasa defines as "Yogaha Samādhihi" (yoga is samādhi).

A definition of God

According to yogic philosophy, human beings and the natural world are steered by a higher power that exists equally in everything and in everyone. In India, this power goes by a variety of names, depending on whether this source has been personified and taken the form of an ishta devata (personal god) or if it remains formless. Some examples of the names are: Brahman, Ātman, Paramātman, Īśvara, Śiva, Viṣṇu, Brahmā, Krishna, Pārvatī, Durgā, Lakṣmī, and Sarasvatī. A note to Western students: Avoid feeling overwhelmed or alienated by all the names and concepts for God, gods and goddesses. Call this energy by whichever name you feel the most affinity for: Jesus, Buddha, Allah, the Holy Spirit, inner bliss, peace, the higher self, the higher power, the soul, universal consciousness. All names for this divine essence are welcome, as yoga is not bound to any religion. It is a philosophy and a systematic training that purifies and strengthens all people who practie it, and its foremost goal is for humanity to uncover discriminative knowledge and to understand the pure nature of spirit, both seen and unseen.

"When the heart is opening, God is coming."
– *Śrī K. Pattabhi Jois*

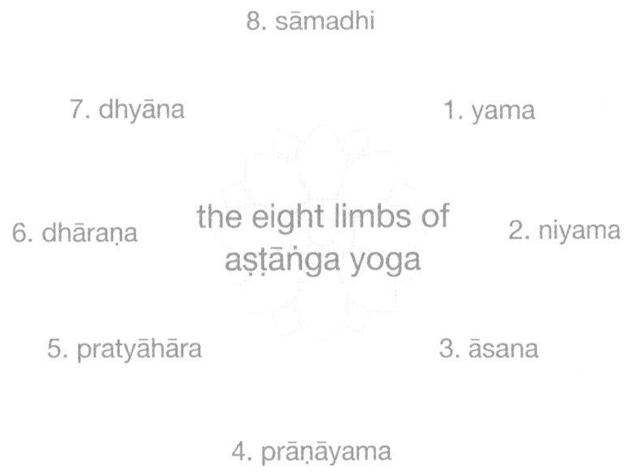

energy flows of the body

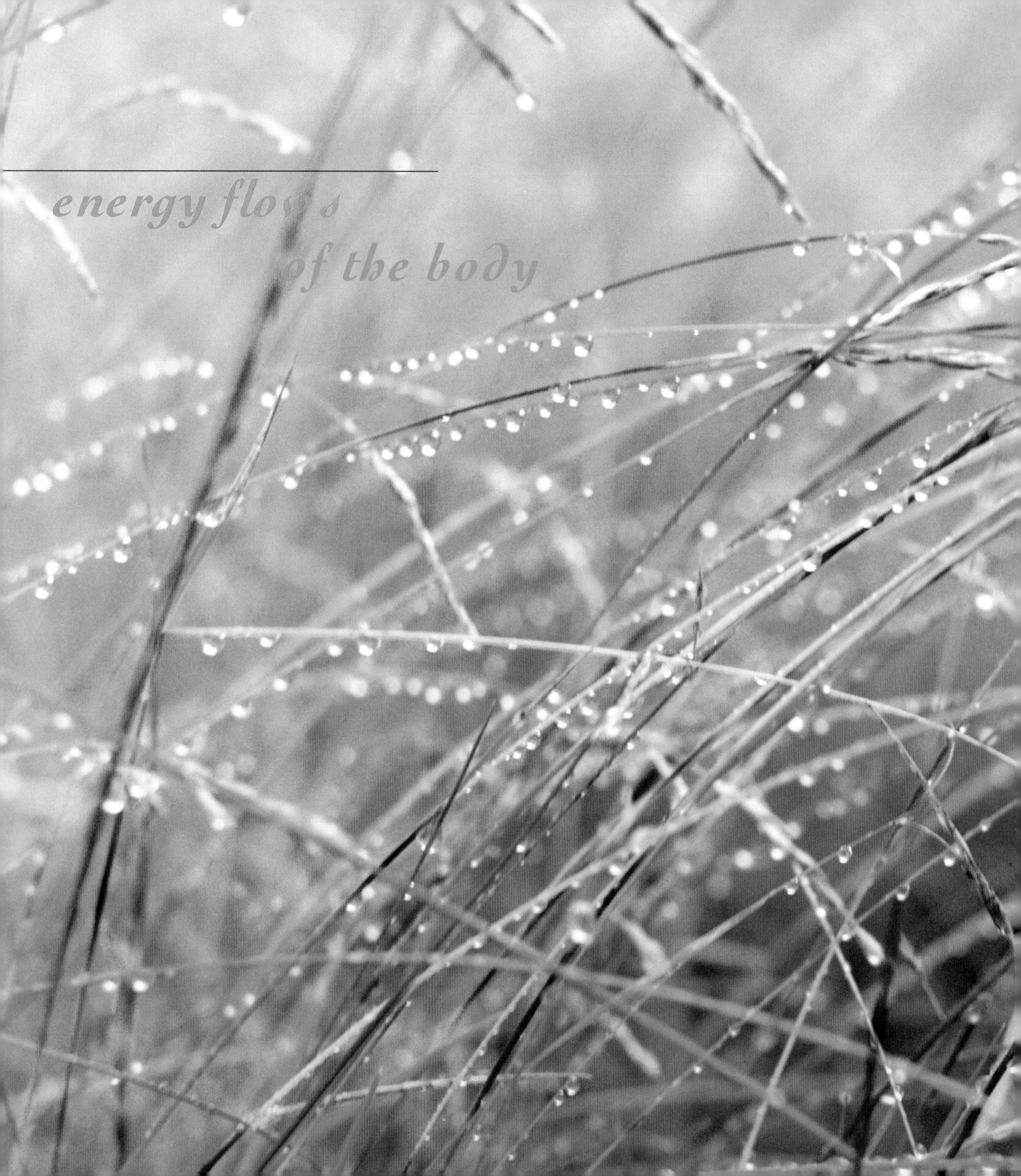

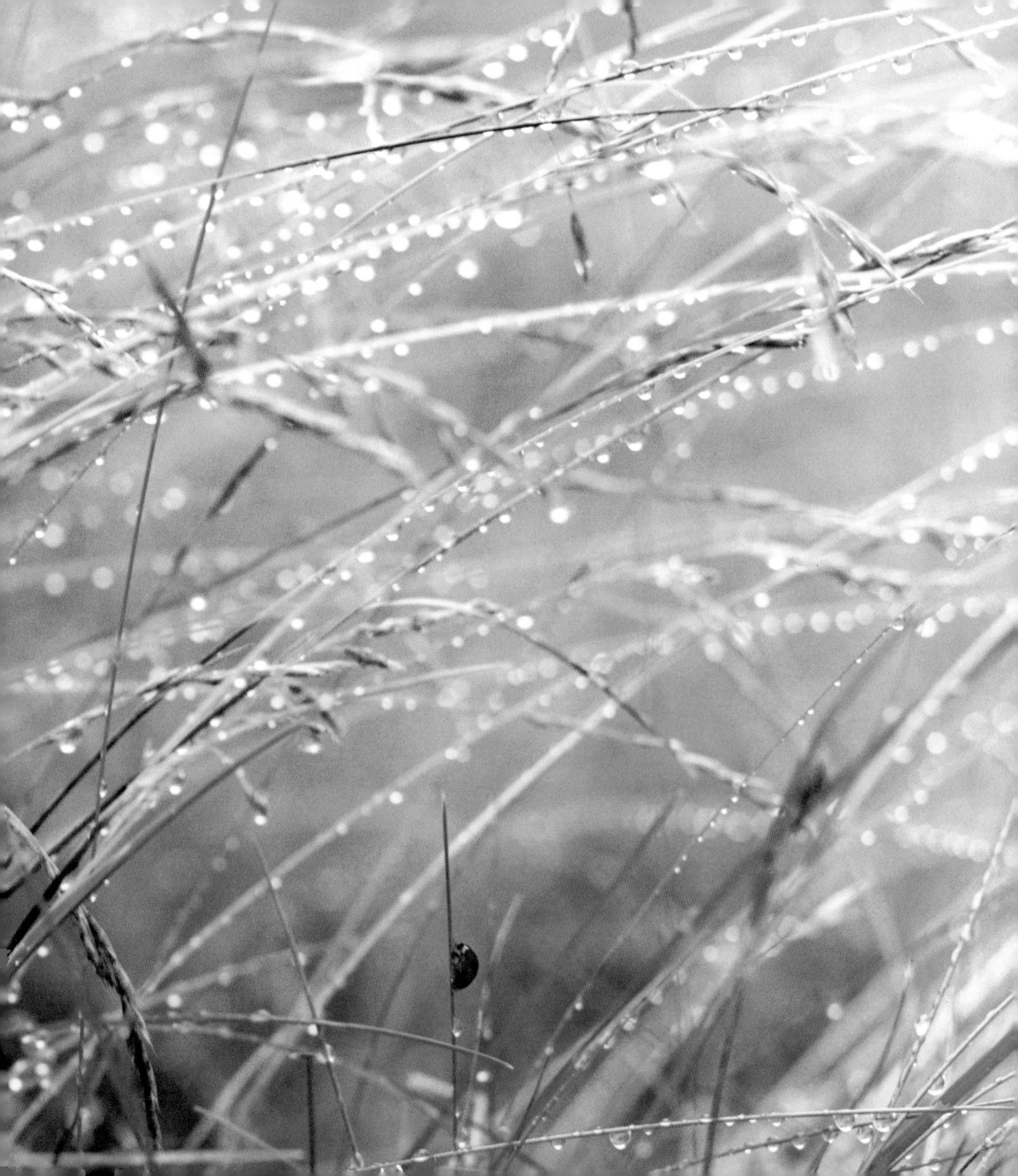

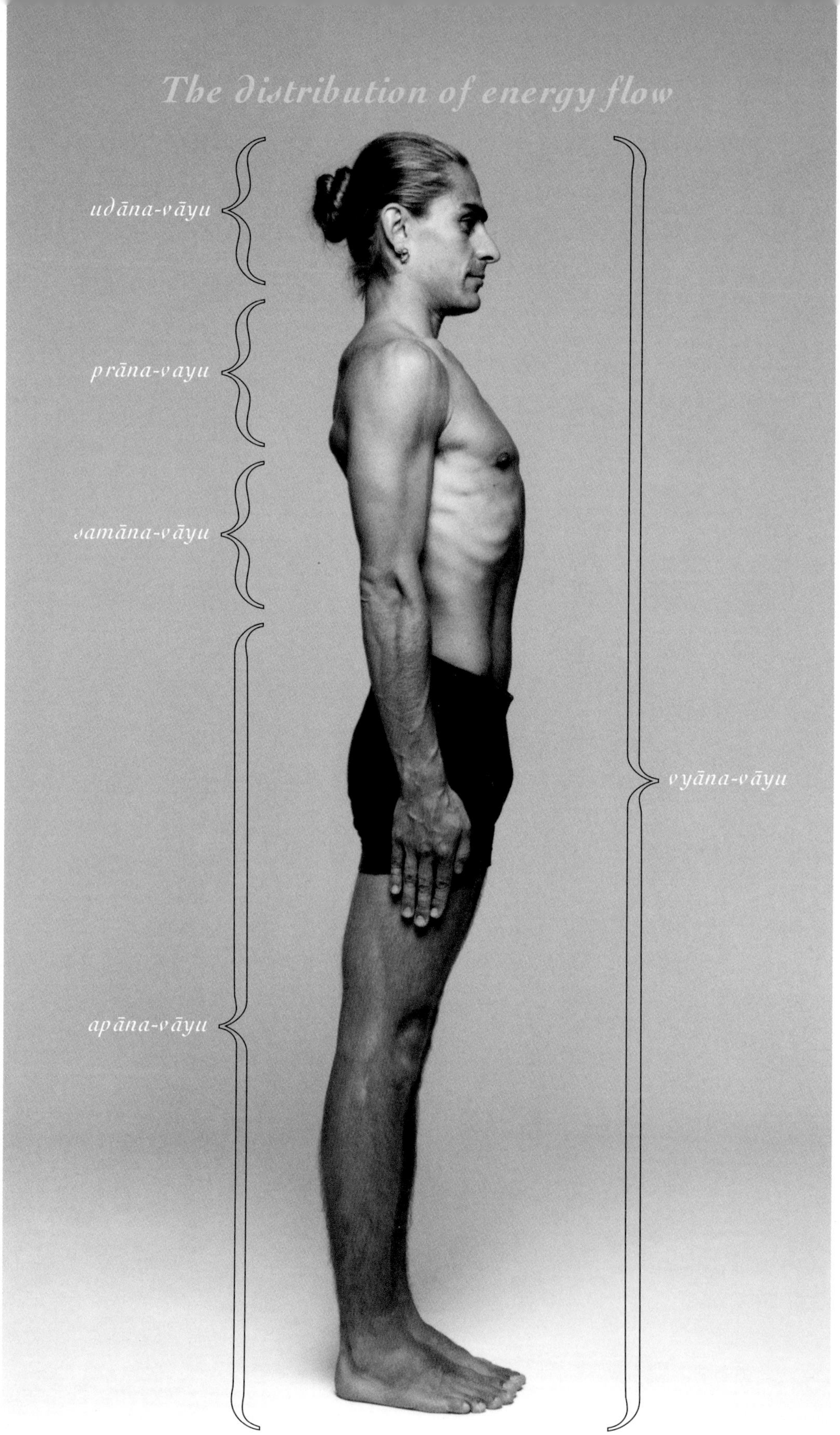
The distribution of energy flow
udāna-vāyu
prāna-vayu
samāna-vāyu
vyāna-vāyu
apāna-vāyu

prāṇa, nāḍī, vāyu & cakra – energy flows of the body

Prāṇa universal spirit; pure energy; cosmic energy; breathing
Nāḍī energy channel; a hollow straw;
Vāyu wind; air, rich with prāṇa
Cakra ring; circle; disk: vibrating energy center

Prāṇa

Prāṇa is the seed of the practice. It is the spiritual fuel. The body and mind start to become purified through the first four limbs of Aṣṭāṅga yoga (yama, niyama, āsana and prāṇāyama), which build the foundation for a deeper state of consciousness to awaken (pratyāhāra, dhāraṇa, and dhyāna). As a result of this, the body's energy flows are strengthened and balanced, which allows for prāṇa to move freely through the energy channels (nāḍīs) and energy centers (cakras) in its most fundamental form. The pure spirit traveling through the nāḍīs makes it possible for the eighth and final limb, samādhi, to manifest.

According to yogic and Ayurvedic principles, prāṇa is an energy that exists primarily in air, but it is also found in the other elements: earth, water, fire and ether. When one inhales through the nose, prāṇa enters the body and is distributed along the īḍā- and piṅgalā-nāḍīs. These nāḍīs join together at the throat, where the viśuddha-cakra, which activates ujjayī (sound) breathing, separates pranic energy from the air. The viśuddha-cakra functions as the body's purification center, where everything that enters the body, in the form of food, drink, air, negative and/or positive energy or emotions, can be processed. From the viśuddha-cakra, prāṇa is lead down to the apāna-vāyu region, where the mūlādhāra-cakra is located. When the bandhas are held properly, the circulation of prāṇa is then reversed; it rises up from the mūlādhāra-cakra, and, once the granthi-traya have been released, travels back up along the main energy channel (suṣumnā-nāḍī) and through every cakra, to the heart's energy center (anahāta-cakra). As prāṇa makes contact with each cakra on its way up, nāḍīs branch off from these and distribute life-energy throughout the body. From anahāta-cakra (the heart center), 101 nāḍīs branch off, and out of these nāḍīs, one in particular, the ātma-nāḍī, leads prāṇa along the suṣumnā-nāḍī to the sahasrāra-cakra (crown's energy center). This causes a "thousand-petaled lotus blossom to open," and is a symbol of spiritual awakening, represented as an aura of white light that shines around the body or head, as Ṛṣi Patanjali is described in the Aṣṭāṅga yoga opening mantra (see pp. 66–67).

Prāṇa is also strongly linked to the mind, and is led wherever the mind directs it. It is thus very important to direct our focus inwards by reciting mantras, practising meditation, gazing at the proper dṛṣṭi, and observing yama and niyama while leading a sattvic (pure and wholesome) lifestyle. A person who leads an unhealthy lifestyle can end up directing prāṇa out of the body and away from the mind, and thus lose vitality. Unhealthy food and drink, too much careless talk and excessive sex can also drain prāṇa out of the nāḍīs and the body, and in this way, one can eventually fall sick. Prāṇa can also be destroyed by too much, or too little, work. Even too much yoga practice is unhealthy, especially if done under stress, or with attachment to accomplishment and other selfish motives.

Nādis

Nāḍīs are channels along which prāṇa travels to the brain, sense organs and various parts of the body. By consistently leading a healthy, yogic lifestyle, the nāḍīs are cleansed from the toxins and impurities that can accumulate in the organs. Yogic philosophy claims that the soul is reincarnated in a new body, for as long as attainment of samādhi and kaivalya is not reached. According to Pattabhi Jois, each individual goes through 22,000 lives before reaching liberation. When one has attained kaivalya, one is free from the poison of delusion (hālāhala) that is found in identifying solely with sense objects and conditioned existence (samsara). In this state of total liberation, one has freed oneself from all prejudice, selfishness and ego-driven karmic tendencies. Thus, the wheel of life, death and rebirth ceases. With the help of āsana, one can stimulate the nāḍīs and build a firm ground for the purification process.

There are three kinds of nāḍīs: dhamani-nāḍī, nāḍī and śira-nāḍī. The thickest one, dhamani-nāḍī, transports blood, water, and air throughout the body. Nāḍī is thinner than dhamani-nāḍī and transports prāṇa, while śira-nāḍī is the thinnest of all three and transports the finer sense perceptions from the universe to the heart center and further to the inner consciousness.

According to yogic philosophy, there are 72,000 nāḍīs running throughout the body. The starting point of this network of energy is the kāṇḍa, an egg-shaped nerve center located just above the anus. The kāṇḍa is more commonly known as mūlādhāra-cakra. Energy rises up from mūlādhāra-cakra along the three main nāḍīs to the other six cakras or energy centers. From each cakra, the nāḍīs branch off, in much the same way as the branches of a tree, and distribute energy throughout the whole body.

Out of the 72,000 nāḍīs, the suṣumnā-, īḍā-, and piṅgalā-nāḍīs are the fundamental ones. The suṣumnā-nāḍī is our most important energy channel, which travels up along the spine (meru-daṇḍa) and targets each of the cakras, starting from the mūlādhāra-cakra and ending at sahasrāra-cakra. The suṣumnā-nāḍī transports spiritual energy from the lower cakras up to the crown of the head. This spiritual energy is often referred to as prāṇa.

Īḍā-nāḍī, also called candra or ha, refers to the moon. This nāḍī winds itself from the kāṇḍa, through the cakras and culminates in the left nostril. The īḍā-nāḍī transports cool, calm and restorative moon energy throughout the body.

Piṅgalā-nāḍī, often called sūrya or ṭha, refers to the sun. This nāḍī winds itself from the kāṇḍa through the cakras up to the right nostril. The piṅgalā-nāḍī transports warm, transformative and dynamic sun energy throughout the body. Prāṇa usually moves through the body via the īḍā- and piṅgalā-nāḍīs, as it is quite rare for the suṣumnā-nāḍī to open itself up.

Vāyu

Vāyu is the cosmic air element found in the form of wind. The life- force that streams throughout the body is divided into five different forms of energy (pañca-mahā). Each energy form has its own name and function, and they provide each part of the body with health and vitality.

The forms of pañca-mahā

Udāna-vāyu

Udāna-vāyu activates the throat and the following areas located above (the throat): the head, back of the neck and the brain. The head includes seven openings: ears, eyes, nostrils and mouth. Udāna-vāyu regulates breathing and the proper intake of food and affects how speech is formed.

Prāṇa-vāyu

Prāṇa-vāyu activates the heart and chest and is responsible for inhalation. In this way, prāṇa-vāyu is also responsible for the body's entire intake of energy and functions to promote longevity. During āsana practice, one tries to join the downwards-flow of apāna-vāyu with prāṇa-vāyu's upwards force, so that energy can distribute itself throughout the body.

Samāna-vāyu

Samāna-vāyu is located between the heart and the navel, and controls the digestive process (agni vaiśvānara). It also activates the functions of the heart, pancreas and liver.

Apāna-vāyu

Apāna-vāyu is the downwards-moving energy that one specifically tries to bring into balance in āsana practice. Too much energy in the area between the navel and the sex organs leads to a feeling of lethargy and laziness, causing multiple health complications and diseases including, but not limited to, obesity, an overactive sex drive, urinary incontinence, low sperm count, hemorrhoids, intestinal problems, and a general loss of energy. Apāna-vāyu manages the body's elimination processes.

Vyāna-vāyu

Vyāna-vāyu encompasses the whole body and sends energy to the limbs, muscles, bones, tendons and nerves. It maintains the body's balance and locomotion.

Cakras

The cakras are inner energy centers, the body's "flying saucers" which vibrate with energy. They are linked via the 72,000 nāḍīs, from the root energy center up to the forehead and crown energy centers.

Cakras receive vibrational energy according to their placement and function in the body. For example, the heart cakra receives mental and sensory stimulation which is then distributed in that specific form of energy throughout the whole body. The śira-nāḍīs at the heart and crown cakras also receive cosmic vibrations from outside the body and disperse this energy through the nāḍīs and dhamani-nāḍī to the energy (prāṇamaya-kośa) and and physical body (annamaya-kośa). In this way, it is possible to be conscious of the interaction between the energy found in the microcosm of an individual body, as well as the surrounding vibrations that make up the macrocosm, the universe.

Yoga āsana, with a focused mind and the proper quality of breath, cleanses the nāḍīs and makes it easier for energy to flow through to the cakras and throughout the entire body. We can affect how this energy flows through breath awareness in prāṇāyama and kumbhaka, holding the bandhas while we do āsana, as well as by maintaining a yogic lifestyle that optimizes our life-force.

The cakras are often depicted as a specific number of lotus petals, which remind us to keep our awareness open in order to experience the unique energy current associated with each cakra. When prāṇa rises along the three main nāḍīs and passes through the cakras, a wave of energy flows through, transforming into the corresponding number of symbolic petals assigned to the specific cakra.

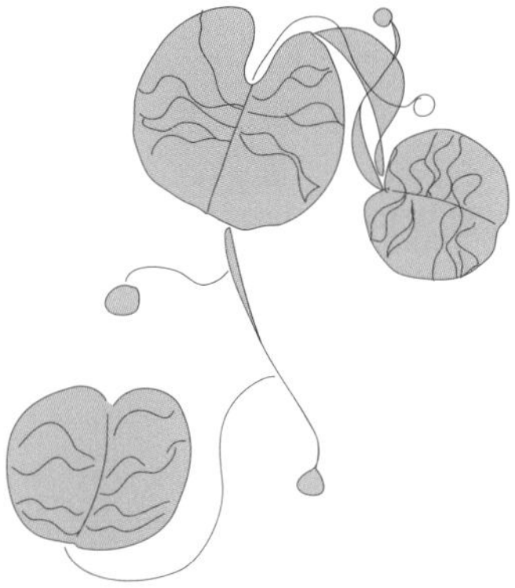

The cakras

Mūlādhāra-cakra

Mūlādhāra means source or root, and is the base from which kuṇḍalinī originates and rises. Kuṇḍalinī is said to be latent and dormant energy located at the base of the spine, which, when awakened, rises up through the spinal column. Mūlādhāra is located in the region of the anus, and is associated with the earth element and the physical body (annamaya-kośa), as well as the digestive system. It plays a role in the downwards-flowing energy (apāna-vāyu), and is therefore associated with the action of excretion, as in urination, menstruation, ejaculation, childbirth and exhalation. As mūlādhāra functions to balance the system, it brings earth-energy, a calming, cleansing, and soul-energizing force to the body. From here, sexual energy (vīrya), can flow upwards and get converted into spiritual energy. Mūlādhāra is represented as a lotus blossom with four petals, and is connected to the nose and sense of smell.

Svādhiṣṭhāna-cakra

Svādhiṣṭhāna is the origin of the inner "I." It is the source of creative energy (prāṇa-śakti) and the desire for pleasure (kāma), such as food and sex. When svādhiṣṭhāna-cakra is in balance, we are full of creative energy, though we must exercise willpower to withstand an excess of desire from interfering with a sattvic lifestyle. Svādhiṣṭhāna is located two inches above the mūlādhāra-cakra and is connected to the body's vital principle (prāṇamaya-kośa), which takes care of processes related to self-propagation, such as blood circulation, digestion, gland secretion and reproduction. This chakra is influenced by the water element and the downwards flow of apāna-vāyu. Svādhiṣṭhāna is represented as a lotus blossom with six petals and is connected to the tongue and sense of taste.

Maṇipura-cakra

Maṇipura means "jewel city" and this cakra works with the sun element (agni) by transporting fire, heat, light and energy via the nāḍīs throughout the body. It also acts as a storage place for prāṇa and is located around the navel. The maṇipura-cakra controls how the organs function and is of rajasic quality: active, willful and strong. Influenced by samāna energy (p. 42) and the fire element, this cakra manages the digestive system and allows for nutrition to be absorbed into the body. Maṇipura is also connected to the prāṇamaya-kośa, in the same way as svādhiṣṭhāna-cakra. Maṇipura is represented as a lotus blossom with ten petals and is connected to the eyes and sense of sight.

Anahāta-cakra

Anahāta means unbeaten, as in an unbeaten drum, and is located along the spine, behind the physical and spiritual heart. It is also called the heart cakra, the feeling center, or the seat of the Divine. The heart cakra is associated with one of yoga's most mystical phenomena: the anahāta-nāda (uncreated sound). This refers to the Vedic idea that one can hear the sound released from all matter and material. It is said to sound like the tinkling of jewels and can be heard only from a state of pure consciousness, rather than on the physical, sensory level of hearing. By purifying the anahāta-cakra, one is freed from selfishness and fluctuating emotional states, boundaries dissolve, there is a strengthening of the inner voice, and a state governed by peace and universal love (bhakti) is imminent. The anahāta-cakra is connected with sahasrāra-cakra and brahma-randhra via the ātma-nāḍī, making it possible for us to perceive god. Anahāta is depicted as a lotus blossom with sixteen petals and is connected to emotion and our ability to feel and sense things outside our physical kośa (layer). It works in collaboration with prāṇa-vāyu, balances our heart and lungs and its element is air.

Viśuddha-cakra

Viśuddha means purifier and this cakra functions on a high level, cleansing both matter and spirit. It works as a filter, purifying what we ingest, draws prāṇa out from the air element and removes toxins. It also develops intelligence in word and clarity of thought, making us conscious of our speech and sharpening our ability of discernment. The viśuddha-cakra is located below the throat, between the collarbones, and works with udāna-vāyu. Its element is ether (ākāśa). When this cakra is in balance, our spirit or soul is similar to the quality of ether: empty and free from excess thought. Viśuddha-cakra is connected to the intellectual body (vijñānamaya-kośa) and deepens our insight and ability to transform our intelligence into wisdom. Viśuddha is depicted as a lotus blossom with twenty petals and is connected with the ears and our speech capacity.

Ājñā-cakra

Ājñā-cakra is often called the third eye. It is also known as Śiva's or Īśvara's eye, wisdom's eye, the guru-cakra, the center for boundless psychic power (siddhi), or, literally, the "command center." It is through this center that we find direct contact with universal knowledge, divine luminance and experience of the self. One might even be able to access one's previous lives. When this cakra is in perfect balance, all sense of ego and dualistic thinking dissolves, the power of insight is strengthened, and the connection with universal creative energy is possible. Ājñā-cakra is depicted as a lotus blossom with two petals; it is located between the eyebrows (bhrū-madhya) and is connected to the center of the brain.

Sahasrāra-cakra

Sahasrāra is the principal cakra, which vibrates with light to all the lower cakras. It is depicted as a thousand-petaled lotus blossom (*sahasra*- thousand). When prāṇa streams through the cakras to sahasrāra-cakra, one experiences spiritual freedom and, it is said, can achieve miraculous powers (siddhis). Sahasrāra-cakra is opened only when prāṇa has passed through the lower cakras. Connected with higher consciousness, the sahasrāra-cakra is located at the crown of the head.

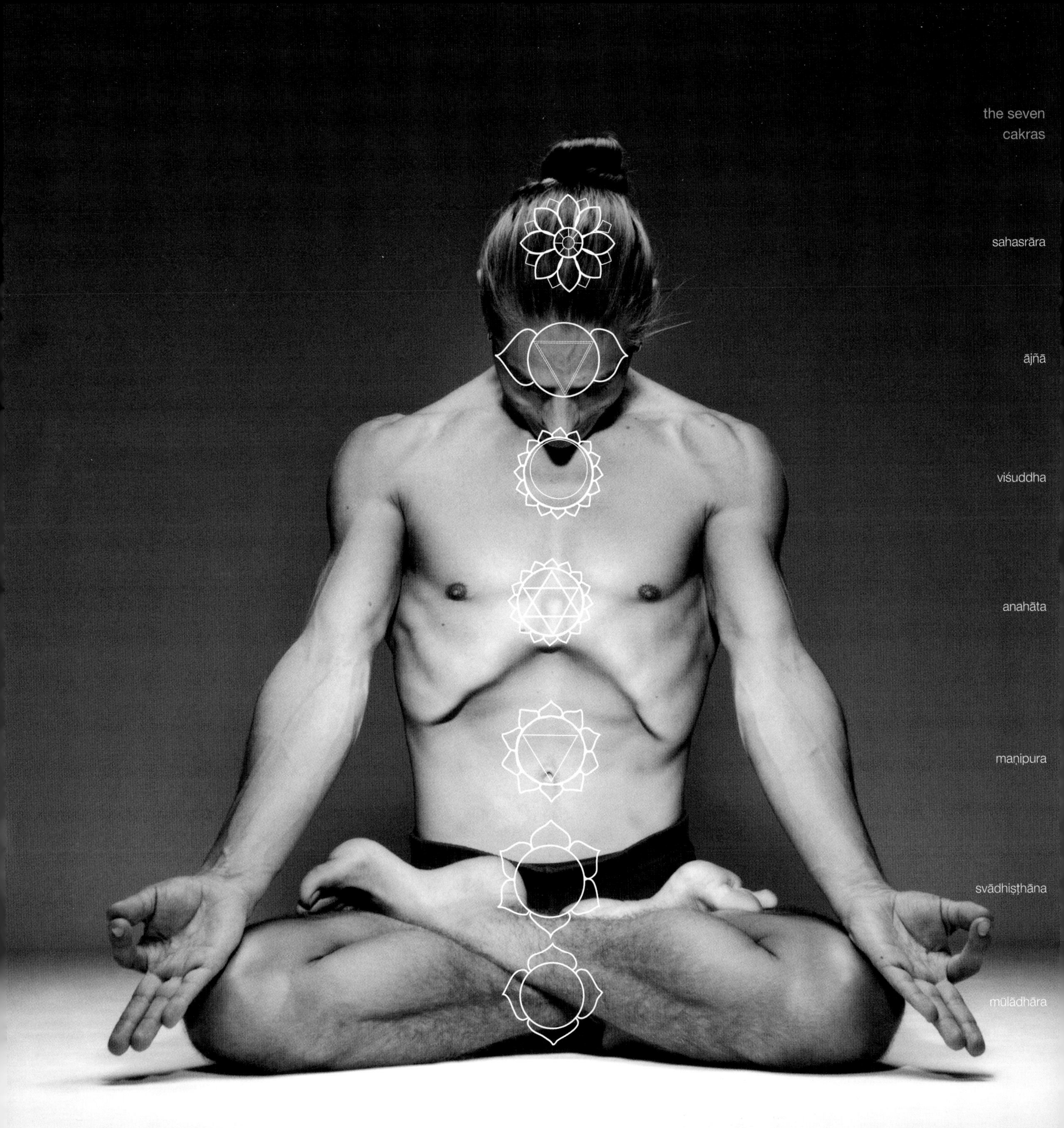
the seven
cakras
sahasrāra
ājñā
viśuddha
anahāta
maṇipura
svādhiṣṭhāna
mūlādhāra

Prāṇāyama practice, engaging the three bandhas after Bhasya kumbhaka

Amṛta-bindu – nectar of immortality

According to the holy texts (śruti- what is heard; smṛti- what is remembered), through practice, the yogi is said to be able to prolong life and reach self-awareness, which is considered unattainable for the common man. If one focuses entirely on the outer world, or is lead by lust and desire, one cannot attain union with this ever-growing energy that yoga provides. Everything that pulls the mind away from the higher self eventually weakens the mind and depletes it of its natural state of purity.

Amṛta-bindu, or nectar of immortality, and how one preserves this vital power is one of the most incredible and ancient insights that yoga offers. The śāstras describe how the formation of amṛta-bindu occurs in the abdomen, through digestion and in a complex process where bile from the liver mixes with food. Bile breaks fat down, so that the absorption of digestive enzymes (produced in the pancreas) can occur, and the bile is then transported back to the liver. In order to get as much nutrition from the food as possible, it is essential that the bile returns to the liver before the liver starts to process our next meal. Therefore, it is said that food eaten in the evening gives more energy than food eaten during the day. During the evening and at night, as the body rests, there is a longer period of time for bile to break down the fat, before it returns to the liver. To be sure that the bile has completely disappeared from the body (i.e. returned to the liver), it is beneficial to practice inversions (viparīta-karaṇi) at the end of the practice. If the bile that remains in the body, still in a highly concentrated form, is carried to the crown of the head during headstand or shoulderstand, some of the brain cells might get damaged and the return of bile to the liver may be weakened. This is the reason why inverted āsanas come at the end of the sequences, after the forward bending and twisting āsanas have heated up the blood. This blood has then circulated through the body and diluted the high concentration of bile.

The transformation of amṛta-bindu: from food to life-force

According to yogic texts, the food that we eat gets broken down into energy, and 32 days after initial ingestion, this food becomes a drop of blood. After 32 drops of blood have been distilled, it takes another 32 days for these drops of blood to be transformed into a single drop of life-force. Once 32 drops of life-force have accumulated, it takes another 32 days for one drop of amṛta-bindu, the nectar of immortality, to be created.

When a drop of (amṛta) bindu has been created, it is then circulated via the blood vessels to the seven functions (dhātus), which keeps the body healthy and youthful. These seven dhātus are comprised of the lymphatic system or plasma (rasa), blood (rakta), flesh or muscle tissue (mansa), fat (meda), bones (asthi), bone marrow (majja), and the sexual fluids (shukra: vīrya, male fluid or semen and śoṇita, female fluid or ova). Through the discipline gained in the fourth yama, brahmacarya, we are able to replenish and increase vīrya and śoṇita, which both contain the elusive bindu.

In addition to the seven dhātus, amṛta-bindu travels from the stomach to the crown of the head, to the sahasrāra-cakra and brahma-randhra (or Brahmā's opening). Brahma-randhra is commonly referred to, in the West, as the fontanelle, the soft spot on the head of a baby. If amṛta-bindu is strong, through brahma-randhra, we can sense god or Brahmā. It is through this opening that the soul leaves the body when we die. It is also said that when a child is six months old, prāṇa travels from the feet, through the body and up to brahma-randhra. When prāṇa reaches the crown of the head, the child begins to move its arms and legs energetically. From the brahma-randhra, amṛta-bindu will typically drop back down to the stomach, and is then burned by the digestive fire (agni). This occurs if an individual is not sufficiently purified enough to contain amṛta-bindu, as the nāḍīs are not able to keep channeling it up.

Living an unhealthy lifestyle and/or mindlessly wasting the body's fluids tires the body and mind and weakens one's life-force. One can become sick more easily, and the mind is susceptible to a variety of usually negative influences. Yoga improves the production of amṛta-bindu and can restore these precious drops to the brahma-randhra. It is essential to preserve these drops, and prevent them from trickling down to agni, where they will get consumed.

Amṛta-bindu is sensitive and reacts to all the functions in the body. The life cycle of amṛta-bindu essentially depends on our health, which in turn depends upon the purity of the food we eat, the quality of the air we breathe and the overall nature of our lifestyle. Āsana increases amṛta-bindu and together with creative and positive action, improves our quality of life while strengthening our spirit.

The final cultivation of amṛta-bindu in the brahma-randhra is a result of viparīta-karaṇi, or inversions, with the headstand being the most effective āsana for the accumulation of amṛta-bindu. Practising inversions daily, and for a significant amount of time, allows for amṛta-bindu to gather inside the crown of the head, where it remains and is prevented from flowing down to the stomach and getting destroyed by agni.

When amṛta-bindu's life-force accumulates in the brahma-randhra, the yoga student begins to feel refreshed and uplifted, mental processes are strengthened, and a youthful energy comes back to life. One can enjoy a long, healthy and happy life. According to Indian thought, Brahmā has given us all 100 years, and if one is able to extend life beyond that normal span this is known as "immortality," overcoming death. According to Pattabhi Jois, a yogi can live up to 150–200 years old by following a dedicated yogic lifestyle and maintaining calm, extended respiration.

Ancient texts stress the importance of amṛta-bindu's life-power, "To lose amṛta-bindu means death, whereas its preservation means overcoming mortality".

"The purpose of a long life is so that we will be able to pray longer."
Śrī K. Pattabhi Jois

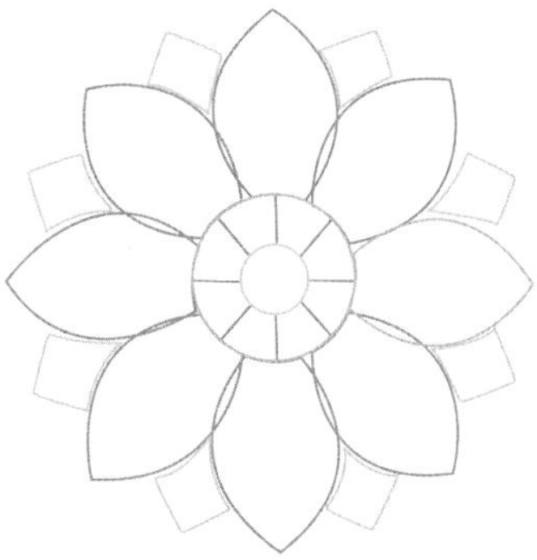

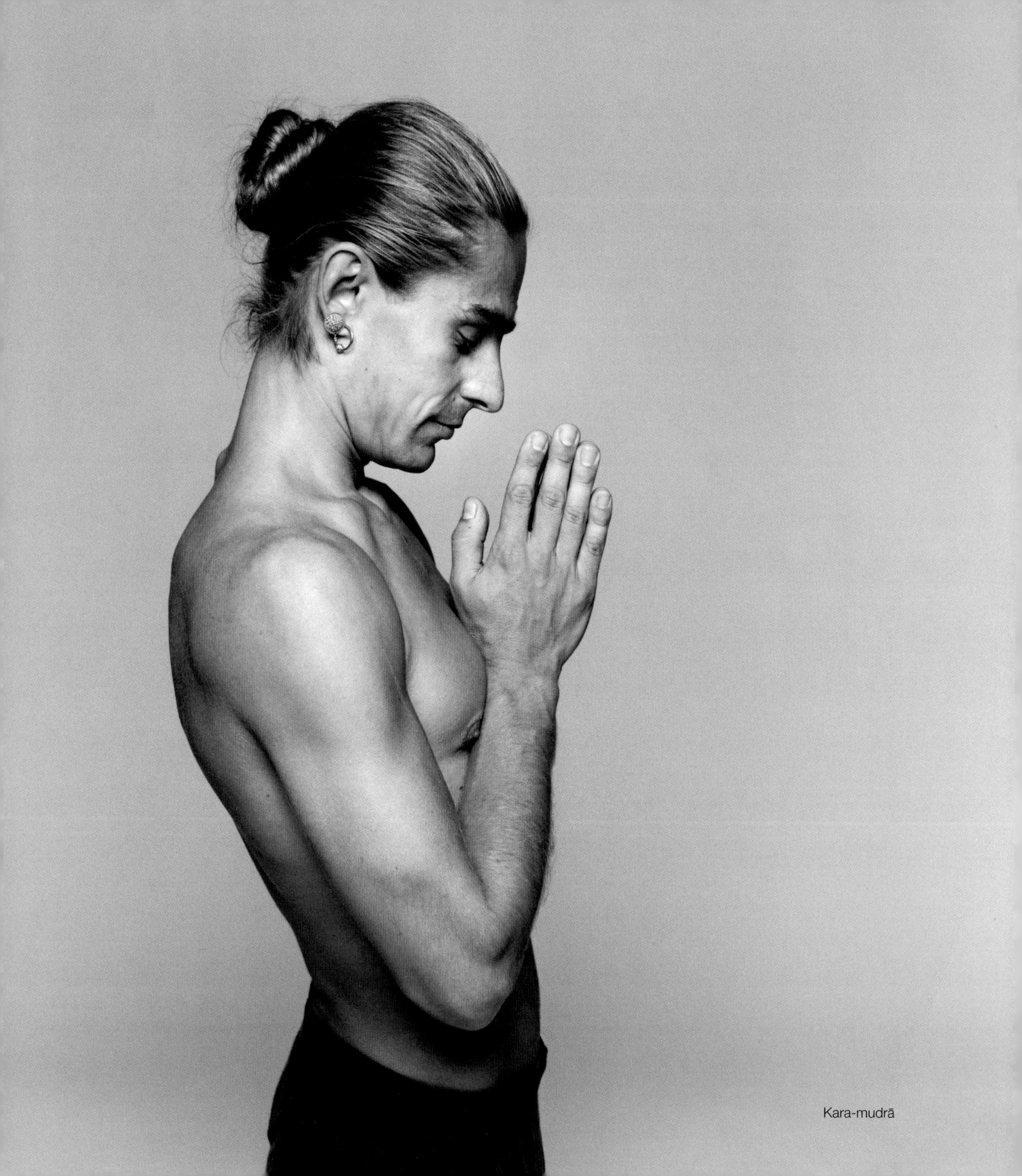

Kara-mudrā

the guṇas

The three guṇas (sattva, rajas, tamas) are the qualities that exist in nature (prakṛti) and have a direct relation with our behavior, tendencies and temperament. Rajas and tamas are opposing qualities, whereas sattva is the state of clarity and balance. These qualities are in constant flux with each other and within nature itself, influencing various aspects of our lives. All the guṇas are needed for everyday life; for example, tamas is the quality of the bones and rajas of the blood circulation. Yoga cleanses the body and mind from opposition and imbalance, and provides us with the tools necessary to bring out our sattvic nature, made up of qualities such as light, love, purity and spiritual awareness. The highest yogic state, which goes beyond the impermanant state of the three guṇas and is beyond nature, is called guṇātīta.

Sattva

Sattva represents clarity and balance, which shows itself as health, purity, cleanliness, clarity, lightness, peace, spiritual awareness, compassion and love.

Rajas

Rajas represents the active and aggressive quality which is constantly shifting and changing. Rajas does not leave people in peace, rather, it constantly fills the mind with thoughts and desires. It has an oppositional, binding and craving nature. The positive side to rajas is that it gives us the impetus to change and transform ourselves, pushing people forwards, away from old habits, illnesses or prejudices that weaken our enthusiasm for life.

Tamas

Tamas is the still, dark, low-energy force, which presents itself as sluggishness, heaviness, ignorance, lack of feeling and selfishness. Pain and illness are also part of tamas, and because of its worrisome nature, these ailments can stay in the body for quite some time. The positive aspect in tamas is that it balances out the active energy of rajas, permitting us to slow down and restore ourselves when needed.

practice methods for body and mind

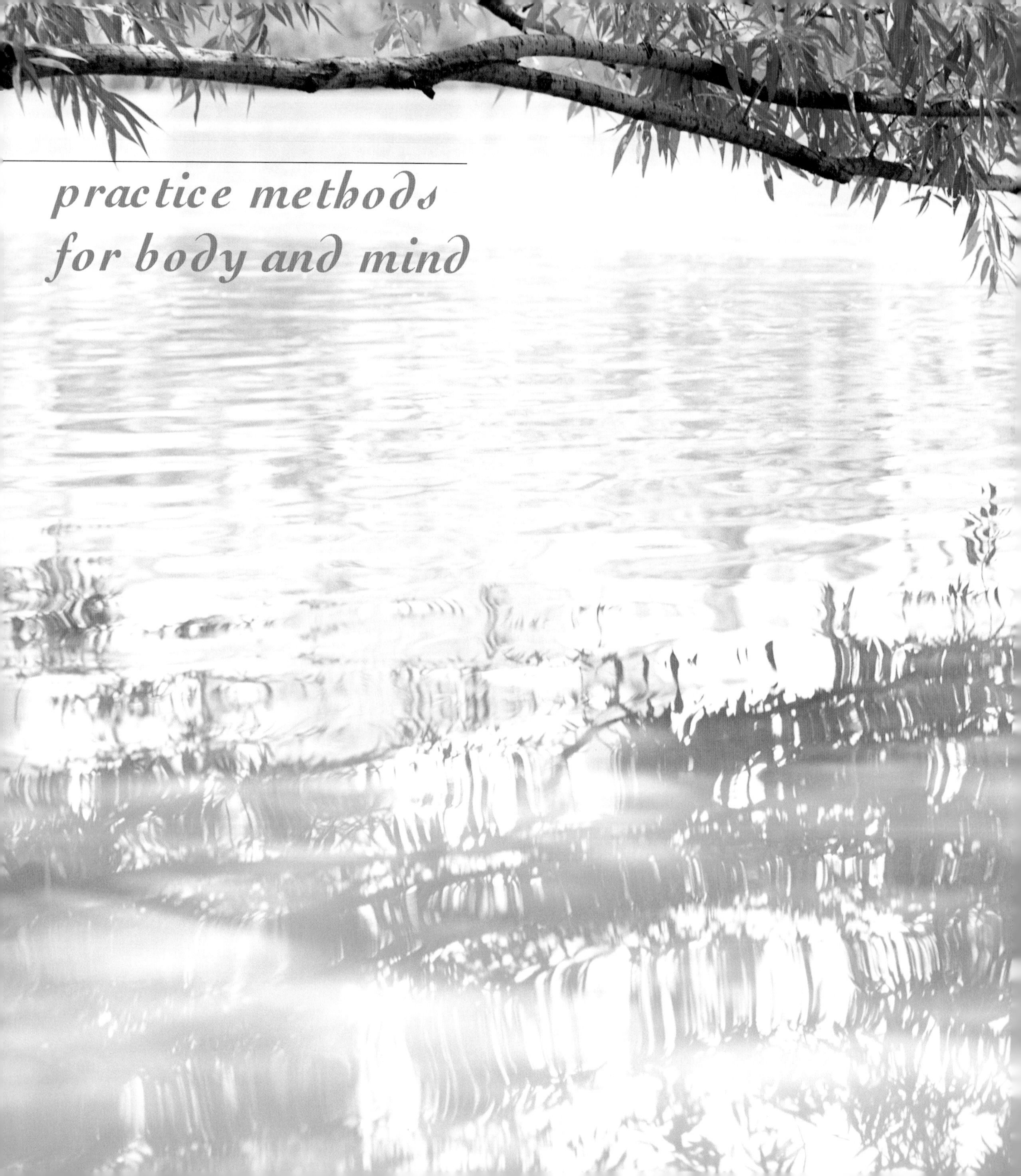

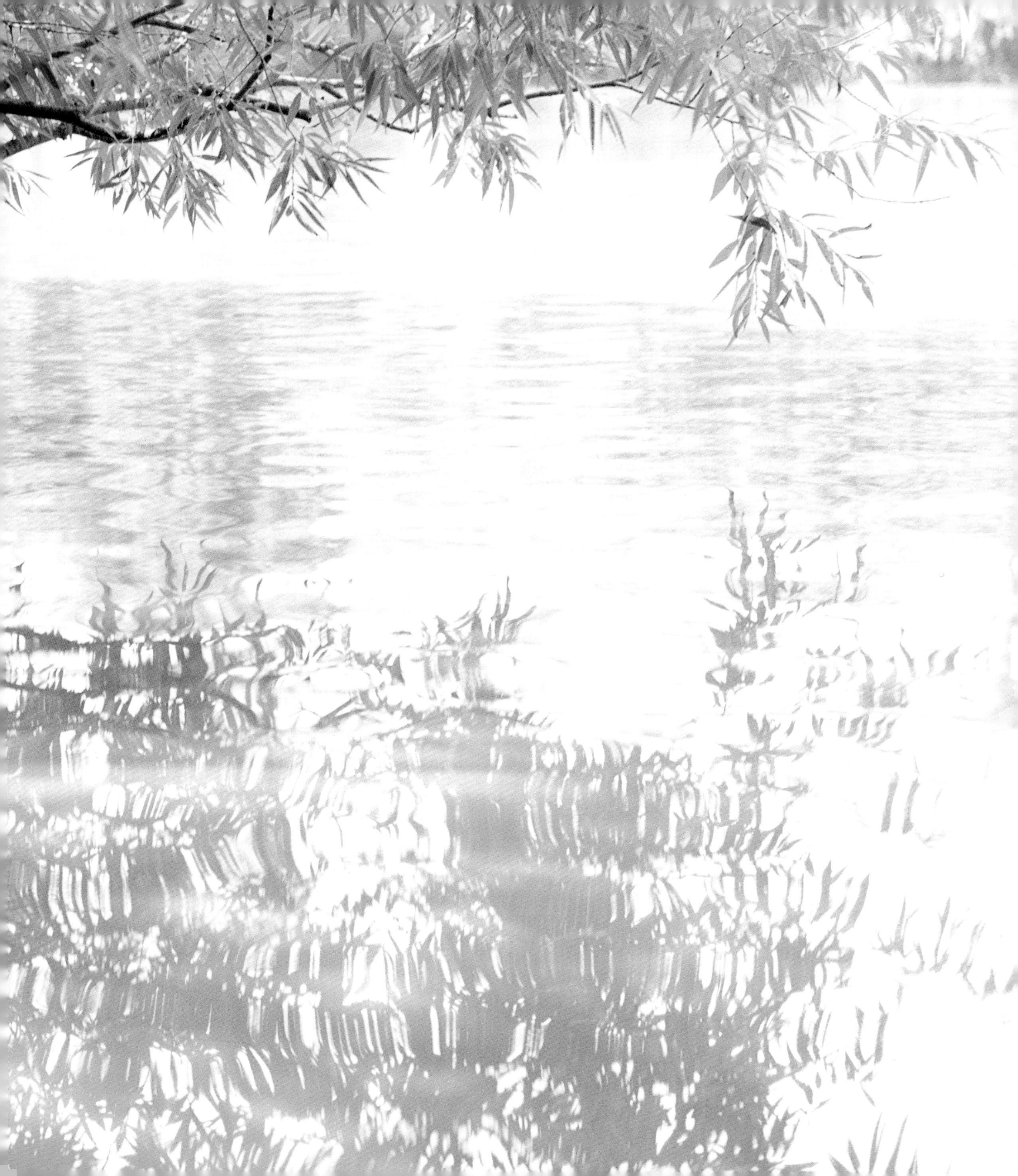

practice methods for body and mind

Aṣṭāṅga yoga contains specific methods, which are done during āsana and prāṇāyama: vinyāsa (linking breath to movement; see p. 61), bandha (muscle and energy locks, p. 54), and dṛṣṭi (gazing points, p. 58). Together these three make up tri-sthāna. Through the use of tri-sthāna, one can deepen the experience of āsana on both the physical and mental level, lessen or eliminate distraction from the outer senses (pratyāhāra), and direct the self inwards, towards a one-pointed meditative state (dhyāna).

Breath

The breathing technique in Aṣṭāṅga yoga is sound breath or audible throat breathing, generally known as ujjayī or victorious breath. Pattabhi Jois frequently called it "sound breathing," to clarify the difference between ujjayī-prāṇāyama, a certain type of prāṇāyama, and this breathing technique, which is used when practising āsana. With this specific technique, one creates a conscious connection between the body, mind and the flow of energy. The body moves in tandem with the rhythm of the breath while deep, even breathing balances and relaxes the mind. One can see the breath as the most vital part of the practice, as it is the foundation of our very being, our health, and eventually our ability to control the mind. In India it is believed that vāyu, or air, is one of God's forms, for without air and breath we would not be able to live. With proper breathing, the body receives enough oxygen even in the more challenging āsanas, the muscles and tendons relax, the mind calms down, and prāṇa can flow through the nāḍīs. In this way, the body becomes light, supple and strong, and the mind concentrated and stable. When the mind grows quiet, connection with the inner self is at hand.

The breathing done with āsana is different from the breathing done during prāṇāyama. The inhalation and exhalation are not as long during āsana and the breath is not retained (kumbhaka). Furthermore, the inhalation and the exhalation should be of equal length during āsana, meaning each inhalation and each exhalation lasts about 5–10 seconds. These will be lengthened during the finishing sequence. Stable and calm breathing during āsana practice creates a suitable and harmonious rhythm for the vinyāsa and ensures a sufficient amount of energy and oxygen for the body. This breathing technique, in addition to strong bandhas, purifies the body and releases tension through the build-up of heat and the process of sweating. Regardless of the length of the breath, the lungs should be filled completely on an inhalation and emptied fully on the exhalation.

During prāṇāyama, the inhalation and exhalation can be of varying ratios and often increase in length considerably. The breath can also be held in certain exercises, often up to several minutes at a time.

Sound (ujjayī) breathing technique

Ujjayī breathing literally translates as victorious breath, although it is more accurately called sound breathing, as one audibly engages the breath at the base of the throat. The breath is not forced in the same way as in ujjayī-prāṇāyama, rather, it is smoother, enabling free movement of prāṇa to take place. The sound of the breath can be described as the sound of waves on a beach, or of the wind in the tree-tops. It is a smooth, even and audible breath that begins at the start of practice and continues throughout, to the last āsana.

1. You can either stand in Samasthitiḥ, sit with crossed-legs or get into Padmāsana, lotus pose. Straighten the spine, expand the upper body and keep the shoulders relaxed and neutral so that the lungs can move freely and it's possible to take a deep breath.
2. Close the mouth gently without tensing the lips. Begin with a calm inhalation through the nose, extending it for slightly longer than your normal inhalation.
3. Direct the breath to the throat and gently engage the muscles of the throat to form a slightly smaller channel for breathing.
4. As you draw the breath in through this smaller channel, a soft roaring sound is created in the throat. If you hear the sound coming through the nasal passage, this is not yet correct. Try to deepen the breathing, keeping the focus in the throat, as opposed to the nose. The proper technique requires that the sound comes from the throat.
5. Try to create this gentle, roaring sound as purely as possible: it should be soft, deep and continuous, without any extraneous sounds such as snorts and whining. Try not to force it by breathing too deeply or heavily, and avoid pressing the air through the throat, as this wastes energy and can make your practice heavy.
6. Even out the inhalation and exhalation so that they are of the same length and quality. The breath should move in and out of the body at the same pace from start to finish, so avoid speeding up at any point during the inhalation or exhalation. Do not hold the breath while doing āsana, as this locks the muscles, preventing them from relaxing, and creates pressure in the head which can lead to headaches or dizziness.
7. Sound breathing is done together with uddīyana- and mūla-bandha. This strengthens the pelvis and abdominal areas and

prevents the lower abdomen from moving as one breathes. During āsana practice, the area from the navel and below do not visibly move in and out with the breath, even if prāṇa streams through these regions.

8. During the inhalation, let the prāṇa flow up from the apāna region (hip area); expand the muscles in the lower back while lifting and engaging uddīyana-bandha, in the lower abdomen. Fill the lungs with air, and expand the chest and upper spine. At the end of the breath, the diaphragm has expanded, giving depth and power to the breath. When the lungs have been filled, lengthen the entire torso in order to give the spinal discs and upper body more space. When exhaling, draw the diaphragm inwards, tightening mūla-bandha towards the end of the breath, but keep lengthening the torso. Empty the lungs before the next inhalation.

Effects of sound breathing

1. By listening to the smooth, even sound, the mind becomes calm and focused.
2. By listening to the gentle, soft breath while inhaling and exhaling evenly, one can be sure that the breath is supporting the āsanas correctly. When the breath is uneven and erratic or too thick, heavy and forceful, this is a sign that the energy is being misdirected by unhelpful thoughts, or that energy is being wasted.
3. By listening to the breath and adjusting the āsana (and the movements between) to the rhythm of the breath, the practice becomes precise, smooth and meditative.
4. The prāṇa that is collected through sound breathing fills the body with energy and gives the strength needed for āsana.
5. Observing and calming the breath directs the mind inwards to a meditative state.
6. This technique slows respiration down while bringing about powerful and enriching qualities to our breathing process. In this way, one is guaranteed to take in the maximum amount of oxygen for the body and bloodstream.
7. Even and calm breathing gives the body and mind time and space to understand the āsana's inner alignment (inner feelings, peace and movement of energy) as well as a feeling for the outer alignment.
8. By calming and relaxing the breath, the muscles and tendons in turn also relax, and it becomes easier to move through the āsana series free of pain.
9. The subtle friction created at the back of the throat in order to make the breath audible strengthens and refines the throat muscles.
10. Through sound breathing, and the application of bandhas, the inner organs are lifted up, which supports the flow of oxygen to the crown of the head. In this way, the crown becomes clear and energized. Similarly, when engaging the bandhas and breathing with sound during daily activities, one is benefited with an increase in energy.
11. Sound breathing balances the thyroid gland, which is connected to the viśuddha-cakra, functioning as the body and mind's filter, purifying the air and drawing prāṇa out from the air.
12. Strong, controlled breath cleanses the throat, air passages and lungs, clarifies the voice and strengthens the heart.
13. The deep breathing that is developed transforms the way we breathe when we are not engaged in āsana, prāṇāyama or other yogic activities. In this way, we naturally learn to breathe through the nose in a calm and conscious way during our daily routine.

Bandhas

Bandhas direct the body's inner energy flows, prāṇa and vāyu, to the proper nāḍīs and function as support mechanisms for the physical body. Bandha means lock, which works as a physical and energetic support for the body. They bring lightness and strength to the body, so that āsana and prāṇāyama can be performed properly and with less forceful effort. They also stabilize and strengthen the body, while facilitating its flexibility and alignment. In addition, bandhas protect the inner organs as well as balancing and cleansing the digestive system.

There are two bandhas in the Aṣṭāṅga yoga āsana practice: mūla-bandha (root lock) and uddīyana-bandha (abdominal lock). The third bandha, jalandhara-bandha (throat lock) is used only during prāṇāyama, when retaining the breath. In some āsana, i.e. shoulderstand, the chin is tucked down in order to touch the collarbones. However, this is not considered to be jalandhara-bandha. Engaging jalandhara-bandha for the purposes of prāṇāyama is a different matter altogether. In prāṇāyama, these three locks work in conjunction with each other. During āsana, mūla-bandha and uddīyana-bandha are activated by lifting mūla-bandha up, towards the navel, where it meets uddīyana-bandha, which in turn, is lifted upwards and pulled in towards the spine. When one applies jalandhara-bandha during prāṇāyama, this completes the link with the two previous bandhas.

It is important to note that the bandhas are engaged in varying degrees depending on which āsanas are being done. One should work on controlling the bandhas throughout the practice. Occasionally, they are released, sometimes they are only slightly lifted, and at other times they are fully and actively engaged. These differences are mentioned in the chapter on āsana and technique. If there is no special mention of bandhas for a particular āsana, with each exhalation the focus should be on holding in mūla-bandha, and with each inhalation the focus should be on holding and lifting uddīyana-bandha.

Beginners

It can be difficult for beginners to sense and engage the bandhas at first. The muscles that control the bandhas may be weak, and it can be difficult to determine their exact location. Often the mind is focused on remembering the technique and sequence of the āsana, and it may be an extra challenge to keep the bandhas engaged. There is no need to worry about this, as the strength and ability needed to use the bandhas develop gradually. Over time, together with āsana, one is naturally more able to focus on the finer details of the practice, such as bandha and dṛṣṭi. Keep holding the bandhas every time you remember, when the mind is not too busy with the other technical aspects of the practice.

Mūla-bandha and technique

Mūla-bandha means root lock. The name describes the origin of energy (prāṇa, kuṇḍalinī, agni), as the energy channels – the nāḍīs, or even their point of origin, kāṇḍa – are activated by the very muscles that are used to engage this bandha. The technique for mūla-bandha is quite simple. While exhaling, one draws in the anal opening with the external and internal sphincter muscles, and lifts it up towards the navel. One can also mentally focus on this area and lift it in the direction of the navel. The muscles in the pelvis's lower region, including the sex organs and perineum, will be activated to a lesser degree when holding mūla-bandha. Be aware that the gluteal muscles – maximus, medius, minimus gluteal muscles – are not contracted during mūla-bandha.

Mūla-bandha's effects

1. Conscious engagement of mūla-bandha, as well as its subsequent cleansing of the intestines and upwards flow of energy, helps calm the mind, which can then stabilize one's level of concentration.
2. It redirects apāna-vāyu's downwards-flow of energy upwards, where apāna-vāyu can join the upwards-flow of prāṇa-vāyu.
3. It strengthens the muscles around the rectum and sex organs as well as the pelvic muscles. Better control of the sexual organs, bladder and intestines is achieved, which means that bindu and ojas (vigor; life-force) are strengthened.
4. It strengthens and aids in the relaxation of the pelvic area during childbirth, as well as helping to heal and restore the pelvis after delivery.
5. It improves the health and function of the rectum, and eliminates hemorrhoids and other intestinal ailments.
6. It functions as a tremendous support in relaxing and calming the body during challenging āsanas and techniques such as when one lifts the body up and jumps back after the sitting positions, or jumps through to come to a seated position.
7. Drawing mūla-bandha together helps keep the pelvis grounded and in contact with the floor. This is particularly useful in sitting āsanas where the pelvis easily bends forwards with the upper body like in Marīcy-āsana A and B and Baddha-koṇāsana.
8. It cleanses the kāṇḍa (the origin of the nāḍīs) and granthi-trayas (the three energy knots), as well as mūlādhāra-cakra.

Uddīyana-bandha with āsana and technique

Uddīyana means upwards-flying and directs prāṇa upwards through the nāḍīs. It is described as an upwards-flying bird of prāṇa, which provides several health effects for the body. While doing āsana, uddīyana-bandha is located four inches, or four angulas (one angula is the width of one finger) below the navel, and is activated by contracting in and lifting the abdominal muscles up towards the diaphragm and the lungs. Drawing in and lifting up the lower abdomen will cause the whole area around the lower stomach to press into the spine, for the diaphragm to lift up, and for uddīyana-bandha to unite with the engaged mūla-bandha. While inhaling, the entire area of the lower abdomen should remain drawn in, engaged and still, whereas the upper stomach and chest should move freely with the diaphragm and lungs. The lifting up of uddīyana-bandha does not mean that the entire abdomen should be stiff or hard like a boxer's stomach, but rather that the deeper-lying muscles of the stomach are engaged while the outer muscles of the abdomen remain somewhat soft and relaxed. There are some exceptions in certain positions, such as Navāsana, where one needs to engage the larger muscles of the abdomen to perform the āsana. In an advanced prāṇāyama practice, when the breath is held after the exhalation, both the lower abdomen and the diaphragm are lifted up and held still.

Uddīyana-bandha's effects

1. Along with mūla-bandha, uddīyana-bandha helps release and direct apāna-vāyu's energy up towards prāṇa-vāyu, and draw prāṇa into the suṣumnā-nāḍī and up to the crown of the head. At the same time, apāna-vāyu's downwards flow draws toxins into the abdomen where agni, the digestive fire, burns them up.
2. It protects the abdomen and lower back by strengthening the muscles and keeping them engaged throughout āsana practice.
3. It relieves tension and works in the stomach, cleaning and massaging the organs and intestines; it also corrects the alignment of the lower back by supporting the spine and lower back muscles.
4. It protects the inner organs by directing the practitioner to use

the strength of the abdomen and sacral region, as well as by lifting the inner organs upwards.

5. It improves balance and control by keeping the core of the body strong, bringing consciousness into that area.
6. It stretches and strengthens the muscles around the spine and creates expansion in the chest.
7. It dissolves unnecessary fat around the hips and develops the stomach muscles.
8. It lifts the inner organs and chest up, which helps open the passage for fresh oxygen to travel up to the head, keeping it clear and energized.
9. Uddīyana-bandha functions as an important part of the sound-breathing technique. This deeply engaged yet relaxed attention through the diaphragm, chest, abdomen and lungs helps both to deepen and strengthen the breath as well as to broaden one's breathing capacity.
10. It improves blood circulation throughout the stomach and abdomen and aids in generating digestive fluids.
11. Uddīyana-bandha activates and purifies svādhiṣṭhāna-cakra (the second cakra which follows mūlādhāra-cakra).

Jalandhara-bandha and technique

Jalandhara-bandha means chin lock and is engaged by lengthening the back of the neck and pressing the chin half way down towards, against or just below the collarbones. The throat lock is held so that the flow of air in the throat and the movement of the breath stops after an inhalation or an exhalation. For this reason, jalandhara-bandha is only applied in separate breathing exercises (prāṇāyama) and not during āsana, even if the position of the neck appears similar in certain poses such as in Sarvangāsana (shoulderstand).

Jalandhara-bandha's effects

1. It lifts and straightens the spine and helps expand the lungs and chest fully while the breath is retained.
2. It acts as an inner lock, along with mūla- and uddīyana-bandha, making it easier to hold the breath.
3. It creates pressure that pushes prāṇa into the nāḍīs and thus cleanses these passageways.
4. It activates and purifies viśuddha-cakra.
5. It releases pressure from the head, aiding the unrestricted flow of prāṇa along the spine and the suṣumnā-nāḍī, up to the crown of the head.
6. It improves blood circulation in the area of the chest, throat and head.
7. It cleanses and strengthens the air passages, the throat and the heart.
8. Jalandhara-bandha balances the thyroid.

bandha

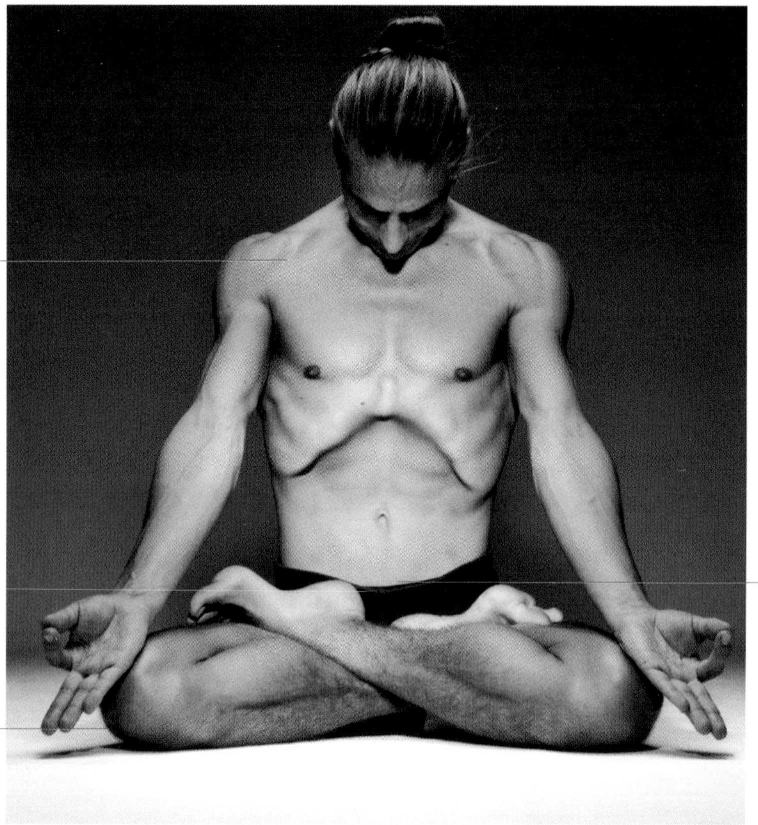

jalandhara-bandha*

uddīyana-bandha*

*{as in prāṇāyama when one holds the breath after the exhalation, bahya or recaka kumbhaka}

mūla-bandha

The bandha and dṛṣṭi symbols are used in the quick-reference guides within the pages of the āsana description.

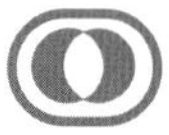

jalandhara-bandha

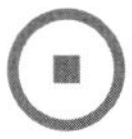

uddīyana-bandha

mūla-bandha

drṣṭi

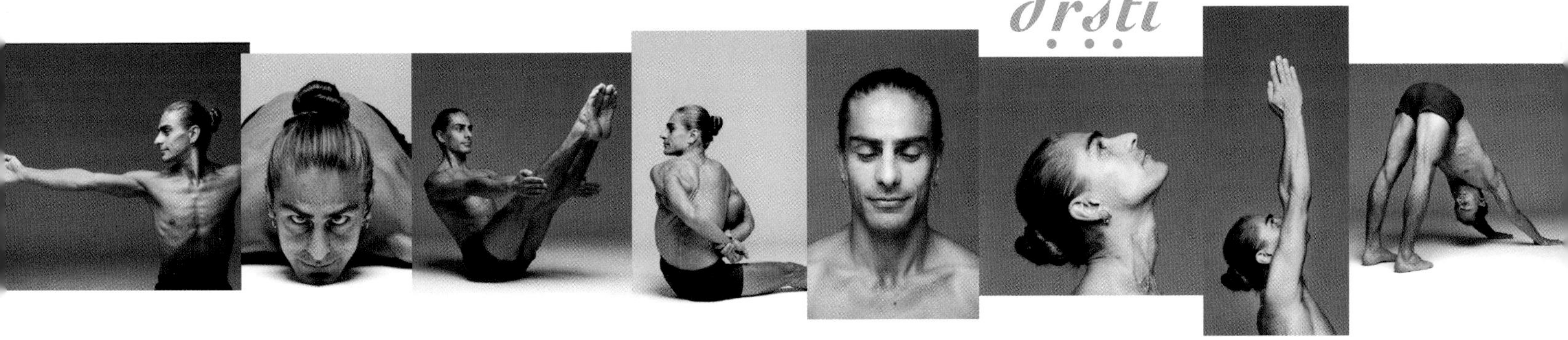

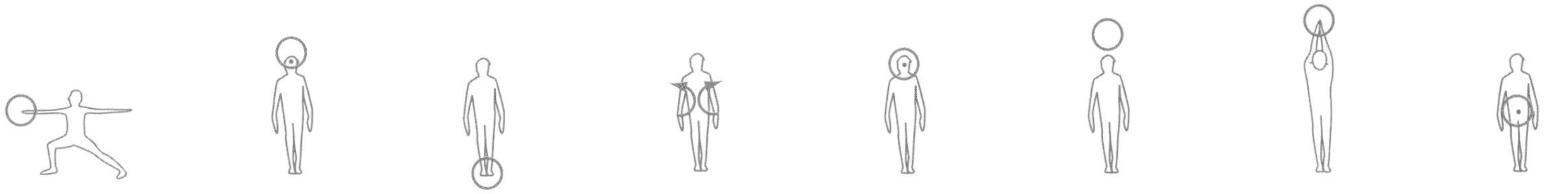

hastāgra

bhrumadhya

pādhayor-agra or pādāṅguṣṭha

parśva (right and left)

nāsāgra

ūrdhva or antara

aṅguṣṭha madhya or angushtha

nābhi chakra

dṛṣṭi – gazing point

In Aṣṭāṅga yoga, dṛṣṭi, or gazing points, are an important tool to incorporate with the āsana. One of the main purposes of dṛṣṭi is to fix one's attention and focus inwards in order to cultivate deep concentration in the āsana, while filling and maintaining the body with radiating prāṇa. Despite the fact that there is often a lot going on in the shala, dṛṣṭi helps the student stay present during āsana practice. While dṛṣṭi is used to keep one's attention from wandering, the student must remain aware of his or her surroundings and be considerate of others, while simultaneously understanding and following the teacher's instructions. This awareness of one's enviornment is important for everybody's safety, first and foremost, as well as in developing communication and a connection between the teacher and student.

One directs the gaze and flow of energy towards nine various points (nava-dṛṣṭi). The energy which is directed towards the gaze also stimulates the energy channels (nāḍīs), the energy centers (cakras), and encourages prāṇa to flow through the nāḍīs.

Dṛṣṭi is most fundamental in the state (sthiti) of the āsana (when a pose is held), and can be released during transitions from one āsana to the next. Always ensure that you can perform a movement safely, especially when you encounter a disorienting pose, such as the backwards roll (Cakrāsana). Simply follow the movement with the gaze and re-establish the dṛṣṭi once you are back in the state of the pose. In this way, one follows the body's natural movement and gaze, as well as its placement and alignment in the āsana.

Positive effects of dṛṣṭi

Balancing poses – makes it easier to hold one's balance when gazing at a specific point.
Forward-bending poses – draws the body into correct alignment and stretches out the spine and back of the neck.
Back-bending poses – opens the chest, makes it easier to balance and keeps the head properly aligned.
Twisting poses – deepens the twist and helps in holding the pose calmly for the entire duration of the breath.

Nava-dṛṣṭi – the nine gazing points

1. Hastāgra-dṛṣṭi - the fingertips or hand
Example: Utthita-trikoṇāsana A & B

2. Bhrū-madhya-dṛṣṭi – in between the eyebrows
Example: Kūrmāsana and Upavistha koṇāsana

3. Pādayor-agra-dṛṣṭi – the toes
Pādāṅguṣṭha-dṛṣṭi – the big toe
Example: Navāsana (toes) and Ardha-baddha-padma-paścima-tānāsana (the big toe)

4. Pārśva-dṛṣṭi – right and left sides
Example: Marīcy-āsana C & D

5. Nāsāgra-dṛṣṭi – the tip of the nose
Example: Samasthitiḥ and Prasārita-pādottānāsana
Nāsāgra-dṛṣṭi is the most commonly-used dṛṣṭi in the Aṣṭāṅga yoga system. If you are ever in doubt of the dṛṣṭi for a particular pose, gaze at the tip of the nose. Nāsāgra-dṛṣṭi can be referred to as an "all-purpose" dṛṣṭi and is safe to use in all āsana.

6. Ūrdhva-dṛṣṭi or antara-dṛṣṭi – upwards
Example: Vīrabhadrāsana and Ubhaya-pādāṅguṣṭhāsana

7. Aṅguṣṭha-madhya-dṛṣṭi – the thumbs
Aṅguṣṭhāgra-dṛṣṭi – the tips of the thumbs
Example: Sūrya-namaskāra A (1st vinyāsa)
Gazing at the fingertips often simply means to look up, which is why the dṛṣṭi is sometimes called fingertips/upwards.

8. Nābhi-cakra-dṛṣṭi – the navel
Example: Sūrya-namaskāra A (6th vinyāsa - Adho-mukha-śvan-āsana)
This stimulates maṇipura-cakra in the navel region. In Adho-mukha-śvan-āsana, the abdomen is lifted and it can be difficult to see the navel, which is why the direction, towards the navel, is often written as a description of Nabhi-cakra-dṛṣṭi. Rounding the back slightly in Adho-mukha-śvan-āsana, like in early yoga pictures featuring Krishnamacharya and Pattabhi Jois, helps one see the navel and lengthen the shoulders and spine.

9. Adho-mukha-dṛṣṭi – down on the floor
Adho-mukha-dṛṣṭi is used in the intermediate series in Tittibhāsana B (while walking), but it can be helpful for beginners to look at the floor in balancing poses, such as Utthita-hasta-pādāṅguṣṭhāsana or if any dṛṣṭi becomes too intense for the eyes.

Ūrdhva-dṛṣṭi

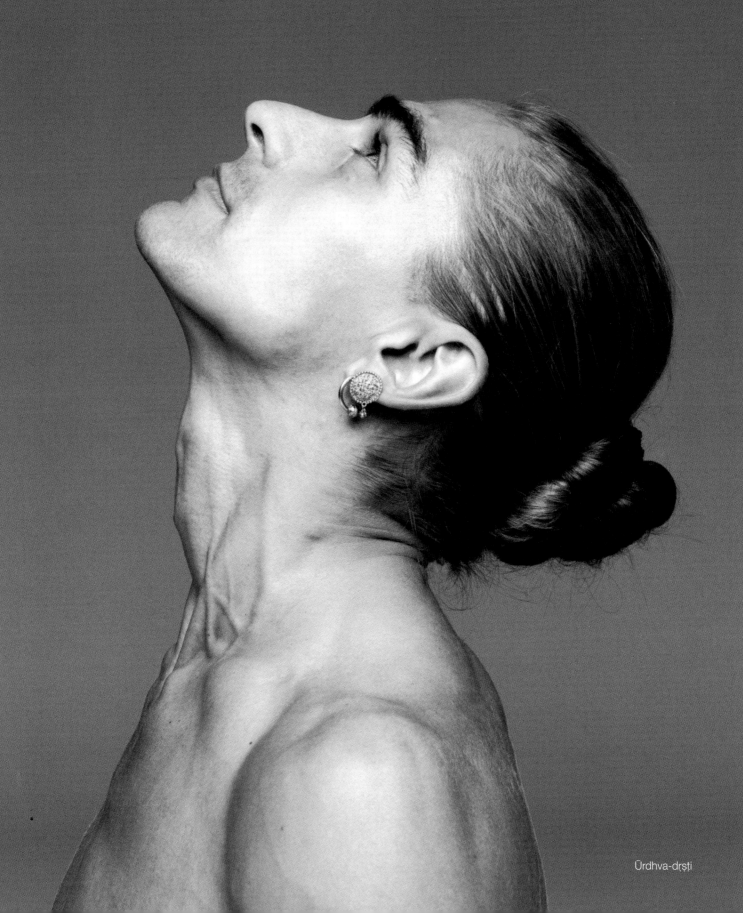

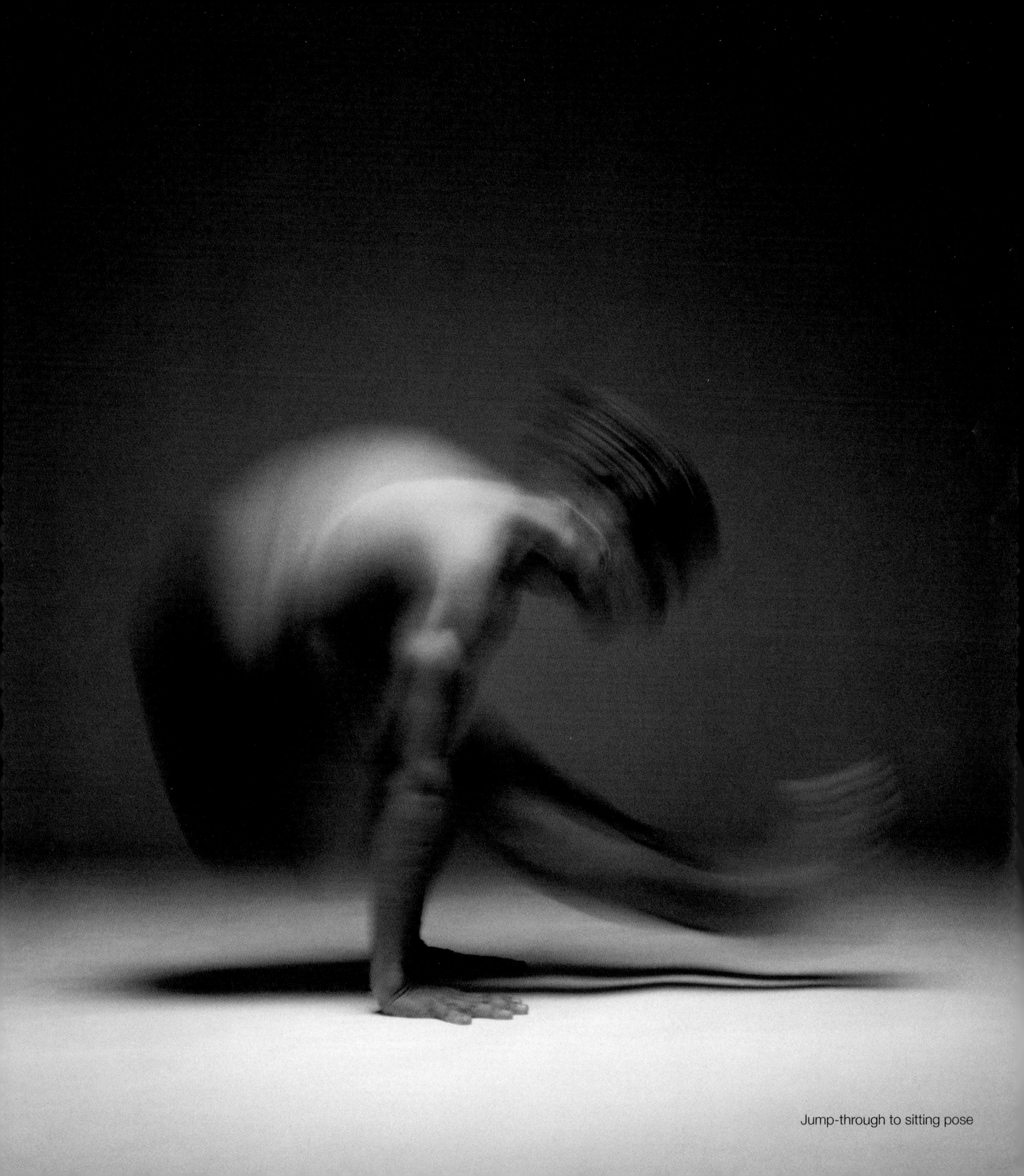

Jump-through to sitting pose

vinyāsa

Vi – to move; nyāsa – to place oneself

Vinyāsa is the essential quality in Aṣṭāṅga yoga's āsana series. It is the art of breathing, moving from one pose to the next, and linking āsanas together with the rhythm of the breath. The combination of breath and āsana enables the stretching and strengthening of the body, while building up heat and sweat. Agni, the inner fire that burns at the navel region, is activated when the bandhas (muscle and energy locks) lift the energy up towards the stomach. In addition, agni activates digestion and encourages an upwards-moving action along the nāḍīs. The heat and sweat are the keys to purifying the muscles, organs and nervous system from toxins and blockages. With the heat that is produced in vinyāsa, one can eventually approach even the most advanced āsana in a safe and protected manner. Another benefit from vinyāsa is its meditative effect, which balances the mind and body's energy systems (e.g. vāyu, prāṇa and nāḍī).

Since the vinyāsa technique in Aṣṭāṅga yoga purifies the mind and body with such totality, it is not necessary to practise other cleansing exercises, such as fasting or the cleansing techniques (kriyās). These are only recommended if you have a particular problem, such as digestive illness or congestion.

Traditionally, in order to move forwards in the teachings, aspirants were required to learn by heart the complete vinyāsa system: dṛṣṭi, āsana names, the number of vinyāsas in each āsana, and how to breathe and move through each vinyāsa correctly.

Vinyāsa in āsana practice

When you apply the vinyāsa technique properly, you can settle into the best possible pose. The meditative flow of the practice is created through well-coordinated breathing in relation to conscious movement. Remember that the calm, even rhythm of sound breathing is the key to a relaxed and supple body.

Vinyāsa in the standing postures

Traditionally, one jumps from Samasthitiḥ to the standing poses. After breathing in the state of the āsana, one jumps back to Samasthitiḥ. When the feet land in the first vinyāsa of the pose, one can sense a subtle vibration, which helps to relax and prepare the body for the next āsana. Different styles of jumping are described for the various standing poses.

Vinyāsa into the sitting postures

The preparation pose to hop or float through to sitting is the same as the 6th vinyāsa (Adho-mukha-śvan-āsana) in Sūrya-namaskāra A. At the end of the 6th vinyāsa, exhale completely, with the gaze directed towards the navel. Inhale, direct the gaze between the hands, hold the root and abdominal locks, lengthen through the shoulders so that the distance between the chest and hands is as wide as possible, press the hands down and straighten the arms. Continuing with the inhalation, bend the knees, and jump between the arms. The legs are either crossed, bent or straight. Land in a sitting position. The feet should stay in the air throughout the entire jump, with the help of the bandhas, the arms and the rhythm of the breath. If one inhalation is not enough to complete the movement, breathe out and in again, and move into the next āsana.

Vinyāsa from a seated position back into Caturaṅga-daṇḍāsana (catvāri)

In many ways, jumping back is similar to the way one jumps forwards into sitting. The last vinyāsa before lifting the body up often ends on an exhalation. For example, one completes the five breaths in Jānu-śīrṣāsana A on an exhalation. The vinyāsa then continues with an inhalation, with the head lifted up and the back and arms straightened. Hold this pose and finish with an exhalation. Continue by placing the hands on the floor on either side of the hips, breathe in, cross the legs with the feet in the air and bring the knees in towards the chest. On the same inhalation, engage both mūla- and uḍḍīyana-bandha, lengthen through the shoulders, and straighten and strengthen the arms. Lift the body up off the floor, then lift the hips up further, so the legs continue on back and through the arms. Gaze at the tip of the nose.

Begin exhaling, straighten the legs out to the back while simultaneously bending the elbows at about 90 degrees, keeping them in towards the sides of the body. Land in Catvāri with a completely straight body (about 3.5 inches or four angulas from the floor). Keep gazing at the tip of the nose and complete the exhalation.

Developing your technique

It generally takes a long time to be able to jump through or back without the feet touching the floor. It requires deep use of the bandhas and the breath. The techniques can be worked on by focusing on the breathing in the vinyāsa, as well as by investigating the movements of the body and their connection to the bandhas. It is of utmost importance that you keep the breath and movements calm and flowing, rather than putting all your energy into lifting the body up off the floor. If one breath cannot last the duration of the jump, take in another breath and finish the movement.

Technique

Step 1 (beginners)

Vinyāsa in the jump-through

Begin the inhalation, bend the knees and lift the heels off the floor. Stretch out the back of the neck and gaze between the hands. Continue with the inhalation, draw the bandhas up and in, and lengthen the shoulders keeping the distance between the chest and the hands as wide as possible. Press the palms into the floor and straighten the arms. Keep inhaling as you bend the knees deeply, take off and jump with crossed-legs in between the arms. If the feet land behind the hands, move the hands in closer towards you, lower yourself down with the legs crossed and sit into the next āsana. If the inhalation ends before the movement is finished, exhale out and inhale back in and complete the jump.

Vinyāsa in the jump-back

Inhale and place the hands on either side of the hips. Cross the legs with the feet in the air while simultaneously engaging both bandhas firmly, and lift the knees into the chest. Continue with the inhalation, hold the bandhas, and lengthen through the shoulders with straight arms. Strengthen the arms and lift the body up off the floor. Lift the legs between the arms. If the legs land in front of the hands, place the hands in front of the knees and lift the hips with the strength of the arms and the help of the crossed legs. Begin to exhale, jump back through the arms, straighten out the legs, bend the elbows in towards the sides of the body and land with a straight body into Catvāri, the weight evenly distributed between the hands and feet.

Step 2 (intermediate)

Vinyāsa in the jump-through
Follow the technique as described in Step 1 (for beginners) until you take off. When you have worked consistently with an āsana series and your jump has developed so that your feet land in between your hands, come to sitting, with crossed legs, and then straighten the legs out for the next āsana. You don't need to continue moving the hands like in Step 1.

Vinyāsa in the jump-back
Follow the technique as described in Step 1, until the body is lifted up on the inhalation, with the legs crossed as they travel through the arms. When the legs touch the floor between the hands, re-engage the bandhas and jump-back on the exhalation, without shifting the hands.

Step 3 (advanced)

Vinyāsa in the jump-through
Follow the instructions in Steps 1 and 2. Now you are ready to jump through on the inhalation, with the legs crossed and lifted above the floor on the way through. Follow the steps described opposite in the "Vinyāsa into the sitting postures" section. Note: The palms should stay firmly on the floor throughout the entire jump.

Vinyāsa in jump-back
Follow the instructions in Steps 1 and 2. When your breathing technique, bandha control and overall strength have improved, you will be able to lift the crossed legs up on an inhalation, carry them through your arms and behind the hands, landing lightly back into Catvāri on the exhalation.

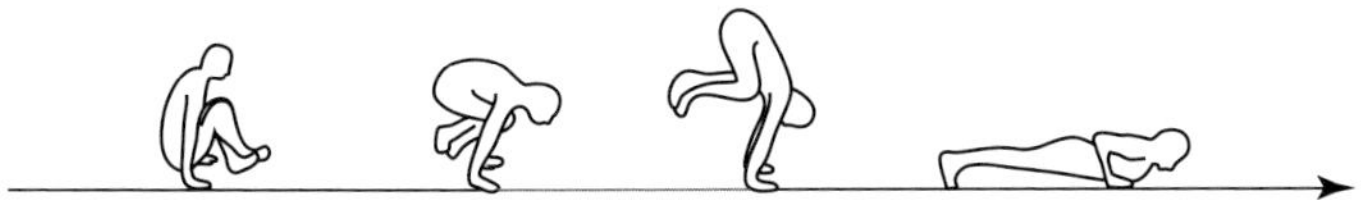

Jump-through vinyāsa to sitting postures

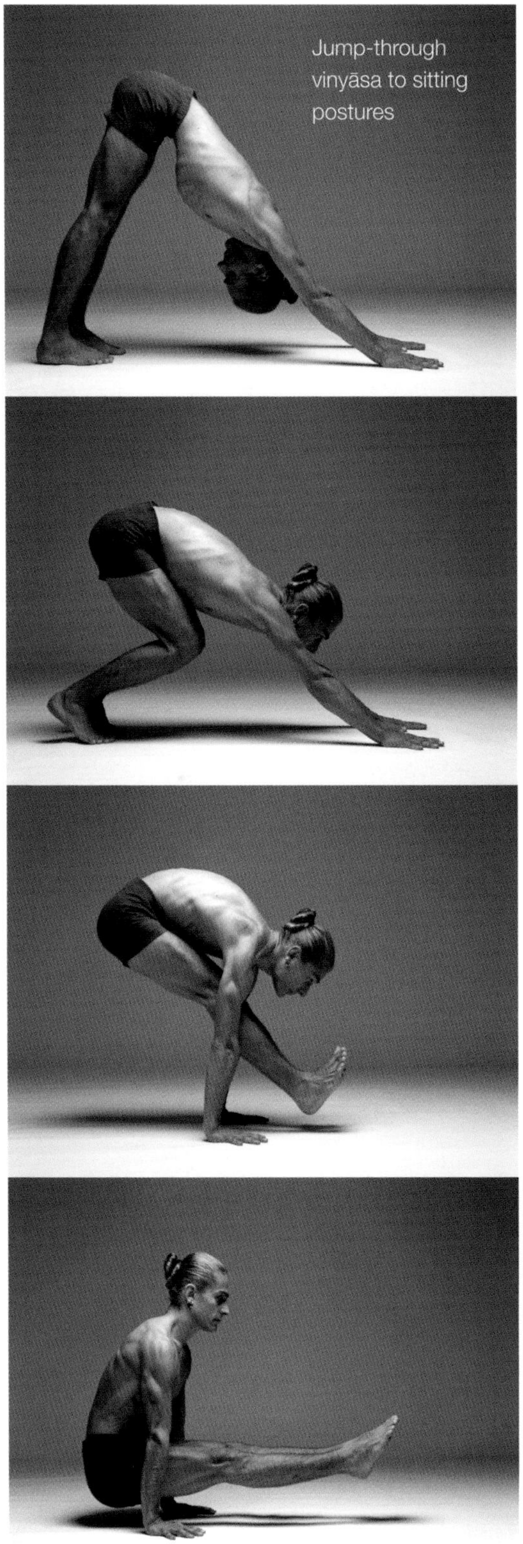

Jump-through vinyāsa to sitting postures

mantra

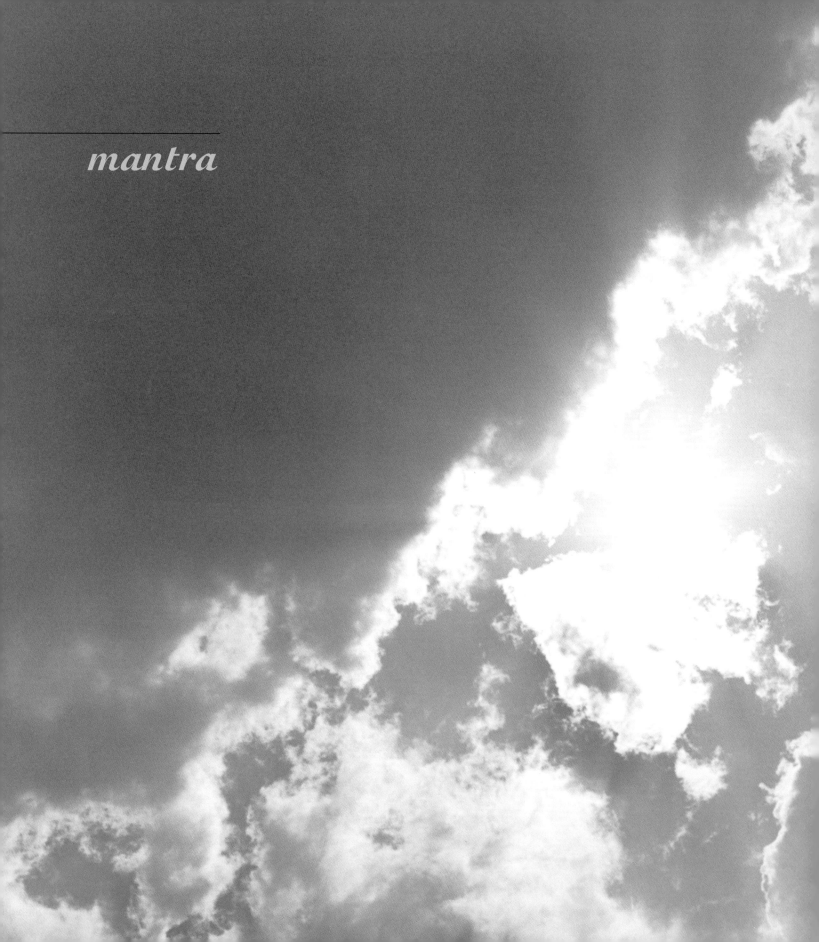

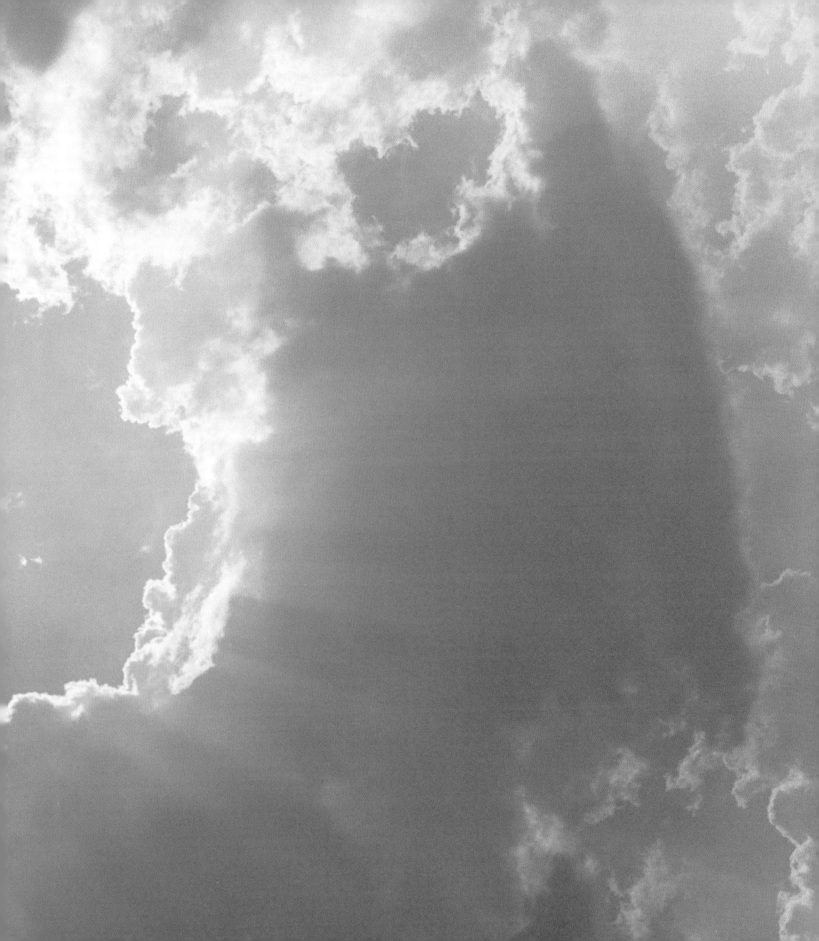

mantra

Man - to think (manas - mind);
tra - tool, instrument, protection
Holy words that serve to protect us from our own minds (the biggest obstacle) and spiritually transform the person reciting them or meditating upon their meaning.

Mantra recitation or chanting is an integral part of religious and spiritual practices in India. One can silently recite mantras, repeat them quietly or say them out loud, as part of a group or alone. Spiritual aspirants often recite prayers, verses from holy texts or passages from mythological epics. The sounds of the letters, syllables and words within the mantras, shlokas (verses), śāstras (explanations) or sūtras (aphorisms), and the rhythm and order are taught with the intention to explain the goals of human life, heal and generate feelings of purity, to increase concentration and to create a connection to the higher powers.

Some letters or combination of letters, when pronounced accurately, will vibrate in a way that can directly affect the organs, blood and energy circulation, and the nervous system. Their function is to help release physical and mental obstacles, such as restlessness, pessimism and energy blockages, which would otherwise hinder the flow of prāṇa through the body and limit one from experiencing clear consciousness and contact with one's inner Self.

Samantrika and Amantrika

Samantrika (with mantra) are the verses from the *Ṛg-veda*, *Yajurveda*, *Sāmaveda* and *Atharvaveda*, which are often recited by the brahmins, the highest class within the Indian caste system, made up of priests and scholars. Samantrika follows strict rules as to correct pronunciation (śikṣā), meter, pitch or tone (svara) and rhythm (mātrā) as well as word or speech (vāk), syllable (akṣara), letter order (varṇa) and sound vibration. Svara is composed of three different tones: higher (svarasudat), lower (anudat) and middle (svarāṭ).

In order to create the accurate sound for mantra recitation, it is also necessary for the Sanskrit scholars, priests and chanting masters (pandits) to be advanced practitioners of prāṇāyama. Through the practice of prāṇāyama both the īḍā- and piṅgalā-nāḍīs are balanced and the oxygen can flow evenly through the right and the left nostrils, providing utmost precision in order for proper recitation to take place.

The slightest mistake in samantrika can change the entire meaning of the mantra, rendering it powerless or, worse still, able to deliver adverse effects. Pattabhi Jois believed that the samantrika-mantras possess significant influence at the micro level, in the body-mind system, as well as the at the macro level, the universe. Samantrika-mantras include the well-known daily ritual chants, Gayatri-mantra and Sūrya-namaskāra-mantra, both dedicated to the sun god.

Amantrika (without mantra) consist of shlokas, "the songs or verses which have been heard." Shlokas typically comprise verses and passages from Indian epics. These do not follow such exacting rules of pronunciation as found in samantrika. Shlokas can also be described as post-Vedic chants that illustrate Hindu mythology, prayers for daily life, philosophical reflections and healing sounds. With the exception of Sūrya-namaskāra-mantra, the shlokas that are chanted before and after āsana or prāṇāyama practice belong to amantrika. Even if amantrika shlokas do not have such strict pronunciation rules, it is still recommended that you learn them from a guru or a well-reputed teacher, ensuring correct rhythm and delivery of the shloka. In this way, one can not only show appreciation for the chanting tradition, but respect for the holy and ancient language of Sanskrit.

Amantrika-mantras include Aṣṭāṅga yoga's opening and closing chants as well as verses from the *Bhagavad-gītā* and the Āditya-hṛdayam, which are chapters found in what are considered to be the two great narratives (itihasa) of India: *Mahābhārata* (Maha - great; Bharata - India) and *Rāmāyaṇa*, translated as Rama's Journey (Rama - a name; ayana - going, advancing).

The *Bhagavad-gītā* (Bhagavad - God; Gītā - song) is part of Sage Vyasa's epic *Mahābhārata* and Āditya-hṛdayam (Āditya - the Sun God; Hṛdayam - that which is particularly healing and nourishing for the heart) belongs to Sage Valmiki's *Rāmāyaṇa*.

Mantras in Aṣṭāṅga yoga

In the Aṣṭāṅga yoga tradition, one can chant both at the beginning and the end of practice.

The opening mantra is the moment when we show our great respect and devotion to the gurus, whose knowledge and wisdom heal us from the poison of ignorance, and who can show us the path to peace and the happiness of our true nature revealed.

The Sūrya-namaskāra-mantra is the prayer to the sun god, a form of the un-manifested para-brahman, that which is beyond Brahman (para - beyond; Brahman - universal self or spirit). Traditionally, one would recite this mantra throughout each sun salutation, building one's concentration and meditative awareness. In Indian tradition the sun has long been considered as the world's health minister, providing us with health, longevity and radiance.

Sūrya-namaskāra-mantras – the 113 verses of Aruṇa-praśna-mantra from *Kṛṣṇa-yajur-veda* – were originally mentally recited during Sūrya-namaskāra A. During Sūrya-namaskāra B, one would devote oneself to mantras from the *Ṛg-veda*.

The closing mantra is a prayer to uplift and maintain the positive energy of the world. With this mantra, one directs the energy, knowledge and experience gained during the āsana and prāṇāyama practice towards generous aims such as understanding, peace and well-being for all creation. The last verse, "*lokāḥ samastāḥ sukhino bhavantu*", is especially well known all over India, and is a symbol of the country's great tolerance towards one's fellow human beings, no matter their cultural backgrounds or religious beliefs.

Given that Aṣṭāṅga yoga's mantras and shlokas are based on Hindu culture and tradition, when the first Westerners came to the AYRI (Aṣṭāṅga Yoga Research Institute) in Mysore in 1964, Pattabhi Jois had to convey the teachings of these chantings in such a way that his foreign students could understand and begin to grasp their meaning. In comparison to the traditional context of yoga, these newcomers viewed yoga as something primarily physical, and perhaps exotic and mystical. Therefore, the more orthodox aspects of Hinduism needed to be adjusted for comprehension. Many Western students, however, have shown interest in studying further, and with great discipline and dedication have committed themselves to memorizing samantrika from the Vedas.

Opening mantra

The opening mantra in Aṣṭāṅga yoga is a prayer and an act of reverence for the guru. One stands tall in Samasthitiḥ, with the eyes closed, and the head bowed towards the hands. The hands are placed in kara-mudrā, or anjali-mudrā – palms together between the chest and the throat, by the heart center.

This is the first shloka from *Yoga-tārāvalī*, written by Śrī Ādī Śaṅkarācārya (788 CE–820 CE), the creator of Advaita-vedānta, the school of non-dualistic philosophy.

In the first verse of the mantra, the student shows respect for the gurus or teachers who have, over the ages and through the parampara (lineage), directly experienced and passed down the godly knowledge, which improves one's quality of life and leads the student to his or her highest path.

The second verse is dedicated to the mysterious embodiment* of Bhagavan Patanjali, and for his invaluable revelations of the mysteries of yoga.

Opening mantra

OM

vande gurūṇām caraṇāravinde

sandarśita svātma sukhāvabodhe

niḥśreyase jāṅgalikāyamāne

saṃsāra hālāhala mohaśāntyai

ābāhu puruṣākāraṃ

śaṅkhacakrāsi dhāriṇam

sahasra śirasaṃ śvetam

praṇamāmi patañjalim

OM

OM
I bow to the lotus feet of the gurus,
who awaken the happiness of one's own self revealed;
who are the ultimate good;
who take the form of medicine men
for curing the delusion of the poison
of birth and death.

Who takes the form of a man
up to his shoulders,
bearing conch, disk and sword,
thousand-headed, white:
I salute Patañjali!
OM

*(Patañjali was born as an incarnation of the thousand-headed serpent, Ādiśeṣa, an incarnation of Lord Viṣṇu, who was sent from heaven to earth to be born as a yogi. His mother, Gonika, was an unmarried tapasvini (ascetic) and yogini who prayed to the Sun God for a son to whom she could pass on her knowledge. Just as Gonika was ready to give her offering, a handful of water, to the sun, a miracle occurred. A little white serpent came splashing down into the water between her hands, which were placed in a half-open prayer position (anjali-mudrā). This is where the name Patañjali came from, as pat means to fall, which is how the serpent arrived from the heavens, into Gonika's hands, which were in anjali-mudrā. Within a few months the serpent had taken a human form up to the shoulders. His head, however, remained in the terrifying form of Ādiśeṣa. Gonika accepted Ādiśeṣa as her son and gave him the name Patanjali).

Sūrya-namaskāra-mantra

The Sūrya-namaskāra-mantra, or sun-salutation mantra, is the opening to a longer mantra (Aruṇa-praśna) which is dedicated to the sun. This comes from the *Kṛṣṇa-yajur-veda*, one of the oldest Hindu texts (circa 1000 BCE). Aruṇa means dawn or, more specifically, "the moment when the rose of the morning sun fills the sky and the air is rich with the prāṇa produced by the trees and nature." It is a prayer to the sun god for strength and sensitivity. In India, the sun typically rises between 4:30 and 5:30am, and so this mantra is recited especially during that time.

This mantra is not usually recited when doing the sun salutations, as it belongs to the samantrika group of mantra and requires that the speaker has studied Sanskrit and has knowledge of Hindu gods and goddesses and of the rituals that accompany their worship. It could be seen as a rite of passage when Pattabhi Jois introduced his most advanced students to this mantra. (Pattabhi Jois's commentary on the Sūrya-namaskāra mantra can be found in *Nāmarūpa* magazine; Winter issue, 2004.)

According to tradition, the Sūrya-namaskāra-mantra is recited quietly to oneself so that the physiological effects of the chanting can take place, as described by Pattabhi Jois, in the empty space at the back of the head while doing Sūrya-namaskāra A. Each line in the mantra corresponds to the length of one vinyāsa.

Those who fulfill the criteria for samantrika-mantra and have learned them from a guru or knowledgable teacher can recite, among other mantras and shlokas, the Sūrya-namaskāra-mantra, and the last part of the śānti-mantra, together with the Āditya-hṛdayam. The Āditya-hṛdayam is one of the mantras which Gurujī recommended that his students chant. These mantras and shlokas can be done after the (final) resting pose, or during sunrise and/or sunset.

Sūrya-namaskāra-mantra

OM

bhadram karṇebhiḥ śruṇuyāma devāḥ

bhadram paśyemākṣabhiryajatrāḥ

sthirairaṅgaistuṣṭuvāgamsastanūbhiḥ

vyaśema devahitam yadāyuḥ

svasti naḥ indro vṛddaśravāḥ

svasti naḥ pūsā viśvavedāḥ

svasti nas tārkṣyo ariṣṭanemiḥ

svasti no bṛhaspatirdadhātu

OM śāntiḥ, śāntiḥ, śāntiḥ

Oh, Sun God,
Please accept my offering.
May we hear auspiciousness with our ears, oh gods!
May we see auspiciousness with our eyes, oh worshipable ones!
May we, having praised them, with strong bodies and limbs,
enjoy the life given to us by the gods.
May Indra of great renown give us fortune!
May all-knowing Pūṣan give us fortune!
May Tārṣkya of the unbroken felly give us fortune!
May Bṛhaspati give us fortune!
Om, peace, peace, peace

Closing mantra: śānti- or mangala-mantra

The śānti (peace) mantra or mangala (auspicious) mantra is done at the end of practice, in the same position as in the opening mantra. After utplutiḥ, follow through with a vinyāsa and come up to stand in samasthitiḥ. Place the hands together in kara-mudrā or anjali-mudrā and recite the mantra.

The second part of the śānti-mantra, beginning with "Kale varṣatu," is not often chanted in class. Rather, the mantra ends with the words "sukhino bhavantu," after which one chants "Om śāntiḥ, śāntiḥ, śāntiḥ". If you are reciting the mantra on your own, carry on with the second verse and chant "Om śāntih, śāntiḥ, śāntiḥi" after "śaradaṁ śatam."

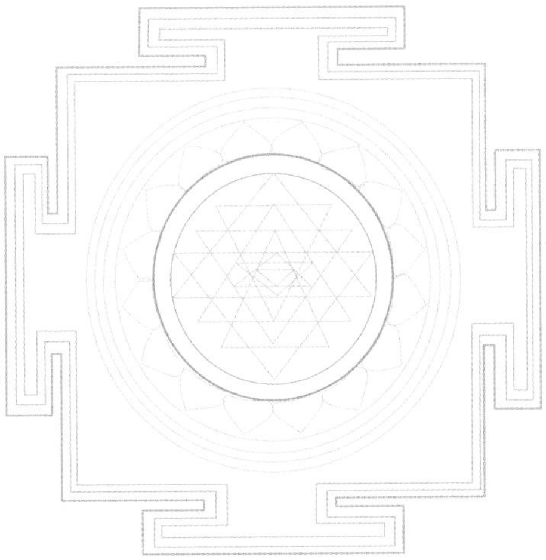

Closing mantra

OM

svasti prajābhyaḥ paripālayantām

nyāyena mārgeṇa mahīm mahīśāḥ

gobrāhmaṇebhyaḥ śubhamastu nityam

lokāḥ samastāḥ sukhino bhavantu

kāle varṣatu parjanyaḥ pṛthivī sasyaśālinī

deśoyam kṣobharahito brāhmaṇā santu nirbhayaḥ

aputrāḥ putriṇas santu

putriṇas santu pautriṇaḥ

adhanās sadhanās santu

jīvantu saradam śatam

OM śāntiḥ, śāntiḥ, śāntiḥ

OM

Fortune to the people,
to the rulers of the earth,
who protect the earth
by following the path of righteousness!

May there always be prosperity
for the cows (peace, wealth, innocence, mother earth)
and the Brahmins (scholars and virtuous people)!
May all the worlds be happy!

May the clouds give timely rain,
may the earth abound in grain,
may this land be free from strife,
may the Brahmins be without fear.

May the sonless get sons,
may those with sons get grandsons,
may the poor increase their fortune,
may they live a hundred years!

Om, peace, peace, peace

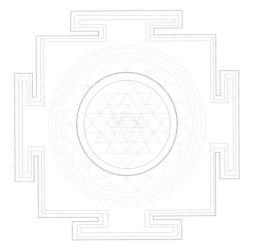

āsana {primary series}
yoga-cikitsā

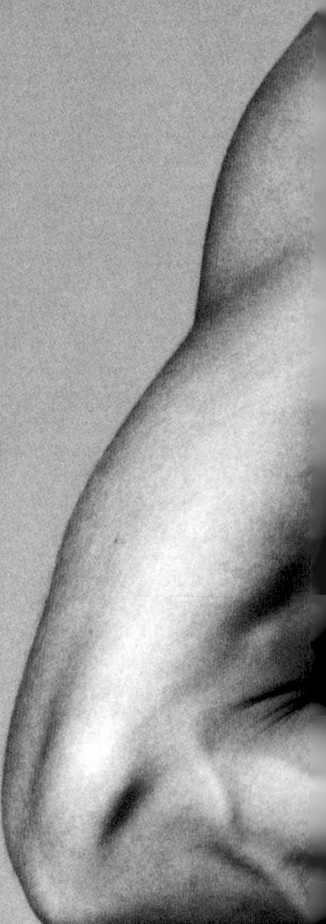

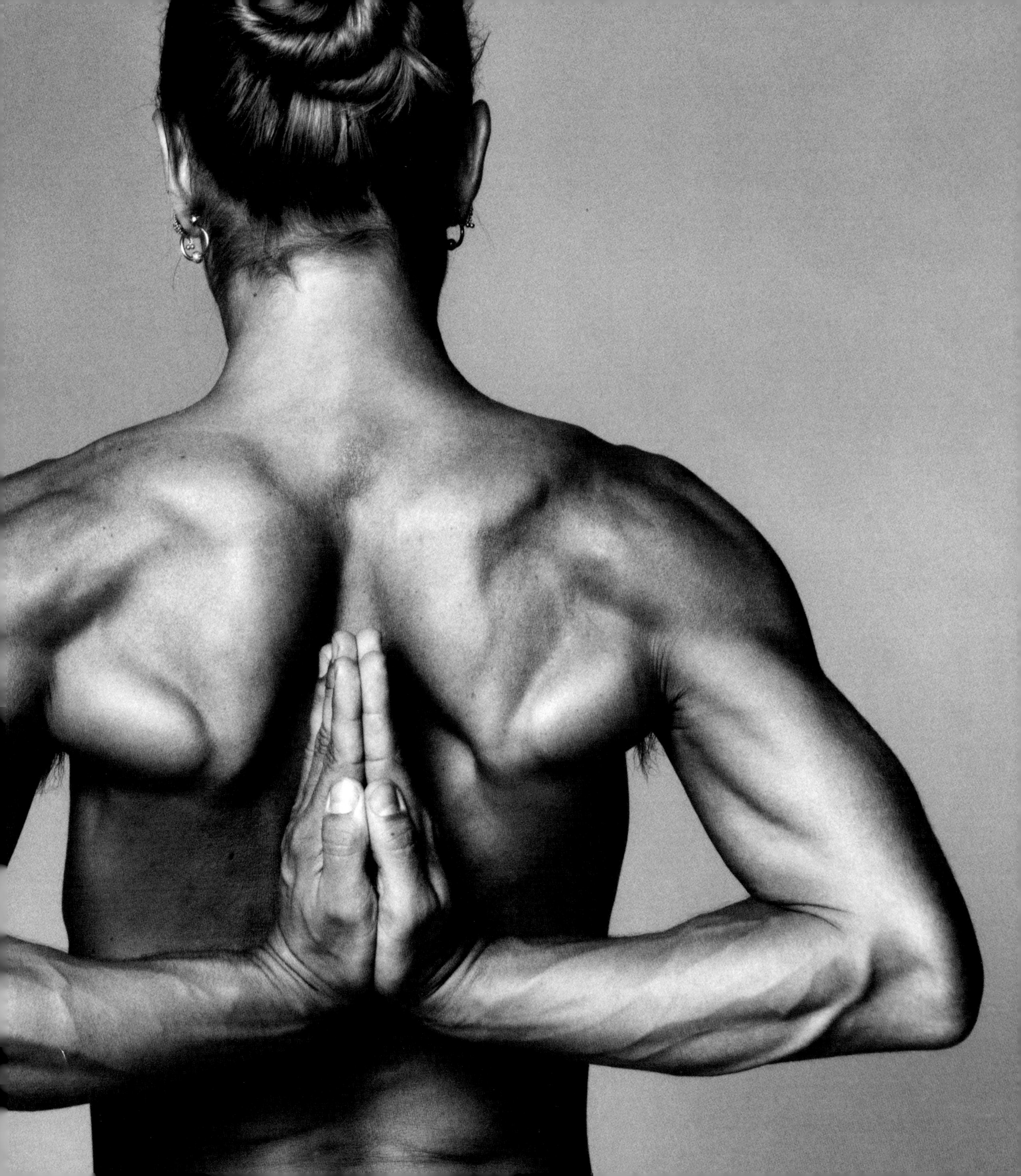

Samasthitiḥ

Sama – same, straight, equal; *sthiti* – in place, state

Samasthitiḥ is the first and last posture in the traditional full-vinyāsa count system. It is beneficial to stand for a moment in Samasthitiḥ prior to the āsana practice. While standing in Samasthitiḥ, begin with sound breathing, draw in and engage the bandhas, and focus on the dṛṣṭi (nāsāgra). Traditionally, one stands in Samasthitiḥ for both the opening and closing mantras.

After each Sūrya-namaskāra, and in between most of the standing āsanas, one returns to Samasthitiḥ. It is not customary to come back up to Samasthitiḥ after each seated āsana, although a few people may still practice the "full vinyāsa" system. This method is not how the practice is currently done in Mysore, India. In this book, the primary series' vinyāsas have been described as "half vinyāsa," meaning without going back to Samasthitiḥ after each seated posture. Notice, however, that the vinyāsa charts on the side of each page have been counted out with the full vinyāsa, enabling one to see where the counting comes from and presenting the aṣṭāṅga vinyāsa method in its entirety.

Technique

Stand at the front of the mat with the feet together or as close as possible, depending on the structure of your legs and feet. Stand evenly on the floor with straight legs. Breathe deeply through the nostrils making an audible sound from the back of the throat. Engage the root lock (mūla-bandha) and lift up the abdominal lock (uḍḍīyana-bandha). Broaden the shoulders, chest and the upper back, and straighten the arms alongside the body with the palms facing in. Do not press the palms against the thighs, but simply try to straighten and lengthen the arms. Lift and lengthen the back of the neck, and lower the chin slightly.

Focus the gaze on the tip of the nose (nāsāgra-dṛṣṭi), straighten the body with a sense of ease while maintaining an energized breath.

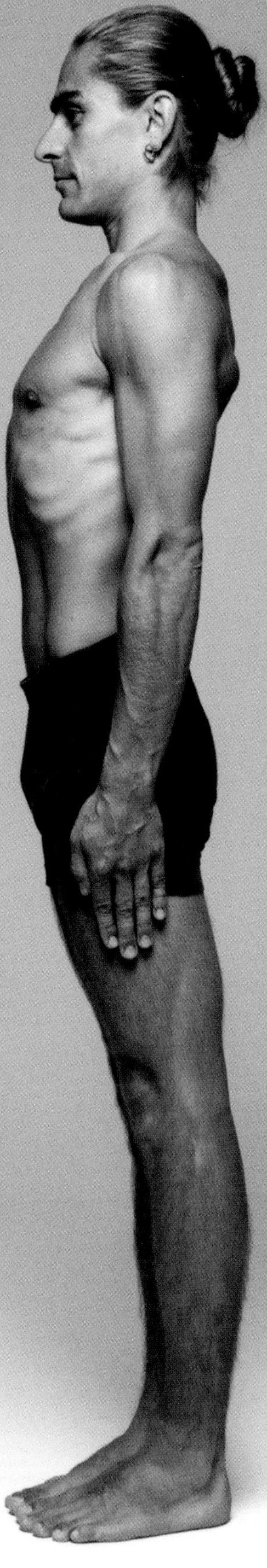

Samasthitiḥ

Sūrya-namaskāra A

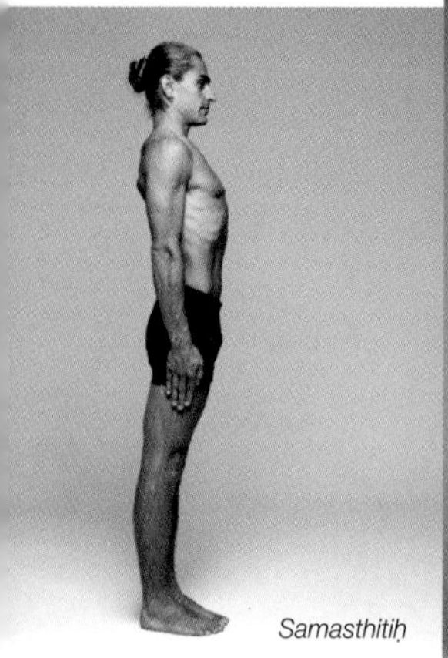

Samasthitiḥ

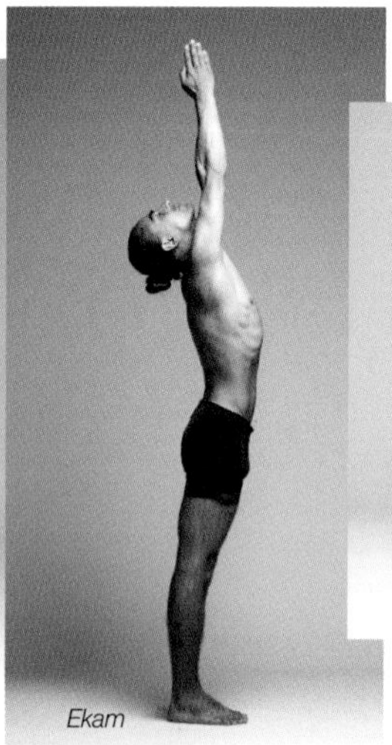

Ekam

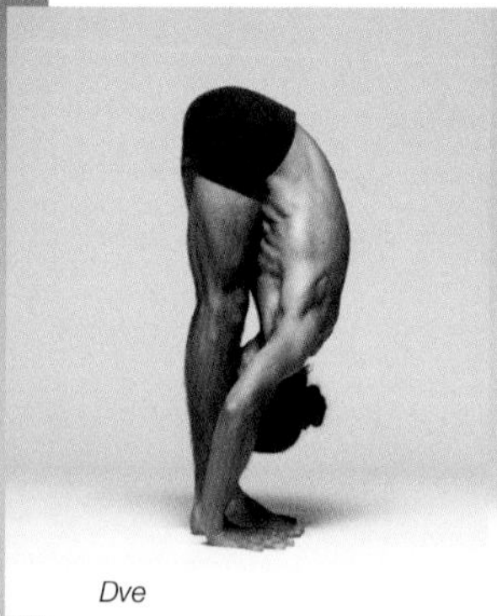

Dve

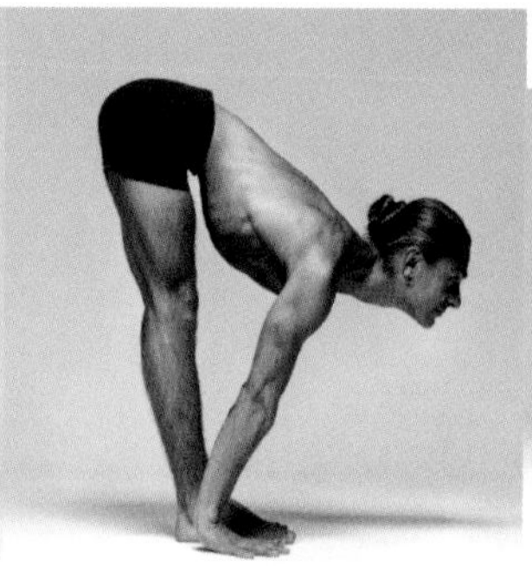

Triṇi

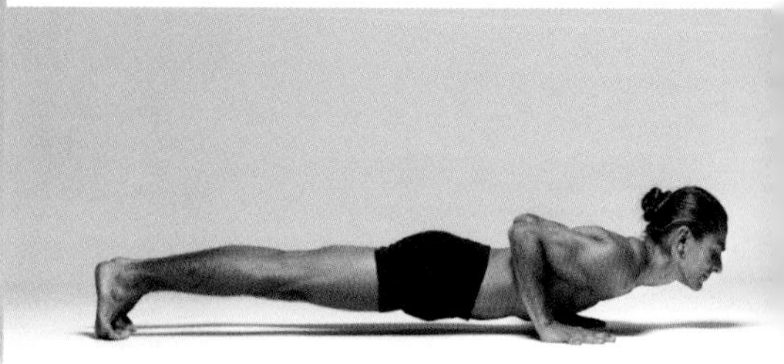

Catvāri

Sūrya-namaskāra *[sun salutation]*

Sūrya – sun, the Sun God; *namaskāra* – salutation

Sun worship is one of the most important rituals in India, which has been documented in both the Vedas and the Purāṇas. Over the millennia, people have developed several varieties of worship to the sun. The sun salutations in yoga are not only done to cleanse the body and mind, but also to pray to the Sun God, "the health minister of the world," for health, prosperity and longevity.

Having been given life, it is our responsibility to respect it by using our time productively and remaining healthy, in both thought and action. Through yoga, we can open up the mind to wisdom and joy. According to *Yoga Mala* and other yogic texts, through practising the sun salutations and doing āsana correctly, we can heal the body from physical (deśika), mental (mānasika), and spiritual (adhyātmika) illnesses and lead a happy life.

Aṣṭāṅga yoga begins with two similar sun salutations. The first, Sūrya-namskara A, has nine vinyāsas, or combinations of breath and movement. The second, Sūrya-namskara B, has 17 vinyāsas. In the sun-salutation sequence, we establish the physical and mental techniques (vinyāsa, sound breathing, dṛṣṭi and bandhas) that continue throughout the whole practice. The sun salutations are a simple and safe series of poses that heat up the body and create a sweat that starts the purification process. This heat keeps the body warm, making it safe to move through new āsanas. The breathing initiated in the sun salutations creates a meditative and soothing rhythm for the mind which, in turn, provides space for the sacred dimension of the practice to unfold.

It is recommended that you start with five rounds of Sūrya-namaskāra A and five rounds of Sūrya-namaskāra B, although as you progress, a system of five Sūrya-namaskāra A and three Sūrya-namaskāra B is usually done.

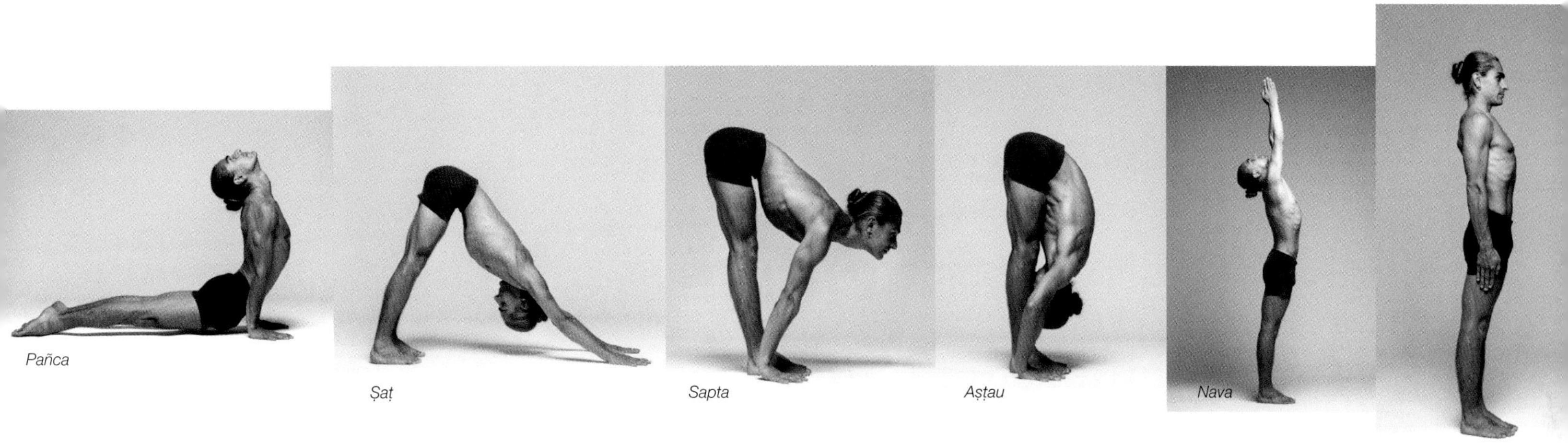

Pañca *Ṣaṭ* *Sapta* *Aṣṭau* *Nava* *Samasthitiḥ*

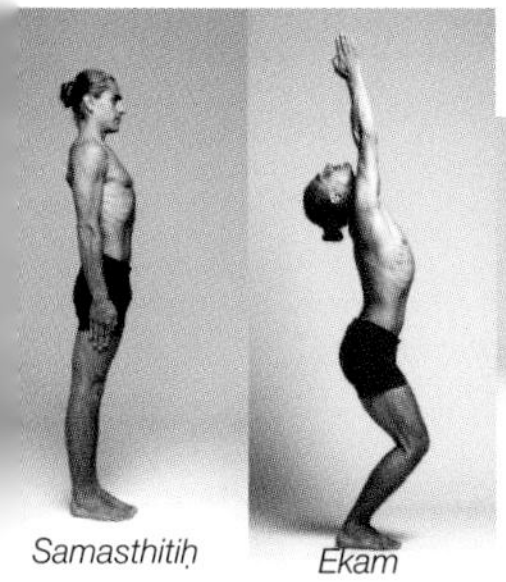

Samasthitiḥ *Ekam*

Sūrya-namaskāra B

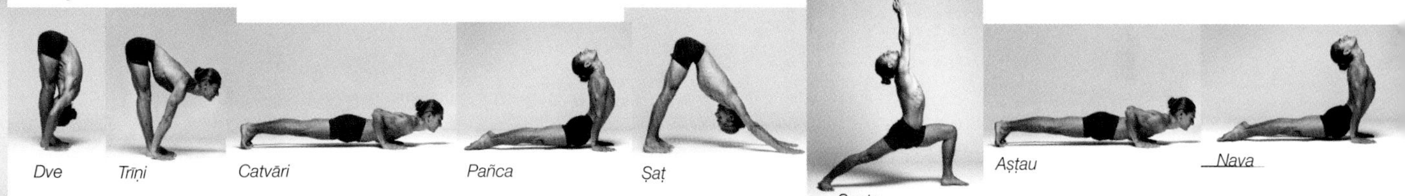

Dve *Triṇi* *Catvāri* *Pañca* *Ṣaṭ* *Sapta* *Aṣṭau* *Nava*

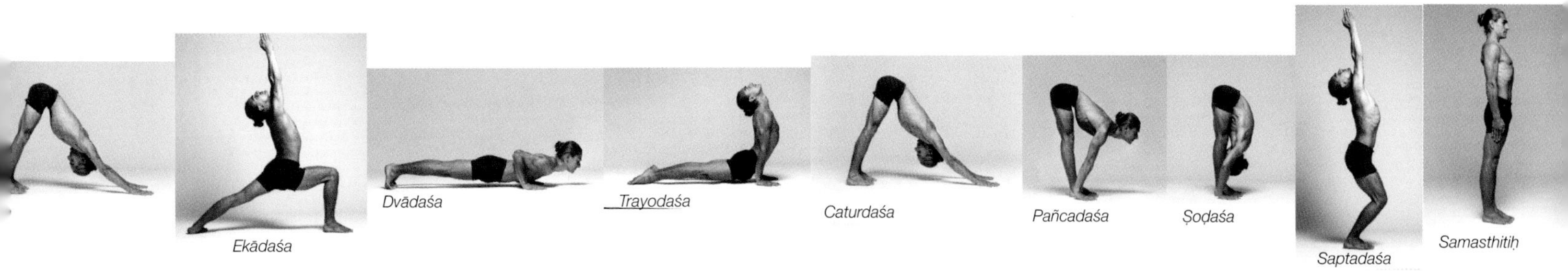

Ekādaśa *Dvādaśa* *Trayodaśa* *Caturdaśa* *Pañcadaśa* *Ṣoḍaśa* *Saptadaśa* *Samasthitiḥ*

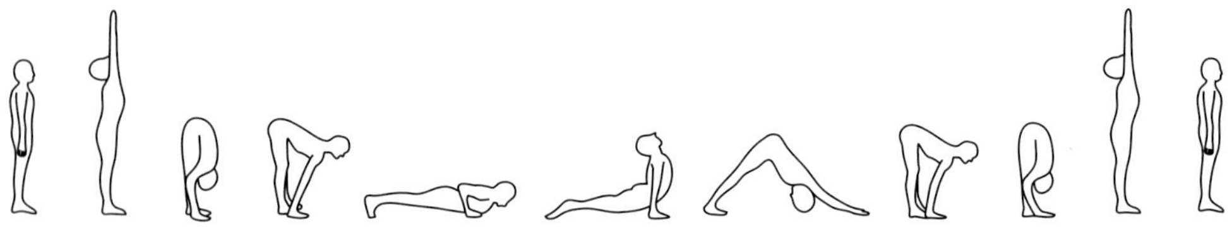

Sūrya-namaskāra A [sun salutation A]

9 vinyāsas

Sūrya – sun, the Sun God; *namaskāra* – salutation

Samasthitiḥ – Stand straight with the feet together, arms by the sides, and gaze at the tip of the nose.

1 Ekam
Inhale, lift the arms up overhead, either out to the side or diagonally in front of you, following the hands with the gaze, and tilt the head back. Let the inhalation broaden the chest and the back, and touch the palms together overhead. Stretch the shoulders and straighten the elbows, lifting the hands up to the ceiling as you ground the feet into the floor. Straighten the back and lengthen the entire body. Direct the gaze to the tips of the thumbs.

2 Dve
Uttānāsana
Uttāna – strong, deep stretch; *āsana* – seat, posture
Exhale, bend forwards from the hips with straight legs and lower the arms towards the floor. Actively draw in uddīyana-bandha, sinking the torso onto the thighs. Place the fingertips in line with the toes, and press the palms onto the floor with fingers spread wide. Relax the back of the neck, press the head into the knees or between the shins. Gaze at the tip of the nose.

3 Trīṇi
Inhale, open the chest, draw the shoulders back and down towards the waist and fully elongate the spine. Lift the head and direct the gaze in between the eyebrows. Straighten the arms and keep pressing the palms onto the floor. (This is the grounding action, working in opposition to the upwards-moving actions of the head, chest and spine). Hold mūla-bandha to support the hips, and apply uddīyana-bandha to open up the chest and straighten the back.

4 Catvāri

Caturaṅga-daṇḍāsana

Catur – four; *aṅga* – limb; *daṇḍa* – stick; *āsana* – seat, posture

Exhale, press the palms firmly onto the floor, hold mūla and uddīyana-bandha, and lift the feet from the floor with the strength of the arms. Float the legs back and land the feet hip-width apart (six to twelve inches). The weight rests only on the hands and the balls of the feet; the legs are straight. Keep the whole body straight with the help of mūla- and uddīyana-bandha, and bend the arms 90 degrees (about four inches from the floor), keeping the elbows in towards the sides of the body. Move the chin forward and gaze at the tip of the nose.

5 Pañca

Ūrdhva-mukha-śvan-āsana

Ūrdhva – upward, ascending; *mukha* – face; *śvana* – dog; *āsana* – seat, posture

Inhale, move the body forwards through the arms, slowly straighten the arms and roll over the toes until the tops of the feet are on the floor. Keep the feet straight, engage the thighs so the kneecaps lift. Keep the knees and the hips raised off the floor the entire time you move through this vinyāsa. Stretch the arms, open the chest and bend the back into an arch. Draw the shoulders back and down towards the waist and lift the head. At the end of the movement, let the head fall backwards and gaze between the eyebrows.*

6 Ṣaṭ

Adho-mukha-śvan-āsana

Adho – downward, descending; *mukha* – face; *śvana* – dog; *āsana* – posture

Exhale, lift the hips up, roll over the toes again so that you are on the soles of the feet, and press the heels onto the floor. While you roll over the toes, keep your arms, back, legs and feet fully extended, as well as the knees and hips off the floor. With the arms shoulder-width apart, press the palms and fingers onto the floor, fingers wide, with the index finger pointing forwards. Broaden the shoulders and lengthen the spine. Draw uddīyana-bandha deeply inwards to facilitate the lengthening and stretching of the entire body. Using mūla-bandha, lift the hips up and find your center of gravity. This lightens the body and makes it easier to press the hands and heels into the floor. Be sure to place the feet evenly, hip-width apart, with the toes in line with each other. Direct the breath to the back to relax the spine. Draw the chin in towards the chest, round the back slightly and gaze at the navel, or towards the navel. Often it is difficult to see the actual navel when uddīyana-bandha is drawn in. Hold this position for a count of five deep breaths.

7 Sapta

Inhale, lift the head up and look for a moment in between the hands. Softly jump forwards and, with straight or bent knees, land the feet between the hands, supporting yourself with the arms. After landing, stretch the arms and legs, keep pressing the hands onto the floor, and open the chest. Draw the shoulders down and back, straighten out the back, lift the head and look up between the eyebrows.

8 Aṣṭau

Uttānāsana

Uttana – strong, deep stretch; *āsana* – seat, posture

Exhale, bend forwards from the hips with straight legs. Relax the back of the neck, press the head into the knees, or in between the shins. Direct the gaze to the tip of the nose.

9 Nava

Inhale, lift the head and come up to standing with a straight back and an open chest. At the same time, extend the arms up overhead and press the palms together. Tilt the head back, keeping control in the neck, and gaze up at the tips of the thumbs.

Samasthitiḥ

Exhale, gently lower the arms down straight to the sides, move the head into a neutral position, and gaze at the tip of the nose.

Note 1:
Repeat Sūrya-namaskāra A five times.

Note 2:
On vinyāsas 3, 5, and 7 you can gaze at either the tip of the nose (nāsāgra) or between the eyebrows (bhrū-madhya).

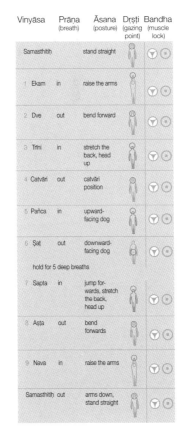

Vinyāsa	Prāṇa (breath)	Āsana (posture)	Dṛṣṭi (gazing point)	Bandha (muscle lock)
Samasthitiḥ		stand straight		
1 Ekam	in	raise the arms		
2 Dve	out	bend forward		
3 Trīṇi	in	stretch the back, head up		
4 Catvāri	out	catvāri position		
5 Pañca	in	upward-facing dog		
6 Ṣaṭ	out	downward-facing dog		
hold for 5 deep breaths				
7 Sapta	in	jump forwards, stretch the back, head up		
8 Aṣṭa	out	bend forwards		
9 Nava	in	raise the arms		
Samasthitiḥ	out	arms down, stand straight		

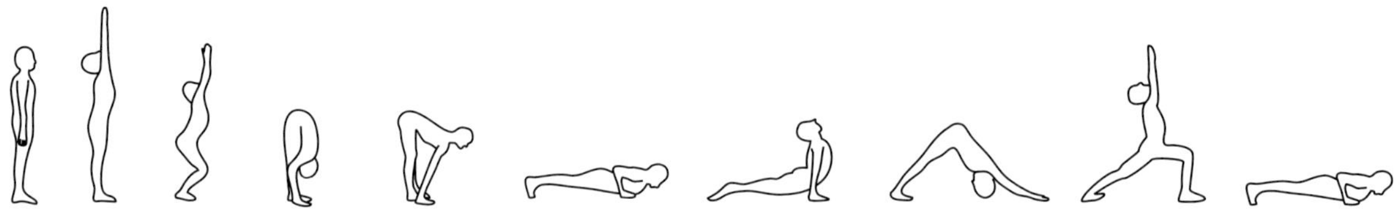

Sūrya-namaskāra B [sun salutation B]

17 vinyāsas

Sūrya – sun, the Sun God; *namaskāra* – salutation

Samasthitiḥ – Stand straight with your feet together, arms by the sides, and gaze at the tip of the nose.

Note 1:
Repeat Sūrya-namaskāra B five times.

Note 2:
On vinyāsas 3, 5, 9, 13 and 15, you can gaze at either the tip of the nose or between the eyebrows.

1 Ekam
Utkaṭāsana
Utkaṭa – powerful, strong, fierce, uneven; *āsana* – seat, posture
Inhale, bend the knees and lower the hips as much as possible while keeping the heels on the floor. Keep the feet and knees pressing together, and the back straight. Lift the hands overhead with straight arms, follow the movement of the hands with the head, tilting the head back when the arms are directly overhead. Let the inhalation expand your chest and back, and press the palms together overhead, with the fingers together. Direct the gaze to the tips of the thumbs.

2 Dve
Uttānāsana
Uttana – strong, deep stretch; *āsana* – seat, posture
Exhale, straighten the legs, release the head, fold forwards from the hips and lower the arms towards the floor. Draw in uddīyana-bandha. Place the fingertips in line with the toes, and press the palms onto the floor with the fingers spread apart. Relax the back of the neck, press the tip of the nose onto the knees or in between the shins. Gaze at the tip of the nose.

Vinyāsas 3–6 are the same as in Sūrya-namaskāra A.

7 Sapta
Vīrabhadrāsana
Vīra – warrior; *bhadra* – good, blessed; *āsana* – seat, posture
Inhale, rotate your left foot 85–90 degrees out, so the sole of the foot touches the floor, and the left heel is facing the right foot. Lean forwards onto the arms and extend the shoulders. Create enough space in order to take a long step forwards, and direct the gaze for a moment in between the hands. Lift your right knee towards the sternum, take a long step with the right leg and place the right foot in between the hands; the palms and the left foot stay grounded. Once your right foot is on the floor, bend the right knee just over 90 degrees, and reach the arms up overhead, pressing the palms together. Let the breath widen the chest and back as you lengthen the shoulders and straighten the elbows. The hips, sternum, and chest should face forwards, in the same direction as the right knee. Engage the left thigh so that the kneecap lifts up and the whole leg stretches out, and press both feet firmly onto the floor. By drawing in mūla-bandha, one creates a strong pelvic floor, which can support the body. Uddīyana-bandha lengthens the spine and sternum. Lean the head back and gaze up.

8 Aṣṭau

Caturaṅga-daṇḍāsana

Catur – four; *aṅga* – limb; *daṇḍa* – staff, stick; *āsana* – seat, posture

Exhale and lower the hands onto the floor, placing them on either side of the right foot. Take the right foot back to meet the left, placing them hip-width apart. Adjust the left foot so you are on the balls of both feet. Keep the body straight with both mūla- and uddīyana-bandha engaged. Bend the arms 90 degrees. Move the chin forwards and direct the gaze to the tip of the nose.

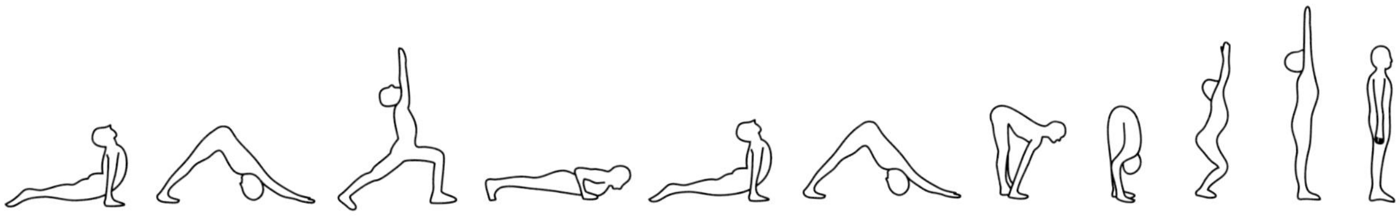

Vinyāsas 9 and 10 are the same as the 5th and 6th vinyāsas in Sūrya-namaskāra A.

Vinyāsas 11 and 12 are the same as the 7th and 8th vinyāsas in Sūrya-namaskāra B, but the step to the front of the mat is taken with the left foot.

Vinyāsas 13–16 are the same as vinyāsas 5–8 in Sūrya-namaskāra A.

Vinyāsa 14 is held for five deep breaths.

17 Saptadaśa

Utkaṭāsana

Utkaṭa – powerful, strong, fierce, uneven; *āsana* – seat, posture

Inhale, bend the knees, lower the hips as much as possible, press the heels onto the floor, squeeze the feet and knees together and elongate the back. Raise the hands, following the movement of the hands with the head, and tilt the head back. Let the inhalation expand the chest and back and press the hands together overhead, palms and fingers together. Gaze at the tips of the thumbs.

Samasthitiḥ

Exhale, straighten the legs, gently bring the head back to a neutral position, lower the arms alongside the body, and gaze at the tip of the nose.

Beginners: Sūrya-namaskāra A and B initiate one into the practice of Aṣṭāṅga yoga. If you have just started Aṣṭāṅga yoga and feel weak or stiff, or if you have an injury or physical limitations, begin slowly and calmly, making small adjustments to the sun-salutation sequence until the movements start to feel familiar and comfortable for your body.

Common adjustments:

- Instead of jumping back to the Catvāri position in the 4th vinyāsa, you can step back, one leg at a time.
- Instead of bending the arms 90 degrees in the 4th vinyāsa, you can bend the elbows and lower yourself down as much as possible, while keeping the body straight. Try to keep the body lifted up off the floor, rather than laying the stomach or legs down on the mat, as you lose the engagement of the bandhas.
- When rolling over the toes, as in the 5th and 6th vinyāsas, keep the feet straight, with the heels facing up to the ceiling. Do not sickle the ankle inwards or outwards.
- In the 7th vinyāsa of Sūrya-namaskāra A, you can step the feet forwards one at a time instead of jumping forwards.
- In the 7th and 11th vinyāsas of Sūrya-namaskāra B, the step forwards is often too short, so step as far forwards towards the hands as possible, leaving the foot where it lands and then lifting the hands up. It is important to remember to breathe consciously while stepping forwards, so that the duration of the physical action and of the inhalation match up. This will develop the breathing technique as well as increase your lung capacity. If one inhalation is not enough for you to complete the stretch within the vinyāsa, breathe out and in again until you complete the āsana. Avoid holding the breath, which creates pressure in the head.

Vinyāsa	Prāṇa (breath)	Āsana (posture)	Dṛṣṭi (gazing point)	Bandha (muscle lock)
Samasthitiḥ		stand straight		
1 Ekam	in	bend the knees, raise the arms		
2 Dve	out	straighten the legs, bend forwards		
3 Trīṇi	in	stretch the back, head up		
4 Catvāri	out	catvāri position		
5 Pañca	in	upward-facing dog		
6 Ṣaṭ	out	downward-facing dog		
7 Sapta	in	warrior pose, right side		
8 Aṣṭau	out	catvāri position		
9 Nava	in	upward-facing dog		
10 Daśa	out	downward-facing dog		
11 Ekadaśa	in	warrior pose, left side		
12 Dvādaśa	out	catvāri position		
13 Trayodaśa	in	upward-facing dog		
14 Caturdaśa	out	downward-facing dog		
hold for 5 deep breaths				
15 Pañcadaśa	in	straighten the spine, head up		
16 Ṣoḍaśa	out	bend forwards		
17 Saptadaśa	in	bend the knees, raise the arms		
Samasthitiḥ	out	arms down, straighten the legs		

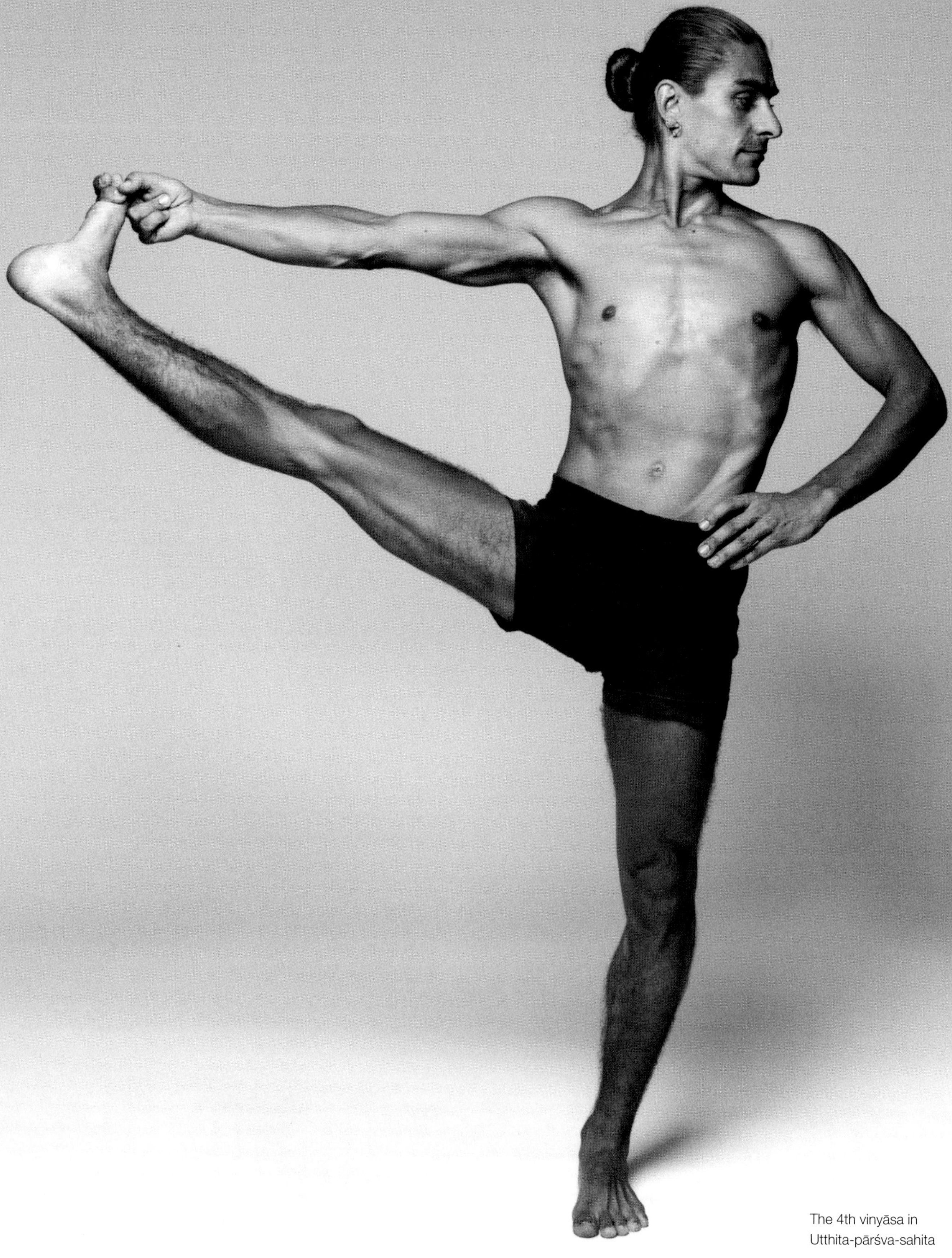

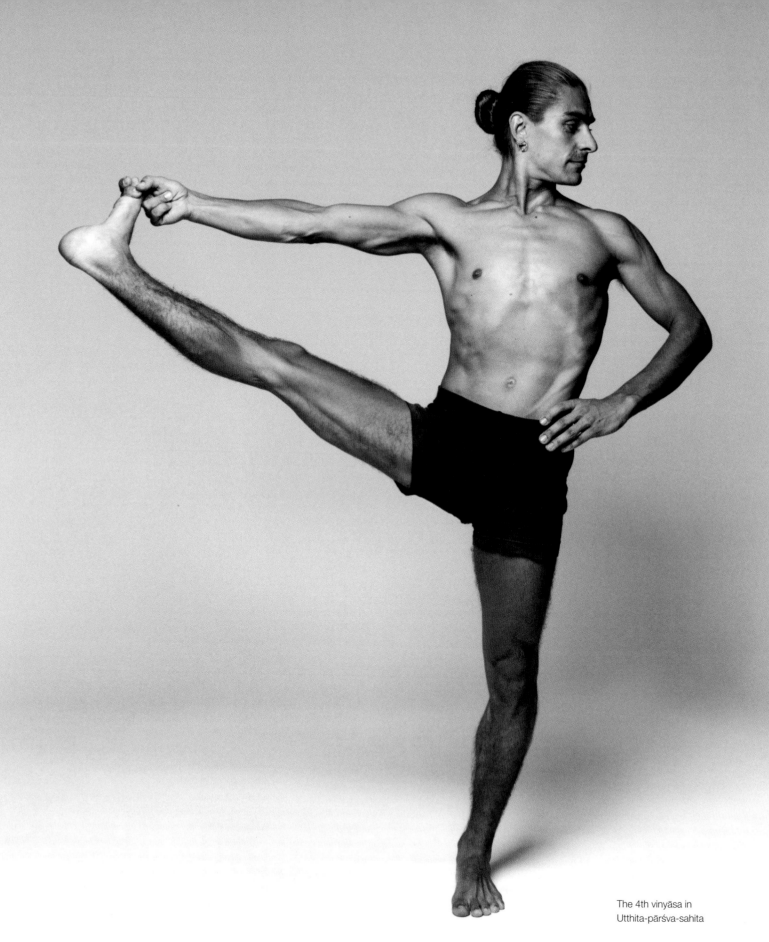

The 4th vinyāsa in
Utthita-pārśva-sahita

standing āsanas

The standing poses follow the sun salutations in the Aṣṭāṅga yoga sequence. The meditative state created in Sūrya-namaskāra A and B, as well as the warmth and flexibility in the body and breath awareness, are necessary in order to proceed further into the standing poses.

The first six standing poses are considered to be foundational āsanas, which start the purification process. They develop flexibility and muscle control and awaken awareness of the bandhas. These standing āsanas are the base for the other āsanas, and, when practised correctly, create a light, healthy body and a strong, alert mind.

The standing postures develop strength in the leg muscles and joints in particular, and increase one's sense of balance. In these postures, one begins to understand and experience how the bandhas, rhythmic breathing, and proper dṛṣṭi work to create a feeling of expansion and relaxation.

Note: One can begin the standing postures with the hands down by the sides, as in Samasthitiḥ, or in kara-mudrā, with the hands pressed together in front of the chest. For many students, this is a calming gesture, a return to prayer between each āsana. The same can be done when you jump back from the standing āsanas and return to Samasthitiḥ, you can either place the hands directly to the sides, or take kara-mudrā for a moment before lowering the arms to your sides.

Pādāṅguṣṭhāsana

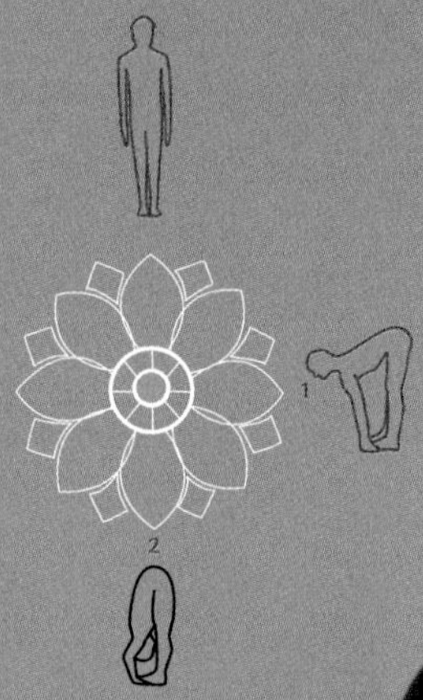

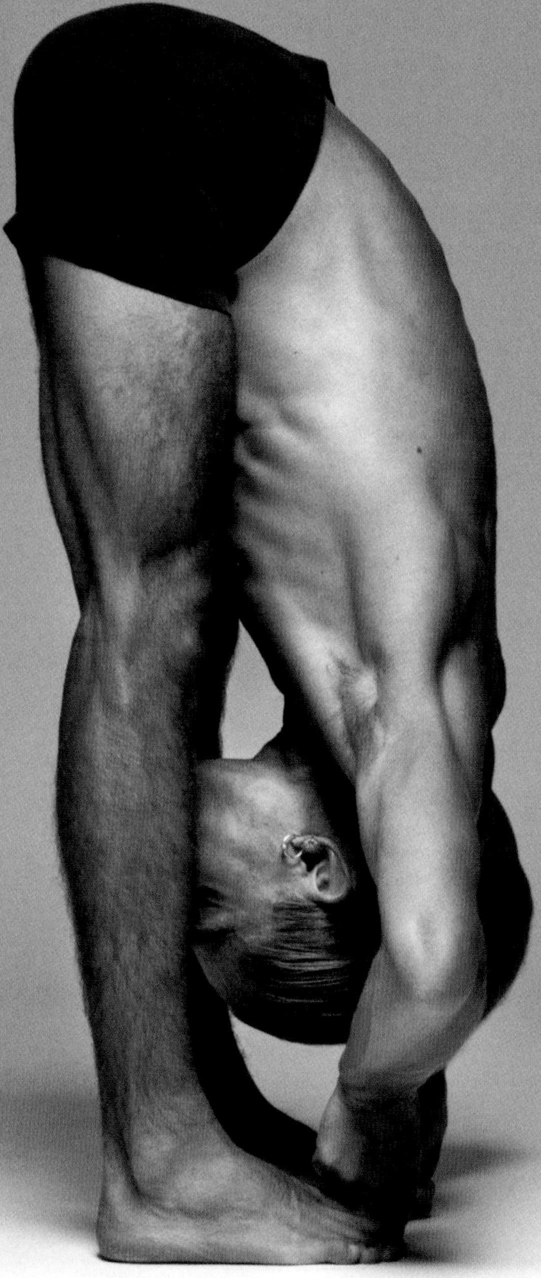

Pādāṅguṣṭhāsana [big toe pose]

3 vinyāsas

Pāda – foot; *aṅguṣṭha* – big toe; *āsana* – seat, posture

Samasthitiḥ – Stand straight with the feet together, arms by the sides, and gaze at the tip of the nose.

Preparation for the āsana:
Option 1: Inhale and jump the feet slightly apart, about half the length of your own foot. Exhale and hold the position.
Option 2: Inhale and exhale as described above. After the exhalation, fold forwards and take hold of your big toes. In this way, folding forwards and taking hold of the toes occurs during the space between the exhalation and the inhalation of the 1st vinyāsa. After taking hold of the big toes, inhale and lift the head up, as described in the 1st vinyāsa.

1 Ekam
Inhale, fold forwards and take hold of the big toes with the first two fingers and thumb. Open the chest and sternum, stretch out the entire back and lift the head. Straighten the arms and pull lightly on the big toes, in opposition to the upwards-moving stretch. Look at the tip of the nose.

2 Dve
Exhale, fold forwards from the hips with straight legs, strongly engage uddīyana-bandha to lengthen the back and create space in order to fold in towards the thighs. Pull on the toes and pitch the weight slightly forwards onto the balls of the feet, keeping the heels and toes on the floor. Relax the back of the neck and press the tip of the nose in towards the knees or between the shins. Relax the hamstrings and lower back, and engage the thighs. This is the state (sthiti) of the āsana. Stay here for five deep breaths, gazing at the tip of the nose.

3 Trīṇi
Inhale, return to the same position as in the 1st vinyāsa. Lift the chest, lengthen the spine and raise the head. Straighten the arms and pull on the big toes. Exhale, hold the pose and gaze at the tip of the nose.

After the third vinyāsa go directly to the 1st vinyāsa of Pāda-hastāsana.

Note 1:
There are two preparatory breaths before the vinyāsa counting begins.

Note 2:
There are two breaths in the third vinyāsa.

Vinyāsa	Prāṇa (breath)	Āsana (posture)	Dṛṣṭi (gazing point)	Bandha (muscle lock)
Samasthitiḥ Preparation	 in & out	stand straight jump, feet apart, hold pose		
1 Ekam	in	place hands under the feet, head up		
2 Dve	out	bend forwards		
state of the āsana; hold for 5 deep breaths				
3 Trīṇi	in & out	head up, hold the pose		
Samasthitiḥ	in & out	come up, jump the feet together		

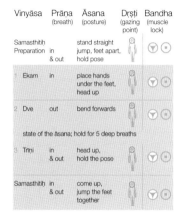

Pāda-hastāsana *[hand to foot pose]*

3 vinyāsas

Pāda – foot; *hasta* – hand; *āsana* – seat, posture

Pāda-hastāsana comes after the third vinyāsa in Pādāṅguṣṭhāsana.

Note:
There are two breaths in the 3rd vinyāsa.

1 Ekam
Inhale, place the palms under the soles of the feet with the toes touching the crease of the wrist. Open the chest, lengthen the spine, lift the head, and gaze at the tip of the nose.

2 Dve
Exhale, lower the head, bend forwards from the hips with straight legs, and engage uddīyana-bandha to help pull yourself forwards onto the thighs. Relax the back of the neck and bring the head towards the knees or between the shins. Press the feet onto the hands while pulling up from the hands. Pitch the weight slightly forwards onto the balls of the feet while keeping the heels on the ground. Relax the hamstrings and the lower back and engage the thighs. This is the state of the āsana. Stay here for five deep breaths, directing the gaze to the tip of the nose.

3 Trīṇi
Inhale, open the chest, draw the shoulders down and back, lengthen the spine and lift the head up. Straighten the arms and press down lightly on the soles of the feet down, in opposition to the upward-moving stretch of the upper body. Hold this position for a full exhalation. Gaze at the tip of the nose.

Samasthitiḥ
Inhale, come up to standing with a straight spine, the arms relaxed against the sides of the body. Exhale, jump the feet together and gaze at the nose-tip.

Beginners:
- Instead of holding the toes or placing the hands under the feet with straight legs, you can bend the knees a little. Keep trying to straighten the legs and engage the thigh muscles.

Vinyāsa	Prāṇa (breath)	Āsana (posture)	Dṛṣṭi (gazing point)	Bandha (muscle lock)
Samasthitiḥ Preparation	 in & out	stand straight jump, feet apart, hold pose		
1 Ekam	in	place hands under the feet, head up		
2 Dve	out	bend forwards		
state of the āsana; hold for 5 deep breaths				
3 Trīṇi	in & out	head up, hold the pose		
Samasthitiḥ	in & out	come up, jump the feet together		

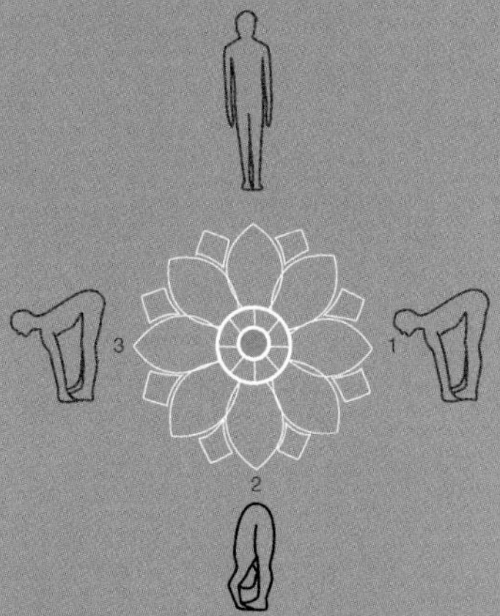
3
1
2

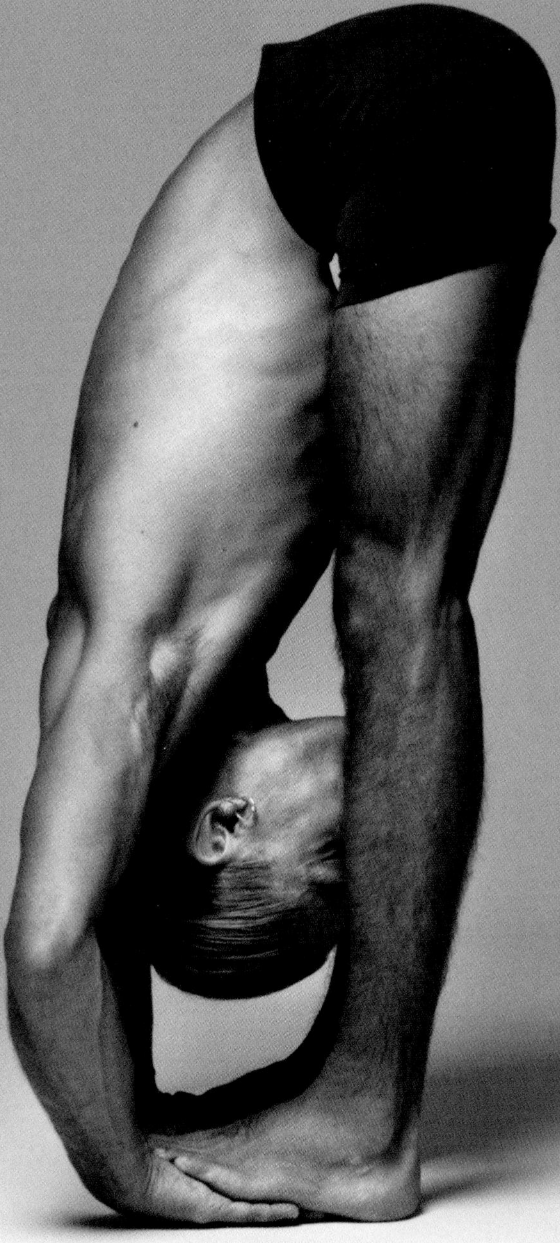

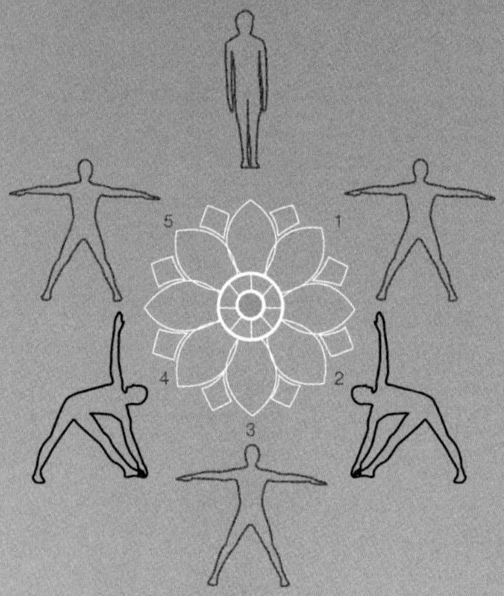

Utthita-trikoṇāsana B

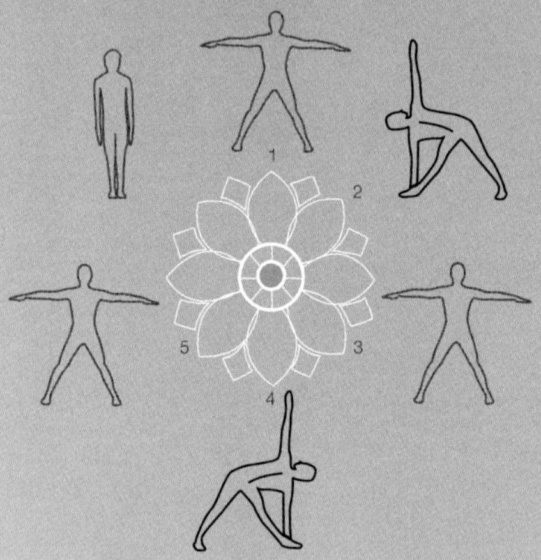

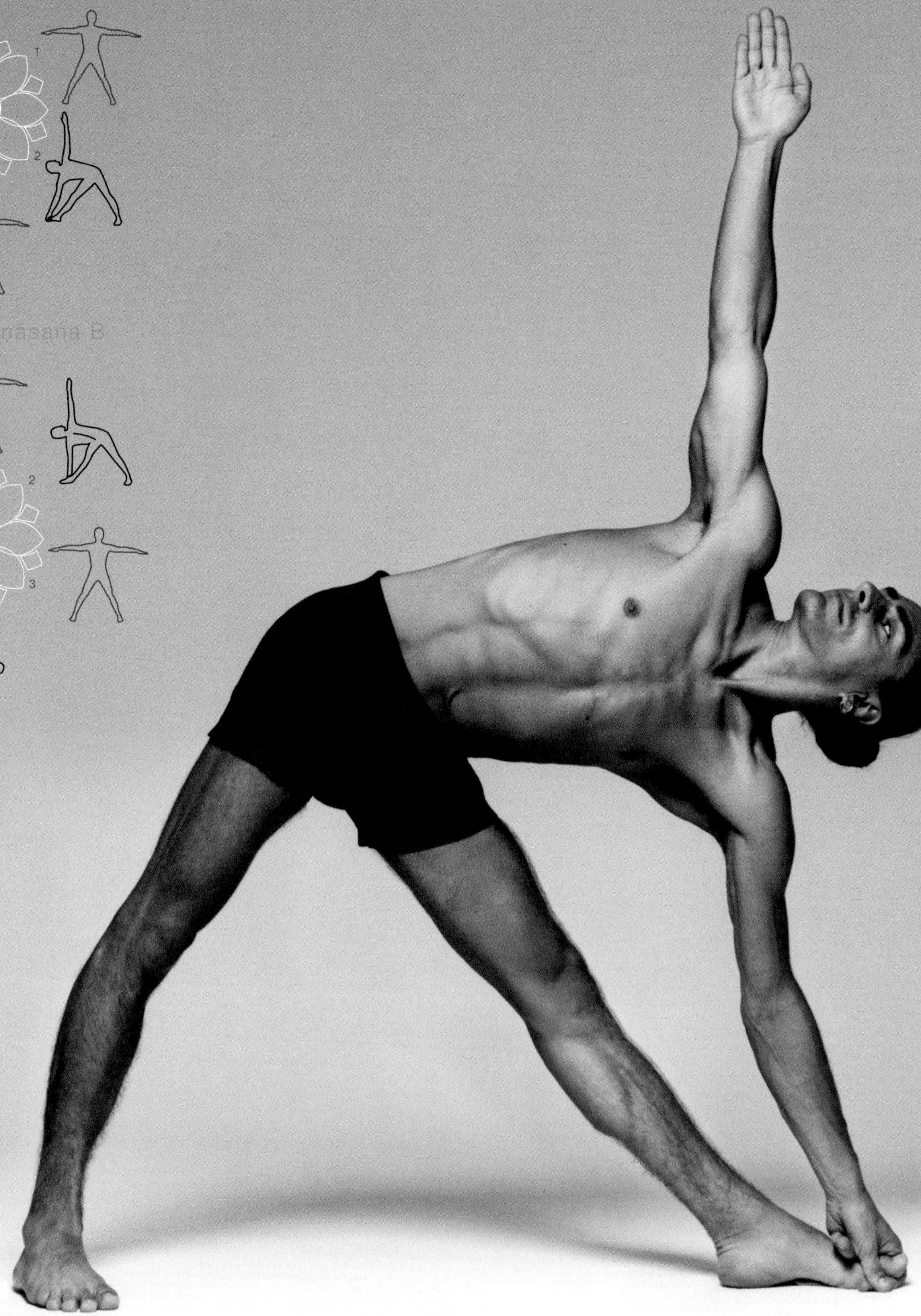

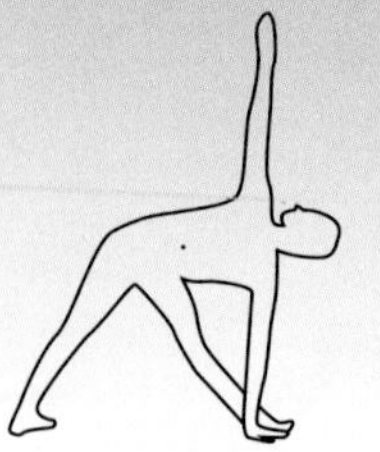

The 2nd vinyāsa in
Utthita-trikoṇāsana B

Utthita-trikoṇāsana A & B [extended triangle pose]

5 vinyāsas

Utthita-trikoṇāsana A

Utthita – extended, intense; *tri* – three; *koṇa* – angle, corner; *āsana* – seat, posture

Samasthitiḥ – Stand straight with the feet together, arms at the sides, and gaze at the tip of the nose.

1 Ekam

Inhale, jump out to the right and separate the legs about three feet from each other (use your own foot to determine the proper length, rather than using the official "foot" measurement). While jumping, extend the arms out to the sides, palms down. Both feet will be facing forwards upon landing. Broaden the shoulders by extending through the arms, open the chest and straighten the spine. Gaze at the tip of the nose.

2 Dve

Exhale, and turn the right foot 90 degrees out, so that the toes point towards the back of the mat. The right heel should remain on the floor and the left foot will point directly to the side of the mat in an 85–90 degree angle. Both feet should be firmly grounded. Note: Unlike many other forms of yoga where the left foot is turned about 45 degrees forwards, in Aṣṭāṅga yoga the left foot remains 85–90 degrees out to the side. This position creates the side and hip-opening effects of the āsana. Reach the right arm out and over the right leg, and take hold of the right big toe with the first two fingers and thumb. Extend your left arm straight up to the ceiling, in line with the sternum, keeping the elbows straight and fingers together. Engage mūla-bandha and uddīyana-bandha to ground yourself in the pose. Lift the left hip up slightly, rotate the chest out towards the side, and turn the head to gaze up at the left hand. The neck should be straight, in a relaxed yet controlled position. Place the right side of the body over the right thigh, so that the body is in line with the legs. Straighten the legs and engage the thigh muscles. This is the state of the āsana on the right side. Stay here for five deep breaths. Gaze at the left hand.

3 Trīṇi

Inhale, and come up with straight arms and a firm body, using the support of the bandhas. Turn the right foot forwards (to face the side of the mat), and stand in the 1st vinyāsa. Direct the gaze to the tip of the nose.

The 4th and 5th vinyāsas are the same as the 2nd and 3rd, but are done on the left side. After the 5th vinyāsa, move directly into the 2nd vinyāsa of Utthita-trikoṇāsana B.

Utthita-trikoṇāsana A

Vinyāsa	Prāṇa (breath)	Āsana (posture)	Dṛṣṭi (gazing point)	Bandha (muscle lock)
Samasthitiḥ		stand straight		
1 Ekam	in	jump 3 feet apart to the right		
2 Dve	out	turn right foot out, take hold of the right big toe		
state of the āsana on the right side, hold for 5 deep breaths				
3 Trīṇi	in	come up, straighten the right foot		
4 Catvāri	out	turn left foot out, take hold of the left big toe		
state of the āsana on the left side, hold for 5 deep breaths				
5 Pañca	in	come up, straighten the left foot		
Samasthitiḥ	out	jump to the front of the mat		

Utthita-trikoṇāsana B follows after the 5th vinyāsa in Utthita-trikoṇāsana A

2 Dve

Exhale, turn the right foot 90 degrees out towards the right, facing the back of the mat. With the arms out to the side, lift up from the left hip to take pressure off the left knee and turn the hips and the chest towards the right leg. Bring the left arm down to the outside of the right foot and stretch the right arm directly up to the ceiling. Place the left palm on the ground, with the fingers spread wide, the middle finger pointing forwards, and the fingertips in line with the right toes. Keep the right hand in line with the sternum, with the fingers pressing together. Open the chest out to the side and rotate the head to gaze towards the right hand, keeping the neck relaxed and straight. The left side is directly above the right thigh and in line with the legs, as you twist the spine deeply. Keep the hips lifted and even. Press the left hand and right foot firmly onto the floor, and stretch the right shoulder and arm up to the ceiling. Straighten the legs and engage the thigh muscles. This is the state of the āsana on the right side. Stay here for five deep breaths, gazing at the right hand.

3 Trīṇi

Inhale and come up, turning the right foot forwards and stand as as in the 1st vinyāsa. Come up with a straight body, fully engaging through the bandhas. Direct the gaze to the tip of the nose.

The 4th and 5th vinyāsas are the same as the 2nd and 3rd, but are done on the left side.

Samasthitiḥ

Exhale and jump to the front of the mat, bringing the feet together and lowering the arms to the sides. Gaze at the tip of the nose.

Utthita-trikoṇāsana B

Vinyāsa	Prāṇa (breath)	Āsana (posture)	Dṛṣṭi (gazing point)	Bandha (muscle lock)
Samasthitiḥ		stand straight		
1 Ekam	in	turn right foot out, left palm on the outer edge of the right foot		
2 Dve	out	turn right foot out, left palm on the outer edge of the right foot		
state of the āsana on the right side, hold for 5 deep breaths				
3 Trīṇi	in	come up, straighten the right foot		
4 Catvāri	out	turn left foot out, right palm on the outer edge of the left foot		
state of the asana on the left side, hold for 5 deep breaths				
5 Pañca	in	come up, straighten the left foot		
Samasthitiḥ	out	jump to the front of the mat		

Beginners:

- When reaching down for the big toe in the 2nd and 4th vinyāsa of Utthita-trikoṇāsana A, to begin with you can lean the body forwards. Over time, the body will open up and you can take hold of the big toe, the torso in line with the front leg.
- If the forwards bend does not help, take hold of your ankle, but keep the legs straight. When the body has become more flexible, you can then reach for the big toe.
- Keep the back foot angled slightly forwards, gradually turning it 85–90 degrees out to the side.
- If you cannot take the hand to the floor in the 2nd and 4th vinyāsa of Utthita-trikoṇāsana B, you can try to touch the fingertips to the floor or take hold of the ankle. Try to keep the body in line with the thighs, and slowly straighten the legs.
- Keep the back of the neck and shoulders relaxed throughout.

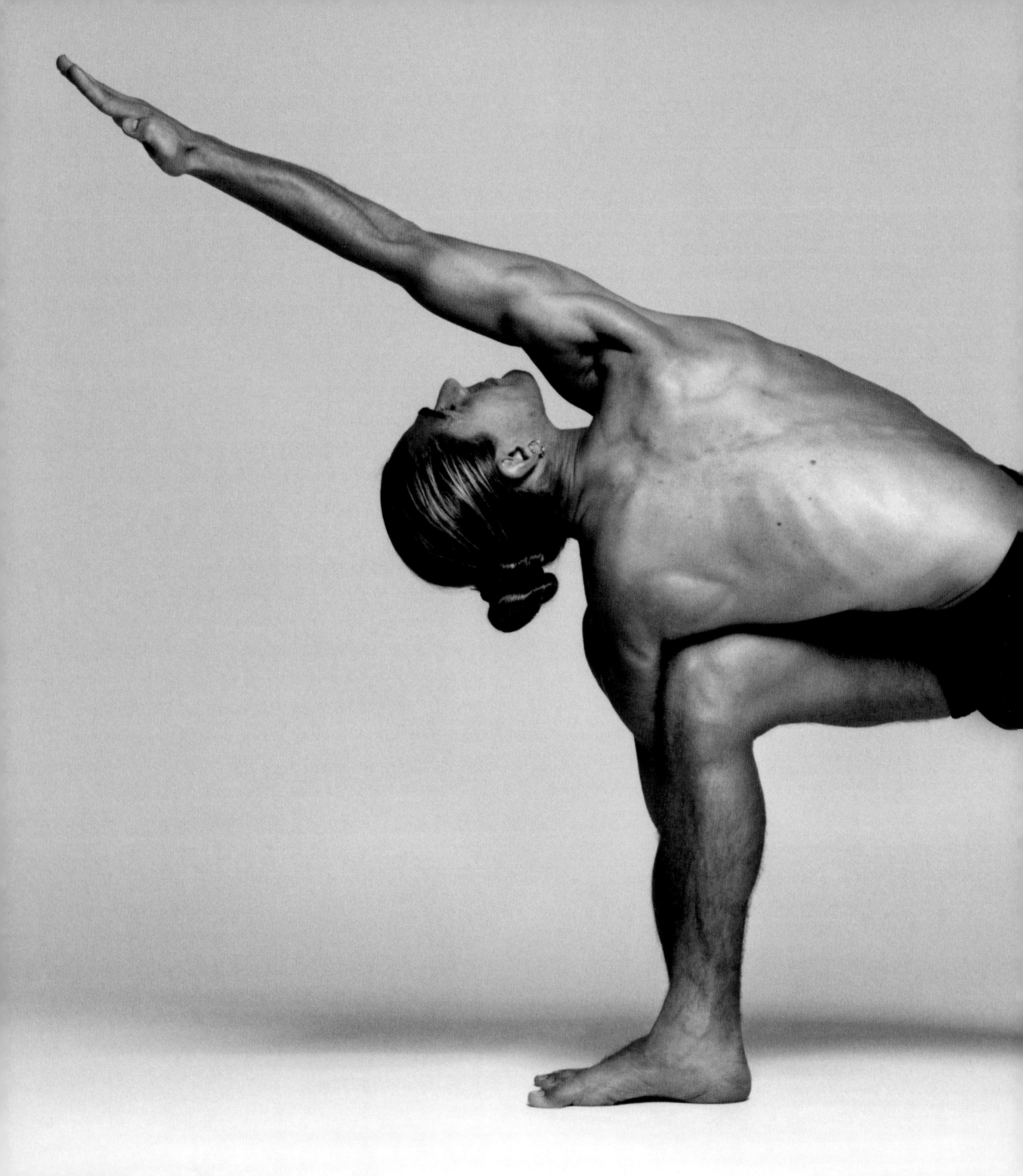

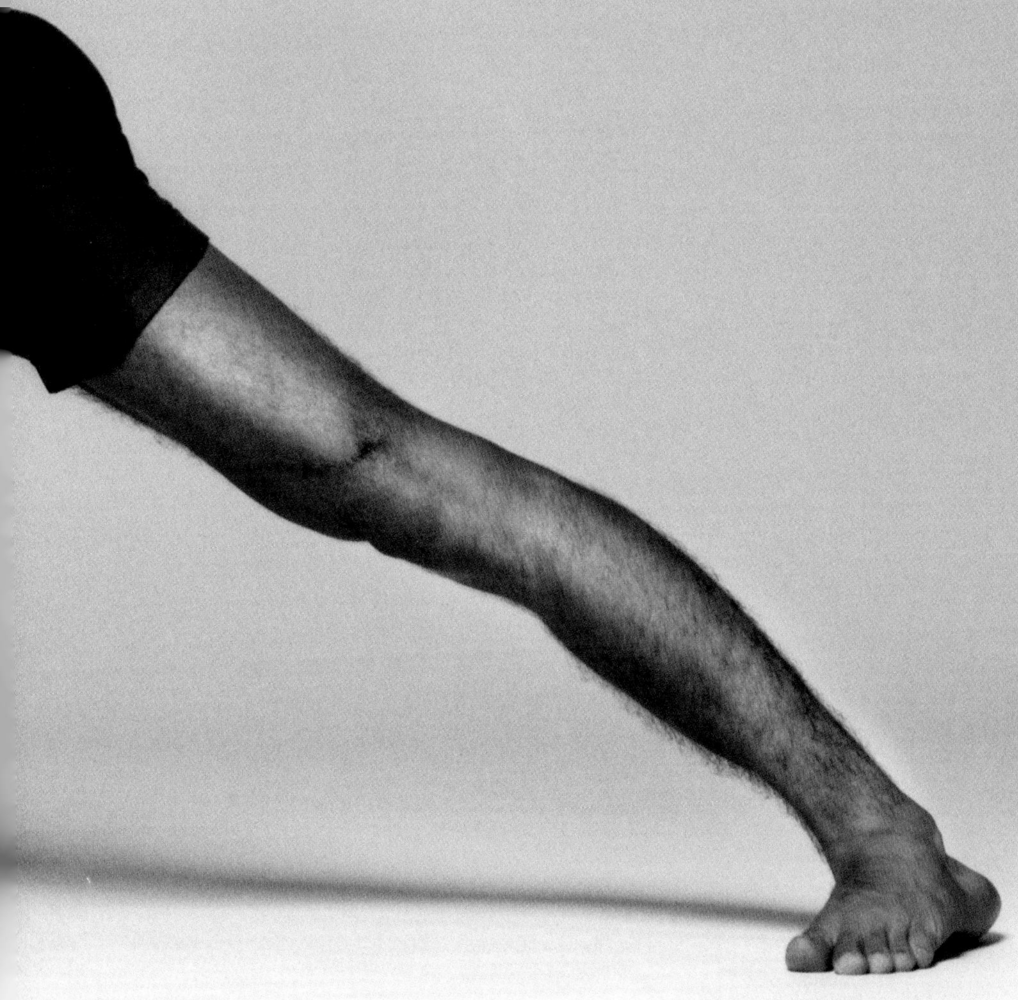

Utthita-pārśvakoṇāsana A

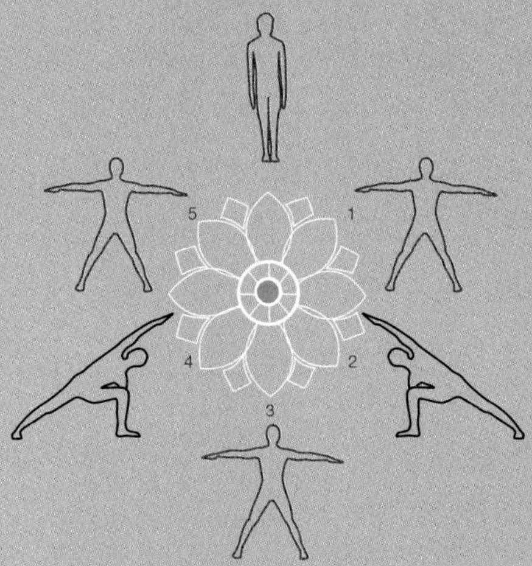

Utthita-pārśvakoṇāsana B

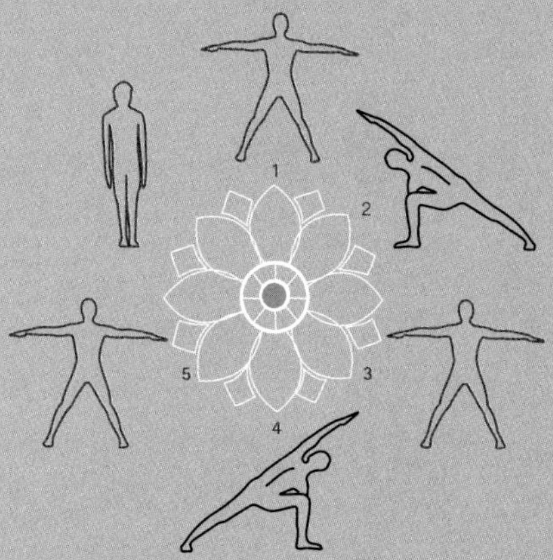

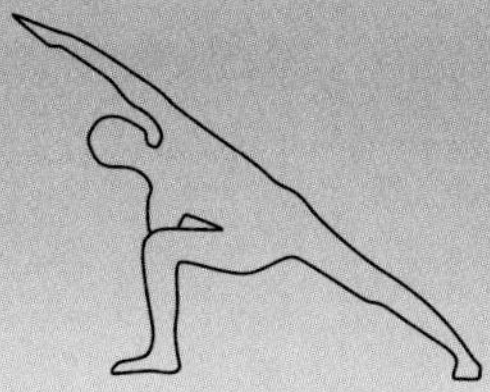

The 2nd vinyāsa in
Utthita-pārśvakoṇāsana A

Utthita-pārśvakoṇāsana A [extended side angle pose A]

5 vinyāsas

Utthita – extended, intense; *pārśva* – side; *koṇa* – angle; *āsana* – seat, posture

Samasthitiḥ – Stand straight with the feet together, arms by the sides, and gaze at the tip of the nose.

1 Ekam
Inhale, jump to the right and land five-feet apart with the toes facing forwards. While jumping, reach the arms out to the side, palms facing down. Stretch the shoulders by elongating the arms away from one another. Gaze at the tip of the nose.

2 Dve
Exhale, turn the right foot 90 degrees out to the right, towards the back of the mat, keeping the heels down and in line with each other. The left foot stays pointing forwards to the side of the mat in an 85–90 degree angle. Note: Contrary to many other yoga styles, in Aṣṭāṅga yoga the left foot is turned out, as this position creates the side and hip-opening effects of the āsana.

Bend your right knee just over 90 degrees and, following the right hand with the gaze, place the palm on the floor, on the outer edge of the right leg. The fingertips are spread wide, in line with the toes, with the middle finger pointing forwards. Extend the left arm straight up over the ear, in line with the left side of the torso and left leg. Open the chest, turn the head up towards the underside of the arm, and relax the back of the neck. Keep the fingers together and gaze at the fingertips of the left hand, with the palm facing you. Press the left foot onto the floor, creating a strong base from which the left side can stretch. Straighten the left leg and stretch the left hip, shoulder and upper body by extending the left arm forwards. Relax through the shoulders and engage mūla-bandha to stabilize the hips and uddīyana-bandha to lengthen the body. This is the state of the āsana on the right side. Stay here for five deep breaths. Gaze at the fingertips of the left hand.

3 Trīṇi
Inhale and with the strength of the legs and bandhas, come up with straight arms and a stable body. Shift the right foot forwards and come to stand as in the 1st vinyāsa. Gaze at the tip of the nose.

The 4th and 5th vinyāsas are the same as the 2nd and 3rd, but are done on the left side. After the 5th vinyāsa, move directly into the 2nd vinyāsa of Utthita-pārśvakoṇāsana B.

Beginners:

- Tension in the body can limit the extent of the arm stretch over the ear. In the state of the āsana, focus on opening the chest out to the side while stretching the arm overhead. Work gradually towards bringing the arm over the ear, in line with the back leg and upper body.

Vinyāsa	Prāṇa (breath)	Āsana (posture)	Dṛṣṭi (gazing point)	Bandha (muscle lock)
Samasthitiḥ		stand straight		
1 Ekam	in	jump 5 feet apart to the right		
2 Dve	out	turn right foot out, bend the right knee, right hand to the floor, left arm over ear		
state of the āsana on the right side, hold for 5 deep breaths				
3 Trīṇi	in	come up, straighten the right foot		
4 Catvāri	out	turn left foot out, bend the left knee, left hand to the floor, right arm over ear		
state of the āsana on the left side, hold for 5 deep breaths				
5 Pañca	in	come up, straighten the left foot		
Samasthitiḥ	out	jump to the front of the mat		

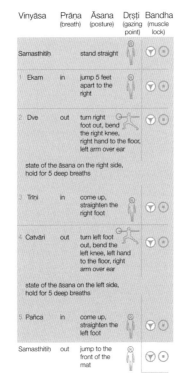

Utthita-pārśvakoṇāsana B [extended side angle posture B]

5 vinyāsas

Utthita-pārśvakoṇāsana B is done after the 5th vinyāsa in *Utthita-pārśvakoṇāsana A.*

2 Dve
Exhale, turn the right foot 90 degrees out to the side, keeping the heels grounded and in line with each other, as in Utthita-pārśvakoṇāsana A. Bend the right knee just over 90 degrees and twist the chest and hips over the right leg. Lift up from the left hip to relieve any pressure in the left knee. Bend down as you twist the spine and chest towards the right. Place the left upper arm over the right thigh, slightly above the knee. Hold it in place, so it doesn't slide over the knee, and place the left palm onto the floor. The fingers should be spread wide, with the middle finger pointing forwards and the fingertips in line with the toes. Follow the left hand with the gaze. Straighten the right arm up and over the ear, in line with the left leg and upper body. Turn the chest and head upwards, relax the back of the neck and gaze at the right fingertips with the palm facing down and fingers together. Press the left foot into the floor, engage the thighs, and straighten the leg. Keep the hips stable by engaging mūla-bandha and let the entire spine release into the twist. Engage uddīyana-bandha to lengthen and open up the body. This is the state of the āsana on the right side. Stay here for five deep breaths. Gaze at the right fingertips.

3 Trīṇi
Inhale, come up with straight arms and a stable body using the support of the legs and bandhas. Shift the right foot forwards, and come to stand as in the 1st vinyāsa. Direct the gaze to the tip of the nose.

The 4th and 5th vinyāsas are the same as the 2nd and 3rd, but are done on the left side.

Samasthitiḥ
While exhaling, jump forwards to the front of the mat, feet together, arms down by the sides, and the gaze at the tip of the nose.

Beginners: Tension in the body can make it hard, at first, to stretch the arm over the ear while pressing the other hand into the floor. In the state of the āsana, try to open the chest in the twisted position while stretching the arm overhead. Work gradually towards bringing the arm over the ear, in line with the back leg and the upper side of the body.

- When moving into the āsana, you can press the thigh of the front leg inwards with your outer hand and bend the back knee. This should make it easier to get the other arm over the knee and thigh. If the palm or fingertips do not reach the floor, leave the hand in the air, but keep reaching it down towards the ground while taking the other arm over the ear.
- If the back leg does not straighten completely, keep it slightly bent.
- Keep the back foot angled slightly forwards, gradually bringing it 85–90 degrees out to the side.
- Avoid doing your own variation of Utthita-pārśvakoṇāsana B. Rather, try to do the posture as much as possible according to the description.

Vinyāsa	Prāṇa (breath)	Āsana (posture)	Dṛṣṭi (gazing point)	Bandha (muscle lock)
Samasthitiḥ		stand straight		
1 Ekam	in	jump 5 feet apart to the right		
2 Dve	out	turn right foot out, bend the right knee, right hand to the floor, left arm over ear		
state of the āsana on the right side, hold for 5 deep breaths				
3 Trīṇi	in	come up, straighten the right foot		
4 Catvāri	out	turn left foot out, bend the left knee, left hand to the floor, right arm over ear		
state of the āsana on the left side, hold for 5 deep breaths				
5 Pañca	in	come up, straighten the left foot		
Samasthitiḥ	out	jump to the front of the mat		

Prasārita-pādottānāsana A [wide-foot forward bend pose A]

5 vinyāsas

Note 1:
There are two breaths in the 2nd and 4th vinyāsas.

Note 2:
If you follow the chart below for your practice, the 5th vinyāsa has in & out, as it is in the āsana description on the right. In the "full vinyāsa" system, there is only an in-breath.

Vinyāsa	Prāṇa (breath)	Āsana (posture)	Dṛṣṭi (gazing point)	Bandha (muscle lock)
Samasthitiḥ		stand straight		
1 Ekam	in	jump 5 feet apart to the right, hands on the hips		
2 Dve	out & in	hands to the floor stretch out, head up		
3 Trīni	out	bend forwards		
state of the āsana, hold for 5 deep breaths				
4 Catvāri	in & out	stretch out, head up hold the pose		
5 Pañca	in	hands to the hips, come up		
Samasthitiḥ	out	jump to the front of the mat		

Prasārita – wide, opened, outstretched; *pāda* – foot; *ut* – deep, strong, intense; *tāna* – stretch, extend, lengthen; *āsana* – seat, posture

Samasthitiḥ – Stand straight with the feet together, arms by the sides, and gaze at the tip of the nose.

1 Ekam
Inhale, jump five feet out to the right, with the toes pointing straight forwards. While jumping, bring both hands to your waist, with the fingertips pointing in towards uddīyana-bandha (i.e. the lower abdomen), and open the chest. Gaze at the tip of the nose.

2 Dve
Exhale and fold forwards from the hips. Place the hands shoulder-width apart on the floor, fingertips in line with the toes. Gaze at the space between the hands, and check the placement of your hands. Spread the fingers wide, with the middle finger pointing forwards, and press the palms into the floor. Inhale slowly, pressing the palms down, straighten the arms and lift the head. Lengthen the spine and expand the chest. Keep the back of the neck relaxed. Apply mūla-bandha to support the hips, as the feet remain grounded into the mat. Draw in uddīyana-bandha to open the chest and straighten the back. Gaze at the tip of the nose.

3 Trīṇi
Exhale, lower the head, strongly engaging uddīyana-bandha and folding forwards with a straight spine down between the legs. Release mūla-bandha slightly here to relax through the hips. Press the hands into the floor to ease the forward bend, lower the crown of the head to the floor with a straight and relaxed neck. Press the feet into the ground, relax the hamstrings, but engage the front side of the thighs. This is the state of the āsana. Take five deep breaths here, gazing at the tip of the nose.

4 Catvāri
Inhale slowly, keep pressing the palms into the floor and straighten the arms. Open the chest, lengthen the spine, and lift the head up, as in the 2nd vinyāsa. Hold this position for an exhalation. Gaze at the tip of the nose.

5 Pañca
Inhale, place the hands on the hips with the fingertips pointing in towards uddīyana-bandha. Come up to standing with a straight upper body, while simultaneously keeping uddīyana- and mūla-bandha fully engaged to support the lower back. Gaze at the tip of the nose and exhale to complete this vinyāsa.

From here, move directly into the next āsana. On the next inhalation, stretch the arms out to the sides. Count this as the 1st vinyāsa in Prasārita-pādottānāsana B.

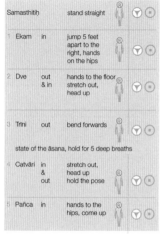

Prasārita-pādottānāsana A

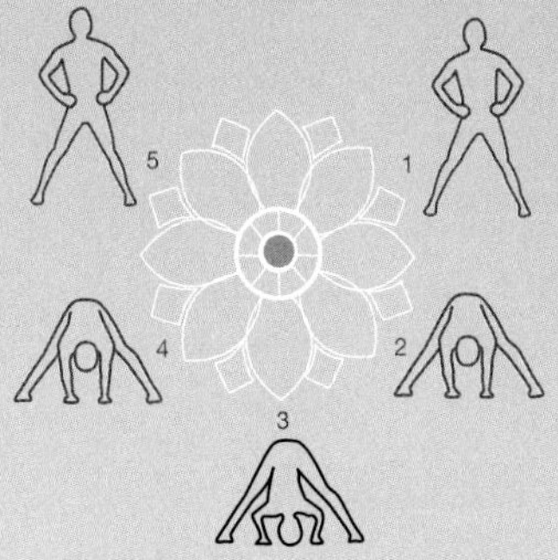

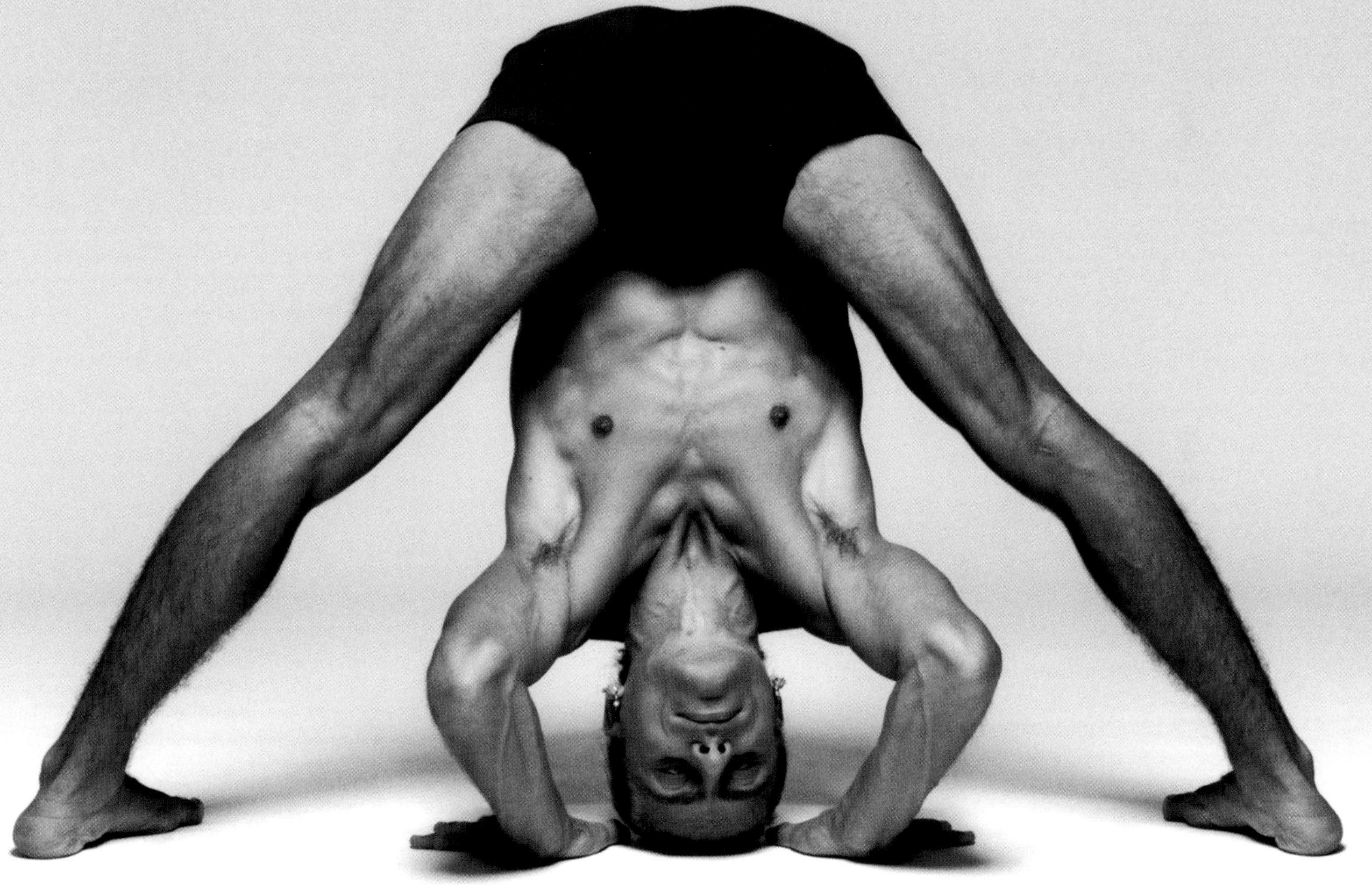

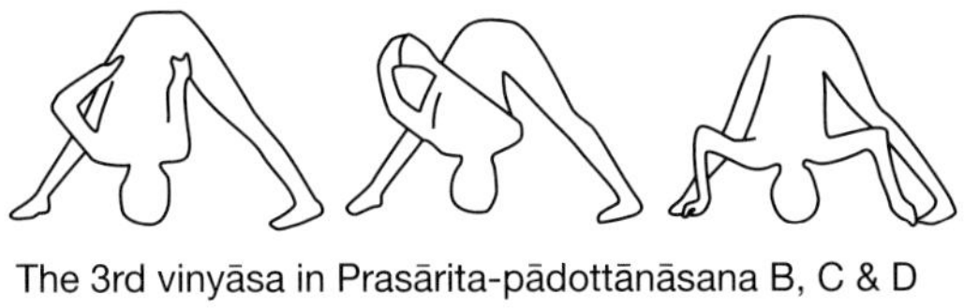

The 3rd vinyāsa in Prasārita-pādottānāsana B, C & D

Prasārita-pādottānāsana B [wide-foot forward bend pose B]

5 vinyāsas

Note:
There are two breaths in the 2nd and 4th vinyāsas.

Vinyāsa	Prāṇa (breath)	Āsana (posture)	Dṛṣṭi (gazing point)	Bandha (muscle lock)
Samasthitiḥ		stand straight		
1 Ekam	in	jump 5 feet apart to the right, hands out to the sides		
2 Dve	out & in	hands on hips, open the chest		
3 Trīṇi	out	bend forwards, keeping the hands on the hips		
state of the āsana; hold for 5 deep breaths				
4 Catvāri	in & out	come up, hold the pose		
5 Pañca	in	extend arms out to the side		
Samasthitiḥ	out	jump to the front of the mat		

1 Ekam
Inhale, extend the arms out to the side, palms facing down and shoulders relaxed. Gaze at the tip of the nose.

2 Dve
Exhale, place the fingertips on the hips, while keeping the chest open. Inhale and draw in uḍḍīyana-bandha as you widen the chest, while engaging mūla-bandha to support the hips. Gaze at the tip of the nose.

3 Trīṇi
Exhale, strongly engage uḍḍīyana-bandha and fold forwards between the legs with the chest open. Lower the crown of the head to the floor in between the feet, relaxing and lengthening the back of your neck. Release mūla-bandha slightly to relax through the hips. Straighten the legs, press the feet into the ground and engage the thighs. This is the state of the āsana. Take five deep breaths here and gaze at the tip of the nose.

4 Catvāri
Inhale and keep hold of your hips as you come up to standing. Fully engage uḍḍīyana- and mūla-bandha to support the lower back. Stay in this posture as you exhale completely. Gaze at the tip of the nose.

From the 4th vinyāsa, go directly to the next āsana, Prasārita-pādottānāsana C. Stretch out the arms from the shoulders while inhaling, counting this as the 1st vinyāsa in Prasārita-pādottānāsana C.

Prasārita-pādottānāsana C [wide-foot forward bend pose C]

5 vinyāsas

Note:
There are two breaths in the 2nd and 4th vinyāsas.

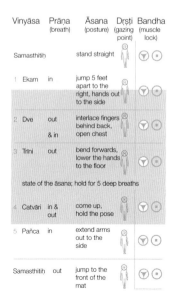

Vinyāsa	Prāṇa (breath)	Āsana (posture)	Dṛṣṭi (gazing point)	Bandha (muscle lock)
Samasthitiḥ		stand straight		
1 Ekam	in	jump 5 feet apart to the right, hands out to the side		
2 Dve	out & in	interlace fingers behind back, open chest		
3 Trīni	out	bend forwards, lower the hands to the floor		
state of the āsana; hold for 5 deep breaths				
4 Catvāri	in & out	come up, hold the pose		
5 Pañca	in	extend arms out to the side		
Samasthitiḥ	out	jump to the front of the mat		

Prasārita-pādottānāsana C follows directly after the 4th vinyāsa of Prasārita-pādottānāsana B.

1 Ekam
Inhale, extend the arms out to the side, palms facing down and shoulders relaxed. Direct the gaze to the tip of the nose.

2 Dve
Exhale, bring the arms behind the back, interlace the fingers, draw the shoulders back and turn the palms outwards. Inhale, stretch the arms and open the chest, sternum and collar bones. Gaze at the tip of the nose.

3 Trīṇi
Exhale, keep uḍḍīyana-bandha fully engaged as the fingers stay interlaced behind the back. Fold forwards with a straight spine and an open chest. Press the crown of the head down into the floor with a straight neck, and reach the hands overhead, towards the floor. Keep the arms straight, shoulders relaxed and lengthened, fingers crossed, and palms turned outwards. Release mūla-bandha slightly to relax through the hips. Straighten the legs, press the feet into the ground, and engage the thighs. This is the state of the āsana. Hold for five breaths, gazing at the tip of the nose.

4 Catvāri
Inhale and keeping the fingers interlaced, slowly come up to standing. Engage uḍḍīyana- and mūla-bandha to support the lower back. Keeping the fingers interlaced behind the back, hold this position and exhale fully. Avoid releasing the hands before completing the exhalation. Gaze at the tip of the nose.

After the exhalation in the 4th vinyāsa, go directly to the next āsana. Place your hands on your hips while inhaling, and count this as the 1st vinyāsa in Prasārita-pādottānāsana D.

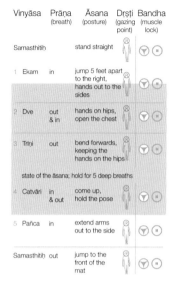

Prasārita-pādottānāsana B

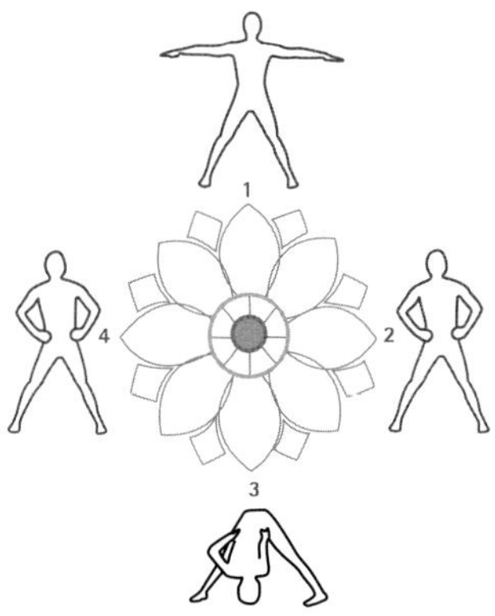

Prasārita-pādottānāsana C

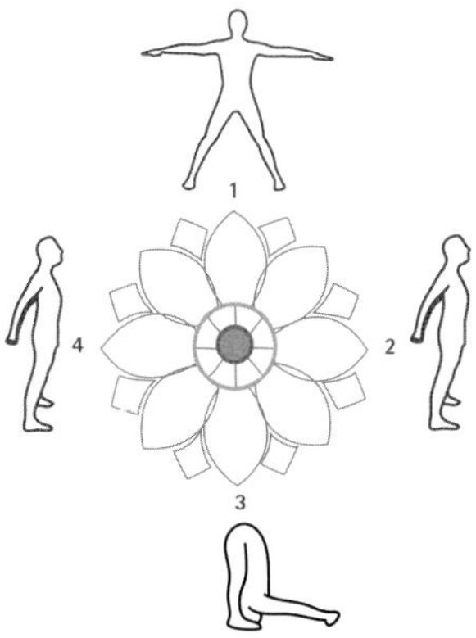

Prasārita-pādottānāsana D

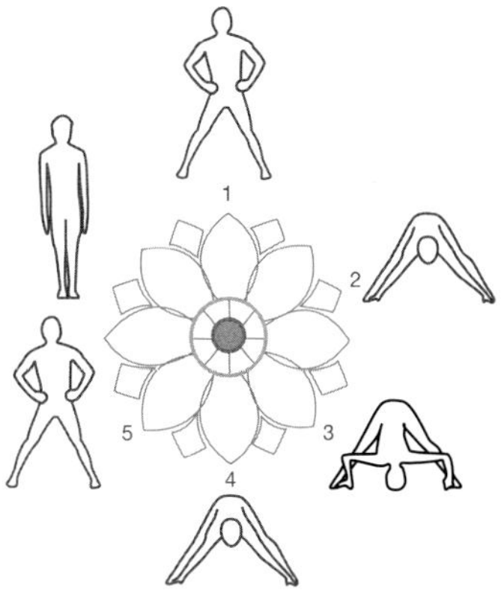

Prasārita-pādottānāsana D [wide-foot forward bend pose D]

5 vinyāsas

Prasārita-pādottānāsana D is done directly after the 4th vinyāsa in Prasārita-pādottānāsana C.

1 Ekam
Inhale, place the hands on the hips with the fingers pointing in towards uddīyana-bandha. Gaze at the tip of the nose.

2 Dve
Exhale and fold forwards from the hips with an open chest. Take hold of your big toes with the first two fingers and thumbs. Inhale and pull slightly on the big toes to maintain the length in the arms. Open the chest, stretch the spine, lift the head and gaze at the tip of the nose.

3 Trīṇi
Exhale, lower the head, folding the upper body down in between the legs. Keep the spine and neck straight and uddīyana-bandha pulled in. Release mūla-bandha slightly to relax through the hips. Pull on the big toes, and place the crown of the head on the floor between the feet. This is the state of the āsana. Take five deep breaths here. Gaze at the tip of the nose.

4 Catvāri
Slowly inhale, pulling on the big toes and straightening the arms. Open the chest and lift the head, keeping the back of the neck relaxed. Gaze at the tip of the nose and exhale here.

5 Pañca
Inhale, place the hands on the hips with the fingers pointing in, towards uddīyana-bandha. With a straight back and an open chest, come up to standing, supported by uddīyana- and mūla-bandha and gazing at the tip of the nose.

Samasthitiḥ
Exhale while jumping to the front of the mat, lowering the arms down to the sides, bringing the feet together upon landing.

Beginners: It often takes some practice, over a period of time, to bring the crown of the head to the floor with a straight spine.

- If the hands cannot touch the floor at first, try widening the legs further, and/or lean forwards slightly into the midline.
- You can lean forwards slightly to touch the head to the floor. As you gain more flexibility, take the head further down, towards the midline of the body, in line with and in between the feet.
- Hold your hands firmly in Prasārita-pādottānāsana C. Try turning the palms to face out, but if this position restricts the shoulders, keep the palms turned in.

Note:
There are two breaths in the 2nd and 4th vinyāsas.

Vinyāsa	Prāṇa (breath)	Āsana (posture)	Dṛṣṭi (gazing point)	Bandha (muscle lock)
Samasthitiḥ		stand straight		
1 Ekam	in	jump 5 feet apart to the right, hands on the hips		
2 Dve	out & in	take big toes, stretch out, head up		
3 Trīṇi	out	bend forwards, head and hands on the floor		
state of the āsana, hold for 5 deep breaths				
4 Catvāri	in & out	stretch, head up, hold the pose		
5 Pancha	in	hands to the hips, come up		
Samasthitiḥ	out	jump to the front of the mat		

Pārśvottānāsana [side stretch pose]

5 vinyāsas

Pārśva – side; *ut* – deep, strong, intense; *tāna* – stretch, extend, lengthen; *āsana* – seat, posture

Samasthitiḥ – Stand straight with the feet together, arms by the sides, and gaze at the tip of the nose.

1 Ekam
Inhale, jump three feet out to the right. Turn the right foot 90 degrees out, so that it faces the back of the mat, keeping the left foot in an 85–90 degree angle. Place the hands behind the back and bring the palms together. Keep the hands facing upwards so that the little fingers touch the spine, and slide the hands up in between the shoulder blades. Turn the hips and chest towards the right leg, and lift the sternum while engaging the bandhas. Lift up from the left hip to relieve pressure in the left knee. Press the palms and fingers together in this inverted prayer position. Draw the shoulders back and gaze at the tip of the nose.

2 Dve
Exhale, fold forwards, and place the chest onto the right thigh, bringing the chin to the knee or shin. Engage the thigh muscles and keep the legs straight. Draw in mūla-bandha to stabilize the hips and uddīyana-bandha to straighten the chest and back while creating space for the stomach to sink into the thighs. This is the state of the āsana on the right side. Stay here for five breaths and gaze at the tip of the nose.

3 Trīṇi
Inhale, keep the legs straight and come up with an open chest. Use the bandhas to support the back and hips. Keep the hands in the same position behind the back, face the feet to the front and change sides. Move the left foot 90 degrees out, so the toes face the front of the mat and leave the right foot as it is, with the toes facing the side of the mat. Bring the hips and chest to face the left leg, and lift the sternum up as you press the outer edge of the little fingers in towards the spine to open the chest further. Engage the bandhas, and gaze at the tip of the nose.

4 Catvāri
The 4th vinyāsa is the same as the 2nd vinyāsa but on the left side. This is the state of the āsana. Stay here for five breaths.

5 Pañca
Inhale, keep the legs straight and come up to standing. Apply the bandhas to support the back and hips. Keep the hands in the same position behind the back, and turn the feet forwards to face the side of the mat. Gaze at the tip of the nose.

Samasthitiḥ
Jump to the front of the mat while you exhale, and bring the arms down to the sides, gazing at the tip of the nose.

Beginners: It can take some time to be able to bring the hands together behind the back and to get the chin to the shin.

- Instead of bringing the palms together behind the back, begin by touching the fingertips together on the lower back and slide the hands up the back as much as you can.
- Keep the back foot angled slightly forwards, gradually bringing it out 85–90 degrees to the side.
- When bending forwards over the leg, first try to bring the head to the knee. As you gain more flexibility you may be able to lower the chin to the knee or shin.

Vinyāsa	Prāṇa (breath)	Āsana (posture)	Dṛṣṭi (gazing point)	Bandha (muscle lock)
Samasthitiḥ		stand straight		
1 Ekam	in	jump 3 feet apart to the right, face the right leg, hands behind the back		
2 Dve	out	bend forwards to the right		
state of the āsana, hold for 5 deep breaths				
3 Trīṇi	in	come up, turn to the left		
4 Catvāri	out	bend forward to the left		
state of the āsana, hold for 5 deep breaths				
5 Pañca	in	come up, turn the feet to the side of the mat		
Samasthitiḥ	out	jump to the front of the mat		

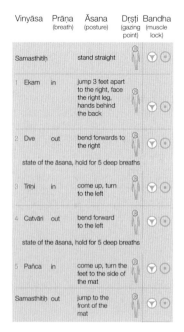

Pārśvottānāsana

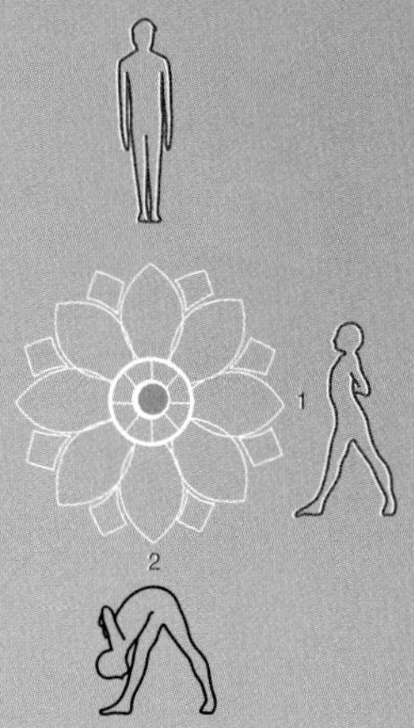

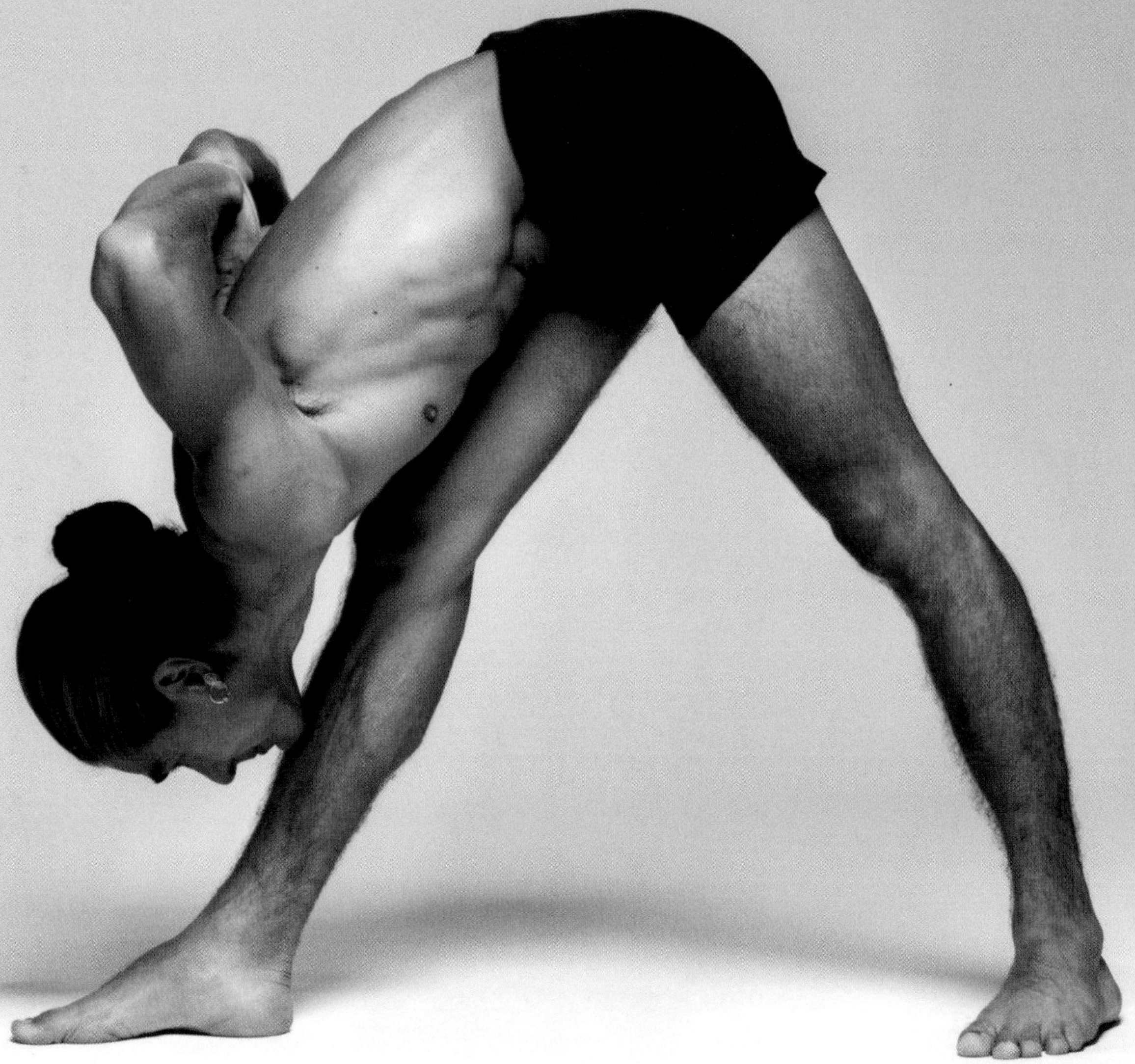

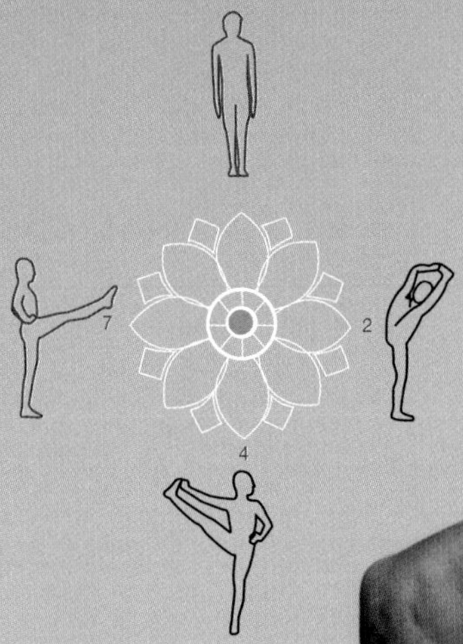

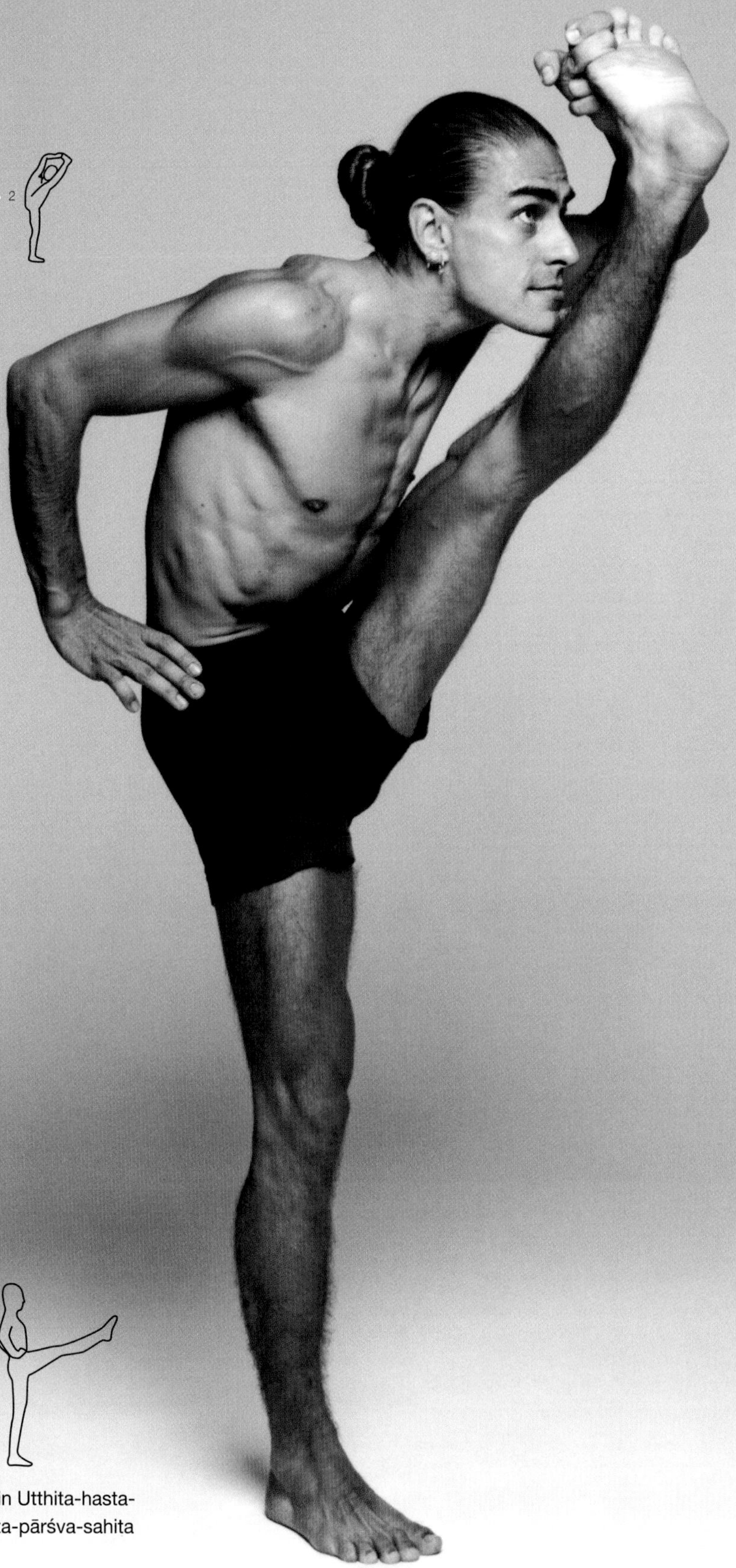

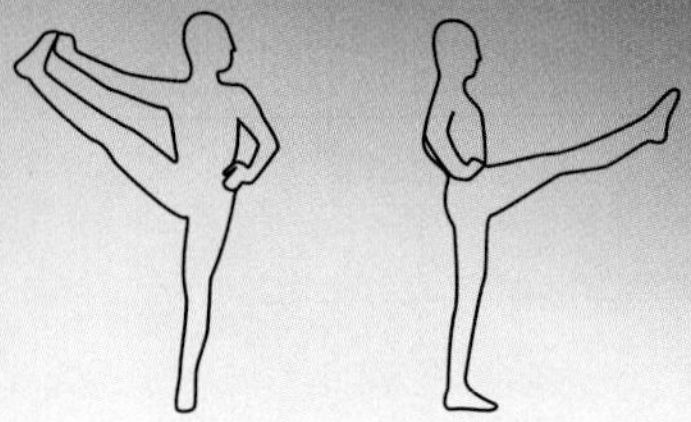

The 4th and 7th vinyāsas in Utthita-hasta-pādāṅguṣṭhāsana & Utthita-pārśva-sahita

Utthita-hasta-pādāṅguṣṭhāsana & Utthita-pārśva-sahita
[extended hand-to-big-toe pose & extended side pose]

14 vinyāsas

Utthita – extended, intense; *hasta* – hand; *pāda* – foot; *aṅguṣṭha* – big toe; *āsana* – seat, posture; *pārśva* – side; *sahita* – fill in, together, to be with, to follow

Samasthitiḥ – Stand straight with the feet together, arms by the sides, and gaze at the tip of the nose.

1 Ekam
Inhale, place the left hand on the waist and lift the right leg up. Take hold of the right big toe with the first two fingers and the thumb of your right hand. Lift the leg up to eye-level, keeping a sturdy grip on the big toe by hooking the fingers and thumb around it. Stand with the left foot firmly on the ground. Straighten both legs and engage the bandhas to maintain balance. Open the chest and lengthen the spine. Gaze at the big toe.

2 Dve
Exhale, fold forwards over the right leg, bring the chin onto the shin while gazing at the big toe. Keep the left foot steady on the floor with the knee straight. Engage mūla-bandha to support both hips and maintain solid contact between the left leg and the floor. Draw in and lift up uddīyana-bandha, which will make it easier to hold the balance and move forwards onto the right leg. This is the state of the āsana. Gaze at the big toe and hold the pose for five breaths.

3 Trīṇi
Inhale, lift the back and come up to the same position as in the 1st vinyāsa, still gazing at the big toe.

4 Catvāri
Exhale, take the right leg 90 degrees out to the side and turn the head to face the left side, with the chin over the left shoulder. Keep the hips balanced, making sure that the right hip isn't higher than the left. Open the chest and straighten the legs and right arm out to the side. Press the left foot firmly into the floor and engage the bandhas to assist with the balance. This is the 4th vinyāsa and is called Utthita-pārśva-sahita. Hold for five deep breaths. Gaze over the shoulder to the left side.

5 Pañca
Inhale, bring the leg back to front, as in the 1st vinyāsa, and gaze at the big toe.

6 Ṣaṭ
Exhale, fold forwards as in the 2nd vinyāsa, but stay here only for the exhalation. Keep looking at the big toe.

7 Sapta
On the next inhalation, lift the torso up from the forward bend, release the fingers and bring the right hand to the right hip. Keep the right leg straight and lifted, pointing the foot. Straighten the back and the legs and open the chest. Engage the bandhas, hamstrings and front thigh muscles to keep the leg elevated and the body balanced. Breathe deeply for five breaths and gaze at the big toe. Exhale, lower the leg and arms and prepare for the left side.

The left side: Repeat vinyāsas 1–7 on the left side, counting them as vinyāsas 8–14. After holding the left leg up in the 14th vinyāsa, exhale and release the leg down. Stand straight with the legs together in Samasthitiḥ, gazing at the tip of the nose.

Beginners: Maintaining the balance throughout the entire sequence requires time and practice.

- To hold the balance, focus the gaze on a point on the floor throughout the entire posture until you are able to use the correct dṛṣṭi for this position.
- Instead of folding forwards in the 2nd vinyāsa, particularly if the balancing is not established yet, bend forwards as much as you can without losing the balance.
- In the 4th vinyāsa, bring the leg out to the side as much as you can, aiming towards 90 degrees.
- It is easier to find and hold the balance if you apply the bandhas and keep the foot of the standing leg firmly grounded into the floor. Try not to move the standing leg during the āsana.

Note:
The last exhalation (when you release the right leg down) is part of the 7th vinyāsa and the last exhalation in the 14th vinyāsa (when you release the left leg down) is Samasthitiḥ.

Vinyāsa	Prāṇa (breath)	Āsana (posture)	Dṛṣṭi (gazing point)	Bandha (muscle lock)
Samasthitiḥ		stand straight		
Right side				
1 Ekam	in	left hand to hip, lift right leg, take right big toe		
2 Dve	out	bend forwards, chin to shin		
state of the āsana, hold for 5 deep breaths				
3 Trīṇi	in	come up, straighten the back		
4 Catvāri	out	take right leg out to the side, look to the left		
this is Utthita-pārśva-sahita, hold for 5 deep breaths				
5 Pañca	in	bring leg back to front		
6 Ṣaṭ	out	bend forwards, chin to shin		
7 Sapta	in	straighten the spine, hands to hips, keep the leg lifted		
hold for 5 deep breaths				
	out	lower the leg		
Left side				
8 Aṣṭau	in	right hand to hip, lift left leg, take left big toe		
9 Nava	out	bend forwards, chin to shin		
state of the āsana, hold for 5 deep breaths				
10 Daśa	in	come up, straighten the back		
11 Ekadaśa	out	take left leg out to the side, look to the right		
this is Utthita pārśva-sahita; hold for 5 deep breaths				
12 Dvādaśa	in	leg back to front		
13 Trayodaśa	out	bend forwards, chin to shin		
14 Caturdaśa	in	straighten the spine, hands to hips, keep leg lifted		
hold for 5 deep breaths				
Samasthitiḥ	out	lower the leg		

Ardha-baddha-padmottānāsana

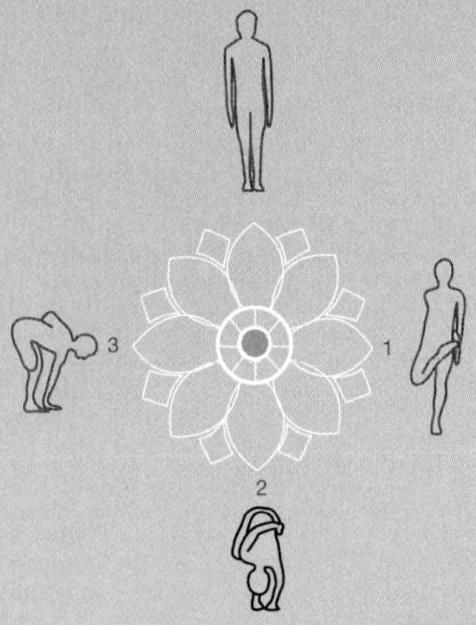

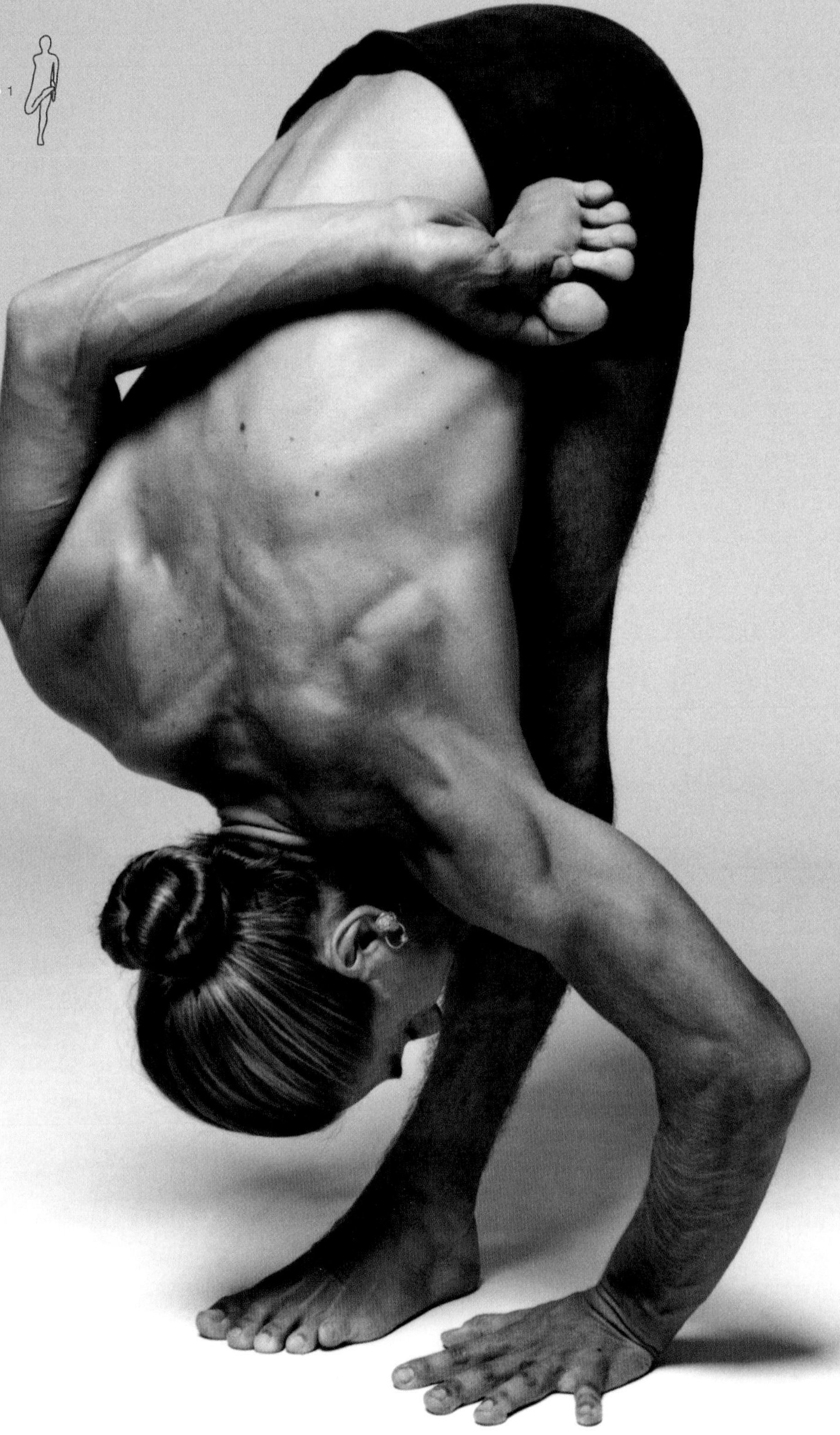

Ardha-baddha-padmottānāsana
[standing half bound lotus stretch pose]

9 vinyāsas

Ardha – half; *baddha* – bound; *padma* – lotus; *ut* – deep, strong, intense; *tāna* – stretch, extend, lengthen; *āsana* – seat, posture

Samasthitiḥ – Stand straight with the feet together, arms by the sides, and gaze at the tip of the nose.

1 Ekam
Inhale, lift the right leg up and take hold of the foot. Turn the sole of the foot upwards and place the outer edge of the foot into the crease of the inner left thigh. Relax deeply through the right hip, and gently drop the right knee down and out to the side, at a 45-degree angle. Be mindful that you don't twist the knee joint itself, but rather move into the half-lotus by releasing in the hip. Reach the right arm around the back and take hold of your right big toe with the first two fingers and thumb of the right hand. The left arm hangs down with the palm facing in towards the thigh. Lengthen the spine and expand the chest by applying the bandhas. Gaze at the tip of the nose.

2 Dve
Exhale, engage the left thigh muscles and hold the bandhas to support the posture. Bend forwards slowly towards the left foot. Place the left hand beside the foot, with the fingers spread and the middle finger pointing forwards. The fingertips should be in line with the toes. Reach the chin down to the shin. Maintain balance by grounding the left foot, pressing the left hand into the floor, and engaging uddīyana- and mūla-bandha. Draw in uddīyana-bandha and flex the right foot, so that the right heel can lift up and press into the abdomen, towards the navel. This massages the intestines and stimulates the digestive system. When performing this āsana on the left side, the liver is massaged and stimulated. This is the state of the āsana on the right side. Breathe here five times. Gaze at the tip of the nose.

3 Trīṇi
Inhale and straighten the left arm as you raise the head and upper body. Keep the left palm flat on the floor and the leg straight. Stay here for a full exhalation. Gaze at the tip of the nose.

4 Catvāri
Inhale and activate the left thigh muscles while engaging the bandhas to strengthen the hips and lower back, and slowly come up to standing. The left arm stays down by the side as you straighten the spine, open the chest and gaze at the tip of the nose.

5 Pañca
Exhale, release the big toe, straighten out the right leg and stand with the legs together. Release the right arm down to the side and gaze at the tip of the nose.

Left side. Repeat vinyāsas 1–4 on the left side, counting them as vinyāsas 6–9.

Samasthitiḥ
After the 9th vinyāsa, while exhaling lower the left foot and place it beside the right foot, both arms down along your sides, and gaze at the tip of the nose.

Beginners: To be able to bring the foot up into half-lotus can take time, as rarely does one start out with such naturally flexible hips. Work towards the pose slowly and gently.

- If you are unable to reach the big toe in the bound position of the 1st vinyāsa, hold the right ankle with the right hand. Keep the left arm down by the side.
- In the 2nd vinyāsa, fold forwards as far as it feels comfortable or place both hands on the floor on either side of the foot.
- If you have recently had knee surgery, or have some other kind of physical limitation, be sure to speak with a qualified teacher.
- If you cannot bend forwards with a straight leg, keep the knee slightly bent.

Note:
There are two breaths in the 3rd and 8th vinyāsas.

Vinyāsa	Prāṇa (breath)	Āsana (posture)	Dṛṣṭi (gazing point)	Bandha (muscle lock)
Samasthitiḥ		stand straight		
1 Ekam	in	right leg up into half-lotus, bind the right toe		
2 Dve	out	bend forward, the left hand on the floor		
state of the āsana on the right side, hold for 5 deep breaths				
3 Trīṇi	in & out	stretch out, head up, hold the pose		
4 Catvāri	in	come up to standing		
5 Pañca	out	release right toe, straighten right leg		
6 Ṣaṭ	in	left leg into half-lotus, bind left toe		
7 Sapta	out	bend forward, the right hand on the floor		
state of the āsana on the left side, hold for 5 deep breaths				
8 Aṣṭau	in & out	stretch out, head up, hold the pose		
9 Nava	in	come up to standing		
Samasthitiḥ	out	undo the left leg, return to Samasthitiḥ		

Utkaṭāsana

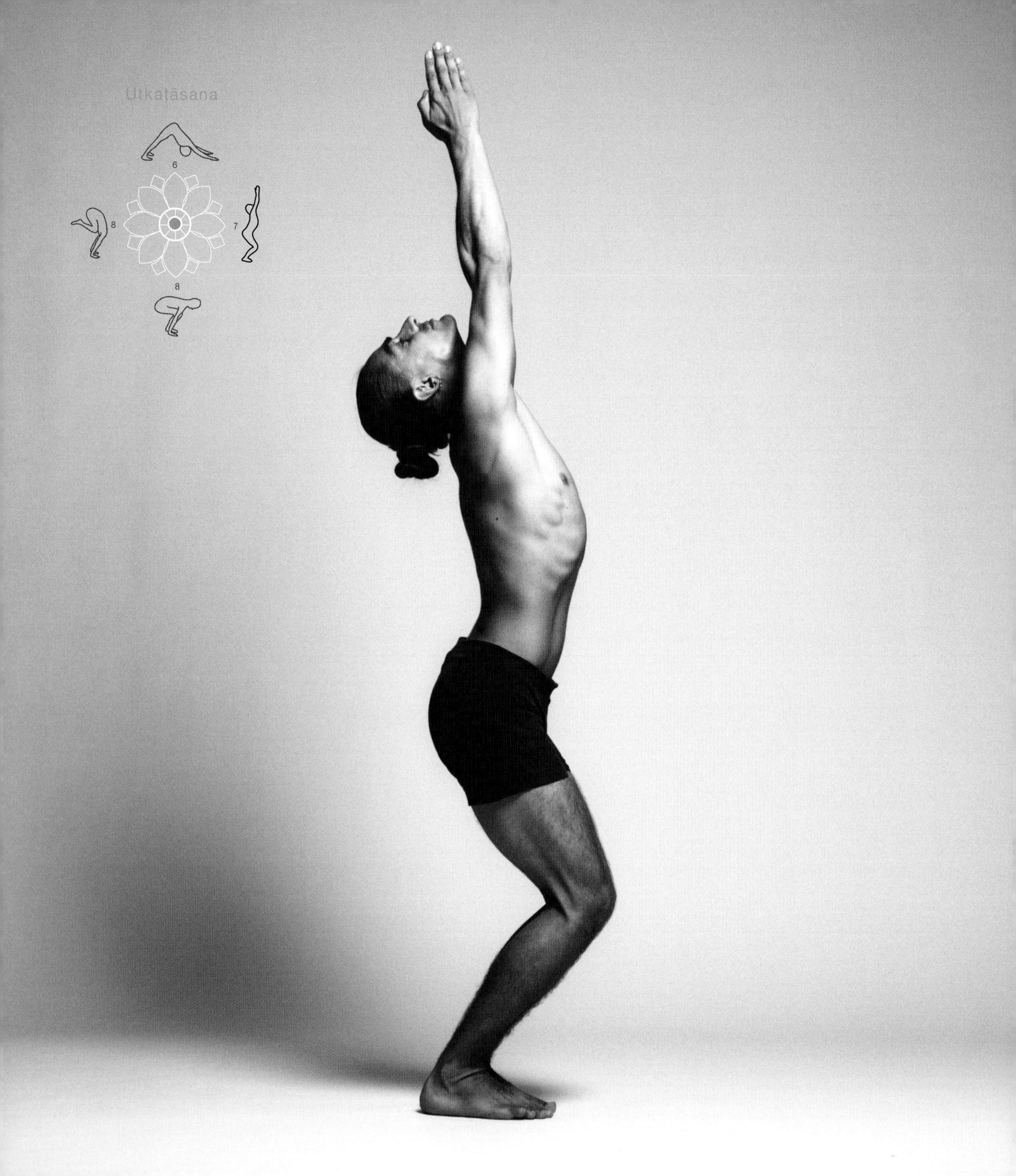

Utkaṭāsana [uneven pose]

13 vinyāsas

Utkaṭa – deep, strong, intense, fierce, uneven; *āsana* – seat, posture

Samasthitiḥ – Stand straight with the feet together, arms by the sides, and gaze at the tip of the nose.

Vinyāsas 1–6 are the same as in *Sūrya-namaskāra A*.

7 Sapta
Inhale, lift the head, lengthen the back of the neck, and look between the hands. Bend the knees and jump softly between the hands, using your arms to support the jump. Keep the legs bent after landing. Lower the hips as much as possible, keeping the heels on the ground with the feet and knees pressing together and the spine extended upright. Lift the arms up, and follow the arms with the head, letting the head tilt backwards on the neck muscles (trapezius and sternocleidomastoid muscles). Use the same inhalation to widen the chest and back, and press the palms and fingers together overhead. Relax through the trapezius muscles, lengthening in the shoulders and drawing the hands up towards the ceiling. Engage mūla-bandha to strengthen the hips. Pull in uddīyana-bandha to open the chest, lengthen the spine and protect the lower back. This is the state of the āsana, and it is held for five breaths. Look straight up, but don't focus on the ceiling.

8 Aṣṭau
Inhale, lower the arms to the floor (this can also be done in between the last exhalation of the 7th vinyāsa and the first inhalation of the 8th vinyāsa). The knees remain bent as you open the arms shoulder-width apart. Focus the gaze for a moment towards the floor and bend the upper body forwards. Lower the arms in front of you, and press the hands down onto the floor next to the feet, keeping the fingers firm and spread wide. Lean forwards on the arms, draw in the bandhas to support the posture, bend the knees and lift the feet about five to ten inches into the air. Don't bring the arms into the legs as in Bakāsana, and do not straighten the legs or lift the body too high up over the arms. This is not a handstand. Gaze at the tip of the nose.

9 Nava
Exhale, straighten the legs back through the air and land in Catvāri position, the 4th vinyāsa in Sūrya-namaskāra A.

Vinyāsas 10 and 11 are the same as the 5th and 6th vinyāsas in Sūrya-namaskāra A.

After the 11th vinyāsa, move directly to the next āsana, the 7th vinyāsa in Vīrabhadrāsana A.

Beginners: Though Utkaṭāsana may look easy, it is a pose that can always be deepened, making it more challenging than it appears.
- In the 7th vinyāsa, which is the state of the Utkaṭāsana, instead of straightening and stretching the arms directly over the head, stretch through the shoulders and try to bring the elbows towards each other. Lift the hands slowly towards the ceiling.
- Do not press, pull or squeeze the head back by tensing the back of the neck. Instead allow the head to relax back, supporting the position with the neck muscles.
- It takes a fair amount of practice before one can lift the body up off the floor in the 8th vinyāsa. Press the hands into the floor, move the weight into the hands, slowly lift the body upwards and lightly spring up and back. Straighten out the legs and come down into Catvāri position on the exhalation.

Vinyāsa	Prāṇa (breath)	Āsana (posture)	Dṛṣṭi (gazing point)	Bandha (muscle lock)
Samasthitiḥ		stand straight	Y	●
Vinyāsas 1–6 according to Sūrya-namaskāra A				
7 Sapta	in	jump forwards, knees bent, lift the arms	Y	●
state of the asana; hold for 5 deep breaths				
8 Aṣṭau	in	hands to floor, lift up	Y	●
9 Nava	out	catvāri position	Y	●
10 Daśa	in	upward-facing dog	Y	●
11 Ekādaśa	out	downward-facing dog	Y	●
12 Dvādaśa	in	jump forwards, head up	Y	●
13 Trayodaśa	out	bend forwards	Y	●
Samasthitiḥ	in	come up, stand straight	Y	●

Vīrabhadrāsana A & B [warrior pose A & B]

16 vinyāsas

Vīra – warrior; *bhadra* - good, blessed, also goddess of the hunt (*Bhadra*); *āsana* – seat, posture

Vīrabhadrāsana continues after the 11th vinyāsa in Utkaṭāsana.

Note:
Vinyāsas 8–10 have reverse breathing patterns in comparison to the other standing positions. At the end of the 8th and 10th vinyāsas, it is also possible to come to standing with an inhalation, then move to the other side with an exhalation.

7 Sapta, Vīrabhadrāsana A
Inhale, turn the left foot 90 degrees out so the heel faces the right foot. Take a long step forwards with the right foot, placing the foot in between the hands. Keep the left foot firmly on the floor. Bend the right knee just over 90 degrees, in line with the right foot. (If you look at the āsana from the side, the tip of the right knee is in line with the middle part of the right foot, making the angle slightly over 90 degrees). Lift the arms up overhead, bringing the palms and fingers together and tilt the head back. Stretch the arms, straighten the elbows and lift the hands towards the ceiling. Turn the hips and chest to face forwards towards the right leg. Engage the thigh of the left leg. Press both feet into the floor and draw in mūla-bandha, deeply engaging the pelvic floor, and uddīyana-bandha to lengthen the spine and lift the chest upwards. This is the state of the āsana on the right side of Vīrabhadrāsana A. Breathe deeply five times. After the fifth exhalation, inhale once and stay in the same position. Direct the gaze straight up.

8 Aṣṭau
Exhale, release the head, straighten the right leg and turn the right foot forwards. Keeping the left heel on the floor, turn the left foot 90 degrees out to the left, so that you are now facing towards the back of the room. The hands remain in the same position as in the 7th vinyāsa. Bend the left knee just over 90 degrees, keeping the knee in line with the left foot, and tilt the head back. This is the same position as in the previous vinyāsa, but now you are facing in the opposite direction. This is the state of Vīrabhadrāsana A on the left side. Hold the pose, gaze upwards and breathe deeply five times. The last breath here is the fifth exhalation.

9 Nava, Vīrabhadrāsana B
Inhale, lower the arms to shoulder-level with the palms facing down. Extend the arms out from the shoulders in a horizontal line over the legs. Turn the chin towards the left shoulder and direct the gaze over the fingertips of the left hand. Open the hips and the chest out to the side of the mat and relax the shoulders. Press both feet into the floor, draw in mūla-bandha and engage uddīyana-bandha, as in the 7th vinyāsa. This is the state of the āsana on the left side of Vīrabhadrāsana B. Gaze at the fingertips of the left hand, hold the pose and breathe five times. After the fifth exhalation, inhale once and stay in the same position.

10 Daśa
Exhale, straighten the left leg and turn the foot to face the side of the mat. Keep the arms and hands as they were in the 9th vinyāsa. Turn the right foot out to the right, so that the toes face the front of the mat. The toes of the left foot remain facing the side of the mat. Bend the right knee just over 90 degrees, keeping the knee in line with the right foot. This is the same position as in the previous vinyāsa, except that it is now done on the right side. Gaze at the fingertips of the right hand, hold the pose and breathe deeply five times. The last breath here is an exhalation.

11 Ekādaśa
Inhale and lower the arms onto the floor. This can also be done during the gap between the last exhalation of the 10th vinyāsa and the next inhalation of the 11th vinyāsa. Reach the left hand forwards to meet the right hand, and place both hands on the floor on either side of the right foot. Spread the fingers wide, keeping the middle finger pointing directly forwards. Using the strength of the arms, lean into them, draw in the bandhas and lift the body up. The arms can be straight or bent. Keep the legs in the same position as they were before the lift: the left leg is straight and the right is bent. Avoid straightening the right leg. Balance in the posture for a moment and gaze at the tip of the nose.

12 Dvādaśa
Exhale, straighten the right leg in the air and land both legs at the same time into Catvāri position. Take the chin forwards and gaze at the tip of the nose.

Vinyāsas 13 and 14 are the same as in the 5th and 6th vinyāsas in Sūrya-namaskāra A. After vinyāsa 14, go directly to the 7th vinyāsa in Paścima-tānāsana A.

Beginners: Although the Vīrabhadrāsana sequence may look like a simple series of movements, it demands particular attention to the positioning of the hips, chest and hands, as well as the correct breathing in each vinyāsa.

- In Vīrabhadrāsana A, turn the chest and the hips forwards to face the front leg. Stretch the arms out, and straighten the elbows completely. Do not press the head back by tensing the neck muscles; instead, relax in this position and lean the head back.
- When moving from the right side to the left in the A pose, you can bring the head up and check that the legs, hips and upper body are properly aligned for the left side.
- In Vīrabhadrāsana B, open both the chest and the hips out to the side, and extend the arms and back leg. Engage mūla-bandha and relax the shoulders, more specifically the trapezius muscles, while engaging through the deltoid muscles.
- It takes practice to be able to lift the body up in the 11th vinyāsa. Press the hands firmly into the floor and strengthen the arms. Lightly jump up while inhaling, with the right leg bent. Straighten out the leg and come down into Catvāri position while exhaling, as described in the 12th vinyāsa.

Vinyāsa	Prāṇa (breath)	Āsana (posture)	Dṛṣṭi (gazing point)	Bandha (muscle lock)
Samasthitiḥ		stand straight		
Vinyāsas 1–6 according to Sūrya-namaskāra A				
7 Sapta	in	warrior A pose, right side		
state of the āsana on the right side, hold for 5 deep breaths plus an extra inhale				
8 Aṣṭau	out	warrior A pose, left side		
state of the āsana on the left side, hold for 5 deep breaths				
9 Nava	in	lower the arms to warrior B pose, left side		
state of the āsana on the left side, hold for 5 deep breaths plus an extra inhale				
10 Daśa	out	warrior B pose, right side		
state of the asana; hold for 5 deep breaths				
11 Ekādaśa	in	hands to the floor, lift up		
12 Dvādaśa	out	catvāri position		
13 Trayodaśa	in	upward-facing dog		
14 Caturdaśa	out	downward-facing dog		
15 Pañcadaśa	in	hop forwards, stretch spine, head up		
16 Ṣoḍaśa	out	bend forwards		
Samasthitiḥ	in	come up, stand straight		

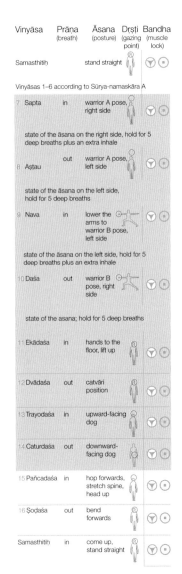

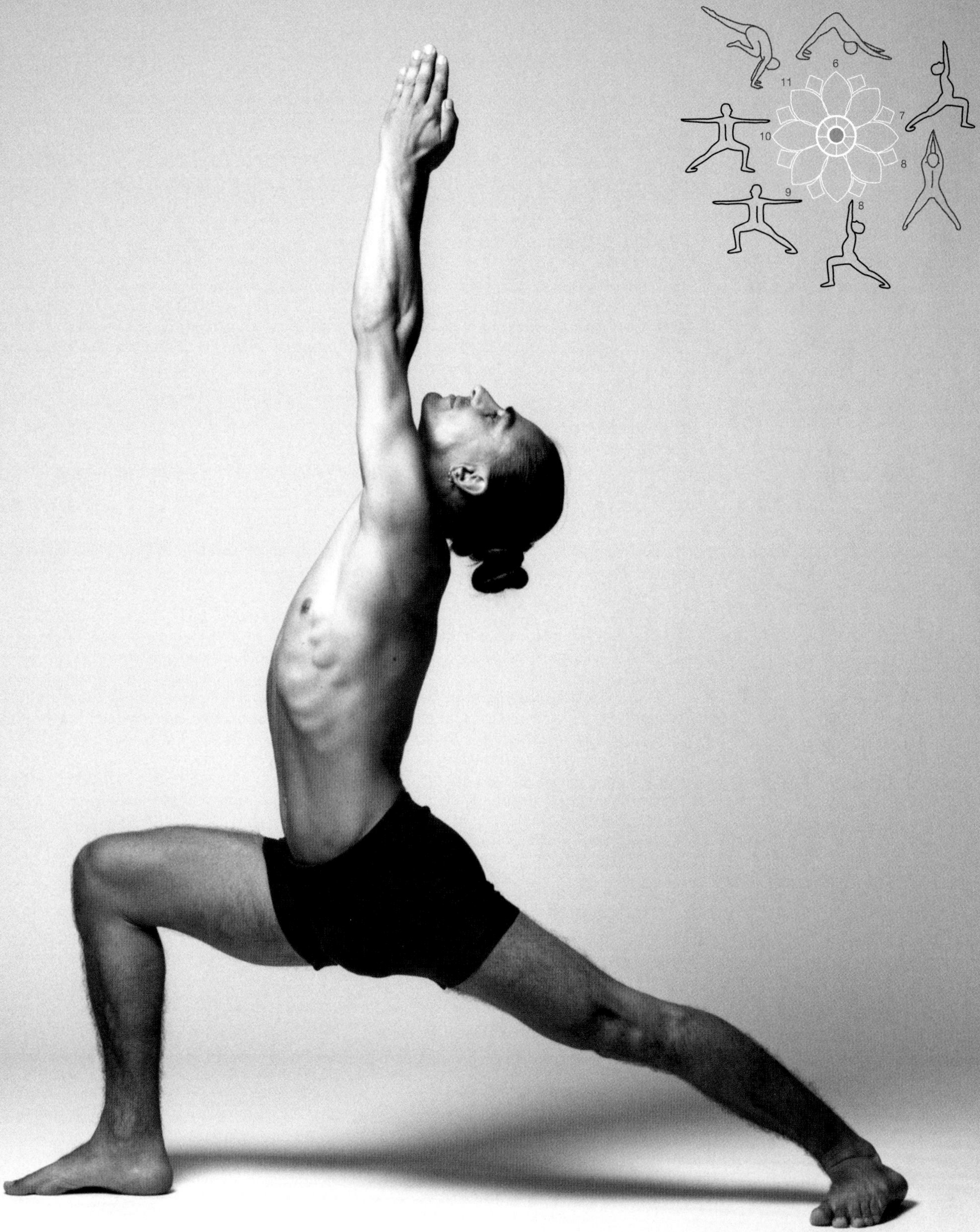
6
7
8
8
9
10
11

Paścima-tānāsana A, B & C [back stretching pose; forward bending pose]

13 vinyāsas

Paścima – western, backside; *ut* – deep, strong, intense; *tāna* – stretch, extend, lengthen; *āsana* – seat, posture.

Paścima-tānāsana A comes directly after the 14th vinyāsa in *Vīrabhadrāsana B*.

Note:
There are two breaths in the 10th vinyāsa.

7 Sapta
Inhale, engage mula- and uddīyana-bandha, press the hands firmly into the floor, straighten and activate the arms and shoulders. Bend the knees and jump through (see p. 62) to sit down without touching the feet to the floor. Sit up with the arms and back straight, and press the palms or fingertips into the mat beside the hips. Expand and lengthen the chest and spine, while tucking the chin in. Straighten the legs and flex the feet, keeping the heels on the floor. Before moving into Paścima-tānāsana A, stay here and breathe five times. Gaze at the tip of the nose.

8 Aṣṭau
Inhale, bend forwards from the hips, and take hold of the big toes with the first two fingers and thumb. This can also be done in between the last exhalation of the 7th vinyāsa and the first inhalation of the 8th vinyāsa. Straighten the arms; engage the bandhas to support the expansion in the chest and spine, and to keep the hips grounded. Lift the head up and gaze at the tip of the nose.

9 Nava
Exhale and fold forwards from the hips with straight legs. Lift and pull in uddīyana-bandha, creating space for the upper body to fold forwards onto the thighs. Release the back of the neck and place the chin to the knees or in between the shins. Relax the hamstrings and engage the front thighs, so that the legs remain straight. This is the state of the āsana. Breathe here five times. Gaze at the toes.

10 Daśa
Inhale, and while still firmly holding onto the toes, open the chest and lift the head up, straightening the spine and arms. Take an exhalation here. Gaze at the tip of the nose.

Note: From here, after the 10th vinyāsa in Paścima-tānāsana A, return to the 8th vinyāsa, and repeat vinyāsas 8–10, changing the position of the hands, as described below. Repeat this vinyāsa sequence again after the 10th vinyāsa in Paścima-tānāsana B. After Paścima-tānāsana C, continue on to the 11th vinyāsa.

In Paścima-tānāsana B, bind the hands by taking hold of the outside edges of the feet. Pull the feet back, slightly pressing the thumbs into the root of the big toes. In Paścima-tānāsana C, extend the arms beyond the feet and bind one hand with the wrist of the other, gently making a fist with the free hand.

11 Ekādaśa
Inhale slowly, place the hands on the floor beside the hips, cross the feet in the air and draw the knees into the chest. Continue with the inhalation as you engage the bandhas and lengthen in the shoulders by straightening out the arms. Press the hands into the floor. Lean the weight into the arms and lift the whole body off the floor. Lift the hips up high enough so that the feet can pass through the arms without touching the floor. Gaze at the tip of the nose.

12 Dvādaśa
With the legs lifted up and in between the arms, begin exhaling and straighten the legs back, landing in Catvāri position. Look at the tip of the nose.

Vinyāsas 13 and 14 are the same as the 5th and 6th vinyāsas in Sūrya-namaskāra A. After the 14th vinyāsa in Paścima-tānāsana C, go directly to the next āsana, the 7th vinyāsa in Pūrvatānāsana.

Beginners: Paścima-tānāsana is the foundation for the forward-bending āsanas.

- The most demanding āsana in this sequence, Paścima-tānāsana C, can be quite challenging in the beginning. If you can't bind the wrist beyond the feet, cross the fingers or reach as far as you can and go a bit further beyond the previous āsana, Paścima-tānāsana B.
- Press the backs of the knees down and straighten the legs; focus on stretching through the hips and lower back as you release the hamstrings. If you cannot touch the feet with straight legs, bend the knees slightly. This should ease the effort needed for the forward bending and binding.
- In the 9th vinyāsa, place the forehead, face or chin towards the knees or shins and gaze at the tip of the nose.

Vinyāsa	Prāṇa (breath)	Āsana (posture)	Dṛṣṭi (gazing point)	Bandha (muscle lock)
Samasthitiḥ		stand straight		
Vinyāsas 1–6 according to Sūrya-namaskāra A				
7 Ṣaṭ	in	jump through to sit, straighten back, hands to floor		
state for sitting āsana; hold for 5 deep breaths				
8 Aṣṭau	in	take toes (A), feet (B) or wrist (C), straighten back, head up		
9 Nava	out	bend forwards		
state of the asana for Paścima-tānāsana A, B, & C; hold for 5 deep breaths				
10 Daśa	in & out	stretch out, head up, hold position		
repeat 8, 9, and 10 for Paścima-tānāsana B & C				
11 Ekādaśa	in	hands to floor, lift up		
12 Dvādaśa	out	catvāri position		
13 Trayodaśa	in	upward-facing dog		
14 Caturdaśa	out	downward-facing dog		
15 Pañcadaśa	in	jump forwards, stretch spine, head up		
16 Ṣoḍaśa	out	bend forwards		
Samasthitiḥ	in	come up, stand straight		

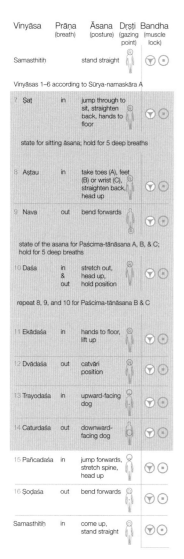

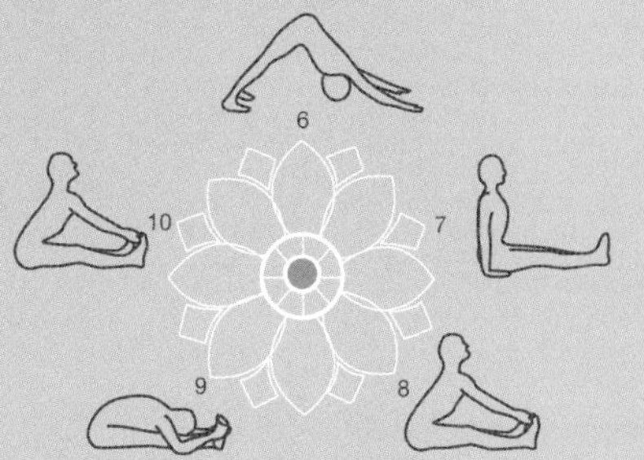

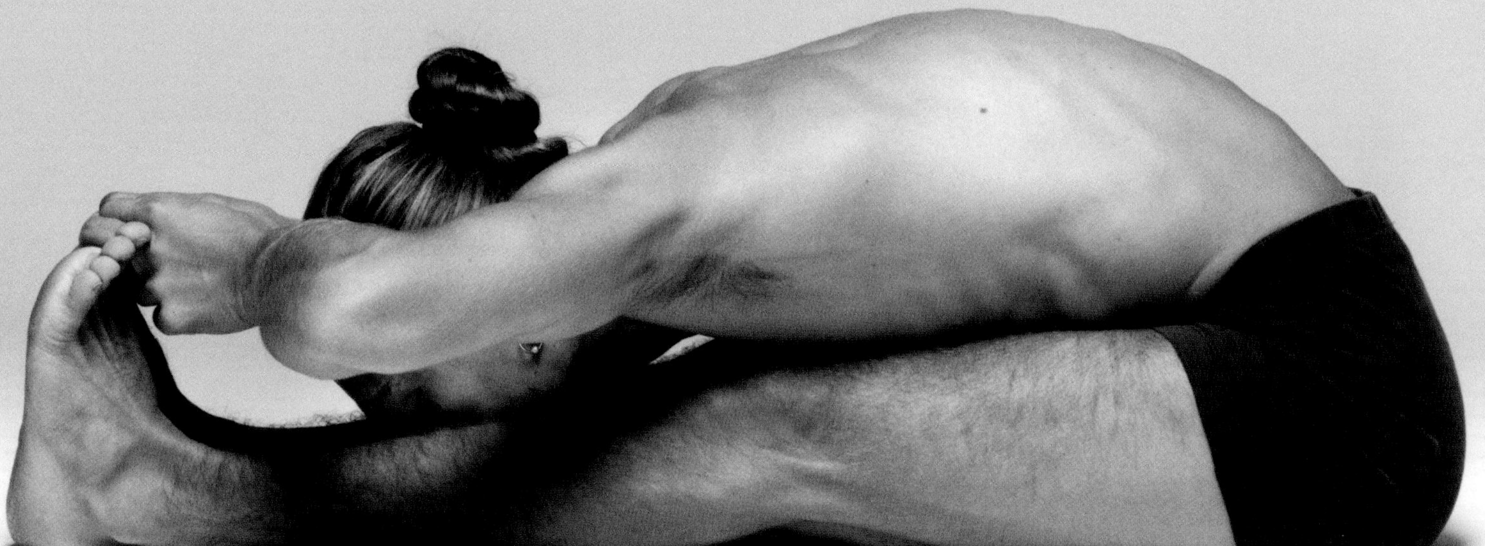

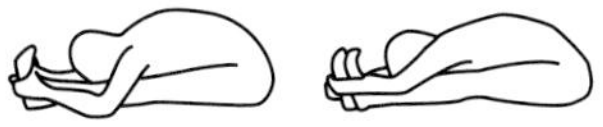

The 9th vinyāsa in
Paścima-tānāsana B & C

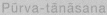

Pūrva-tānāsana

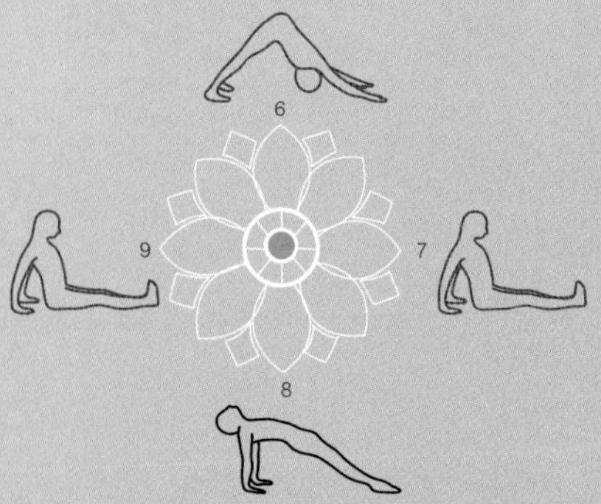

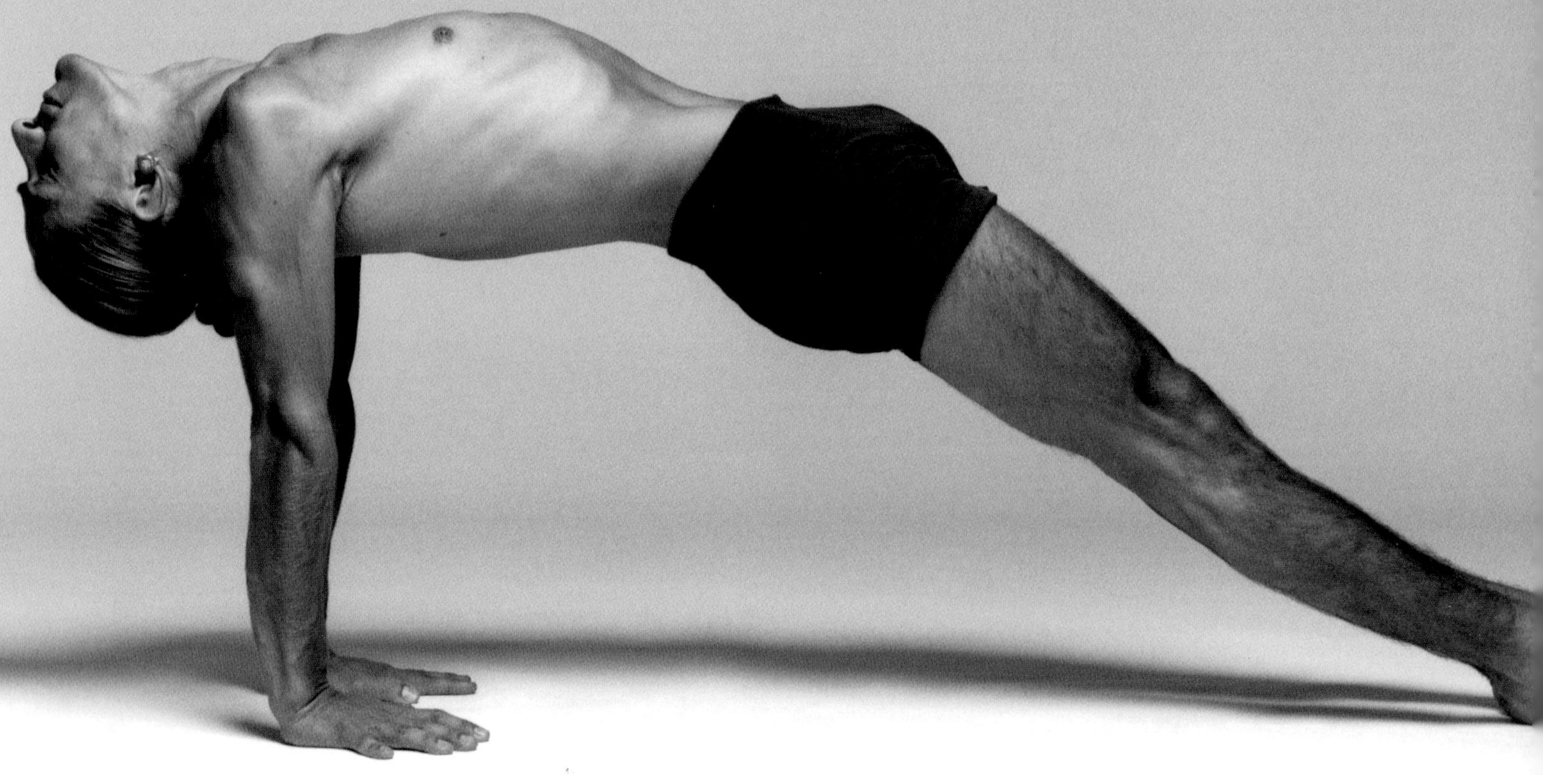

Pūrva-tānāsana [front stretching pose]

15 vinyāsas

Pūrva – eastern, frontside; *ut* – deep, strong, intense; *tāna* – stretch, extend, lengthen; *āsana* – seat, posture.

Pūrva-tānāsana follows immediately after the 14th vinyāsa in Paścima-tānāsana C.

7 Sapta
Inhale, bend the knees and jump through the arms to sitting, keeping your feet lifted. Exhale and place the hands on the floor about a foot behind the hips, with fingertips pointing towards the hips. Straighten the legs and press the feet together. Gaze at the tip of the nose.

8 Aṣṭau
Inhale and keeping the legs straight engage the thigh muscles, point the feet and lift the hips up off the floor. Bring the soles of the feet down to the ground with the heels and big toes together. Support the hips by engaging mūla-bandha. Be sure to maintain uddīyana-bandha as well, as this will be of great assistance and is an often-forgotten detail. Uddīyana-bandha will open the chest and support the lower back. Draw the shoulders back and down, relax the back of the neck and tilt the head back. This is the state of the āsana. Breathe deeply five times. Gaze at the tip of the nose.

9 Nava
Exhale, lower the hips slowly and straighten the back of the neck. Gaze at the tip of the nose.

Vinyāsas 10 and 11 are the same as the 11th and 12th vinyāsas in Paścima-tānāsana.

Vinyāsas 12 and 13 are the same as in the 5th and 6th vinyāsas in Sūrya-namaskāra A.

After the 13th vinyāsa in Pūrva-tānāsana, go directly to the next āsana, the 7th vinyāsa in Ardha-baddha-padma-paścima-tānāsana.

Beginners: It takes some practice to be able to keep the feet and toes together while pressing them down to the floor.

- Keep the legs straight and the feet together while pressing the toes into the floor. Actively engage the inner thighs; this will help keep your legs and feet together.

Note:
There are two breaths in the 7th vinyāsa

Vinyāsa	Prāṇa (breath)	Āsana (posture)	Dṛṣṭi (gazing point)	Bandha (muscle lock)
Samasthitiḥ		stand straight		
Vinyāsas 1–6 according to Sūrya-namaskāra A				
7 Sapta	in & out	jump through to sit down, place hands on the floor behind the back		
8 Aṣṭa	in	hips up, head back, feet to floor		
state of the āsana, hold for 5 deep breaths				
9 Nava	out	lower hips		
10 Daśa	in	hands to floor, lift up		
11 Ekādaśa	out	catvāri position		
12 Dvādaśa	in	upward-facing dog		
13 Trayodaśa	out	downward-facing dog		
14 Caturdaśa	in	jump forward, stretch spine, head up		
15 Pañcadaśa	out	bend forwards		
Samasthitiḥ	in	come up, stand straight		

Ardha-baddha-padma-paścima-tānāsana

[half bound lotus sitting forward bend pose]

22 vinyāsas

Note:
There are two breaths in the 9th and 16th vinyāsas.

Vinyāsa	Prāṇa (breath)	Āsana (posture)	Dṛṣṭi (gazing point)	Bandha (muscle lock)
Samasthitiḥ		stand straight		
Vinyāsas 1–6 according to Sūrya-namaskāra A				
7 Sapta	in	jump through to sit, right leg into half-lotus, head up		
8 Aṣṭau	out	bend forward		
state of the āsana on the right side, hold for 5 deep breaths				
9 Nava	in & out	stretch out, head up, hold the pose		
10 Daśa	in	hands to floor, lift up		
11 Ekādaśa	out	catvāri position		
12 Dvādaśa	in	upward-facing dog		
13 Trayodaśa	out	downward-facing dog		
14 Caturdaśa	in	jump through to sit, left leg into half-lotus, head up		
15 Pañcadaśa	out	bend forwards		
state of the āsana on the left side, hold for 5 deep breaths				
16 Ṣoḍaśa	in & out	stretch out, head up, hold the pose		
17 Saptadaśa	in	hands to floor		
18 Aṣṭadaśa	out	catvāri position		
19 Ekona-viṃśatiḥ	in	upward-facing dog		
20 Viṃśatiḥ	out	downward-facing dog		
21 Ekaviṃśatiḥ	in	jump forwards, stretch spine, head up		
22 Dvaviṃśatiḥ	out	bend forwards		
Samasthitiḥ	in	come up, stand straight		

Ardha – half; *baddha* – bound; *padma* – lotus; *paścima* – western, backside; *ut* – deep, strong, intense; *tāna* – stretch, extend, lengthen; *āsana* – seat, posture

Ardha-baddha-padma-paścima-tānāsana comes right after the 13th vinyāsa in Pūrva-tānāsana.

7 Sapta
Inhale, jump through the arms to sit down, keeping the feet lifted off the ground. Lift the right foot up towards the left inner thigh and take hold of the foot. Using your hands, turn the sole of the foot up and place the outside of the foot into the groin. The heel should point towards the left side of the navel. Relax the right hip and lower the knee towards the floor about 45 degrees away from the body. Be careful not to strain the knee. You should not experience any pain in the knee joint. Wrap the right arm around the back and take hold of the right big toe with the first two fingers and thumb. Reach forwards with your left hand and take hold of the outside edge of the left foot. Open the chest, straighten the spine and the left arm. Pull back slightly on the foot, extending in the opposite direction to the upwards stretch. Engage the bandhas to keep the hips down while supporting the back and chest. Lift the head, gaze at the tip of the nose.

8 Aṣṭau
Exhale and fold forwards onto the left leg, bringing the chin to the shin. Strongly engage the uḍḍīyana-bandha and flex the right foot so there is space for the right heel to press securely into the abdomen. In this position, the heel massages the intestines and stimulates the digestive system. When this āsana is performed on the left side, the liver is massaged and stimulated. Mūla-bandha keeps the hips grounded and is a counter-action to the forwards stretch. Keeping a firm grip on the right big toe, straighten the left knee, and pull back slightly with the hand on the left foot. This is the state of the āsana on the right side. Stay here and breathe deeply five times. Focus the gaze on the left big toe.

9 Nava
Inhale, open the chest and fully lengthen the spine. Straighten out the left arm and draw the left foot back slightly. Lift the head, gaze at the tip of the nose and stay here for an exhalation.

10 Daśa
Inhale, cross the feet in the air and pull the knees in towards the chest. Follow through with the jump-back, as described in the 11th vinyāsa of the Paścima-tānāsana sequence. Another technique is to inhale, keep the right leg in half-lotus while bending and lifting the left knee towards the chest, keeping the foot in the air. With the legs in this position, press the hands down into the floor on either side of the body. Lift the hips up and move the legs back through the arms. Gaze at the tip of the nose.

Vinyāsa 11 is the same as the 12th vinyāsa in Paścima-tānāsana.

Repeat vinyāsas 7-11 on the left side, counting them as vinyāsas 14–18.

Vinyāsas 12 and 13 are the same as the 5th and 6th vinyāsas in Sūrya-namaskāra A.

Vinyāsa 15 is the state of the āsana on the left side. Breathe deeply five times.

Vinyāsas 19 and 20 are the same as the 5th and 6th vinyāsas in Sūrya-namaskāra A. After vinyāsa 20, go directly to the next āsana, the 7th vinyāsa in Tiryaṅ-mukhaikapāda-paścima-tānāsana.

Beginners: It can take some time before you can bring the leg into a comfortable half-lotus with the knee turned out to 45 degrees and resting on the floor.

- Do not use force to press the knee down to the floor. Keep releasing the hip instead, which relieves the pressure in the knee joint.
- If you cannot reach the toe with your arm wrapped around your back, bring both hands forwards and take hold of the ankle or foot of the straight leg.
- Avoid pulling the foot (in half-lotus) onto the front or outer thigh (of the straight leg) as this rotation strains the knee and is of no long-term benefit. Try to keep it on the inner thigh.
- If more than one inhalation is needed to get into the position of the 7th and 14th vinyāsas, calmly breathe out and in again until you have come as far into the posture as you can. Do try, however, to minimize the extra number of breaths you take.
- If you have had knee surgery recently, or have other physical limitations, speak with a qualified teacher before doing this āsana.
- If you cannot bend forwards with a straight leg, keep the knee slightly bent.

Ardha-baddha-padma-
paścima-tānāsana

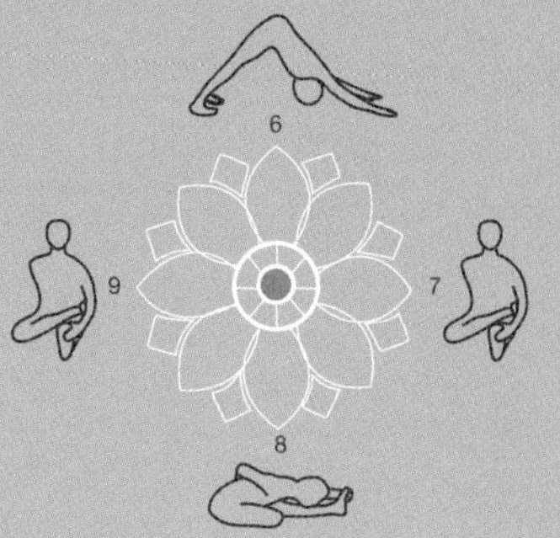

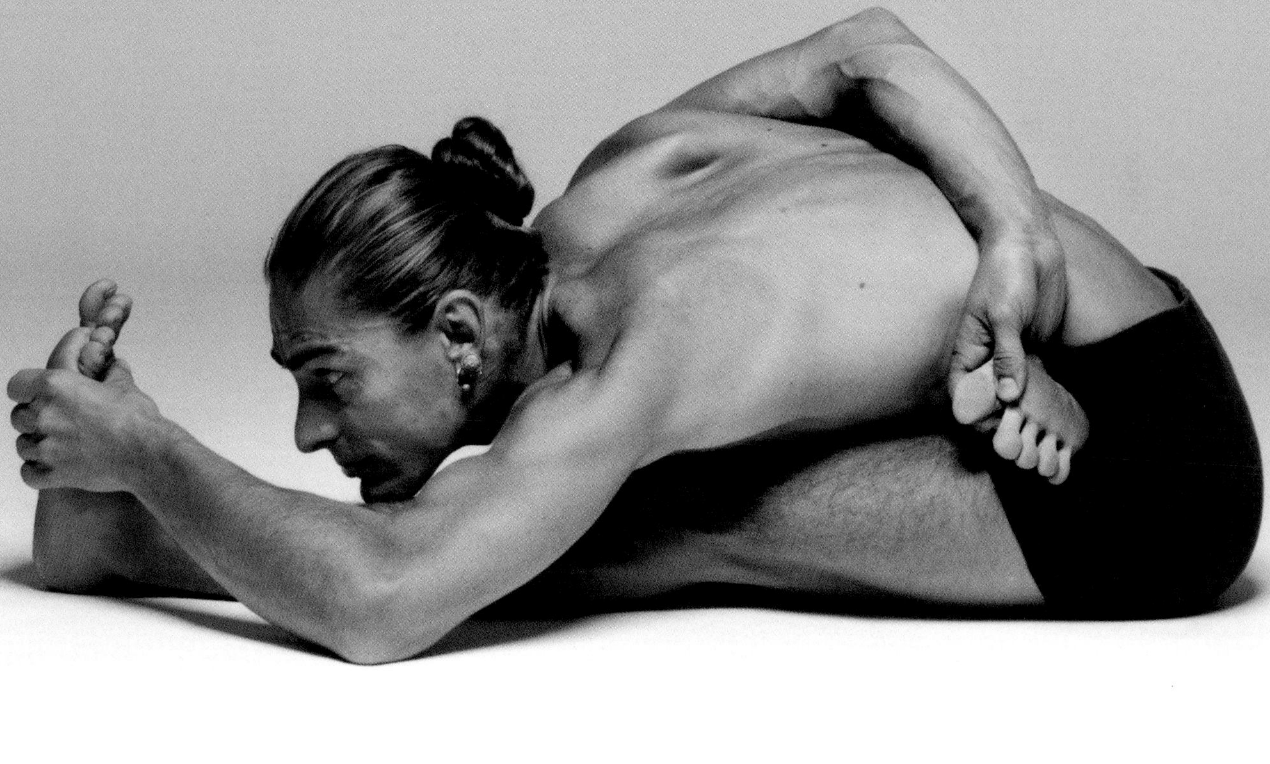

Tiryaṅ-mukhaikapāda-
paścima-tānāsana

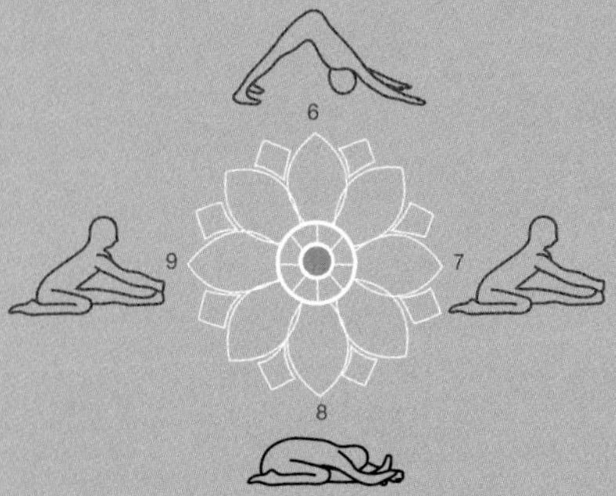

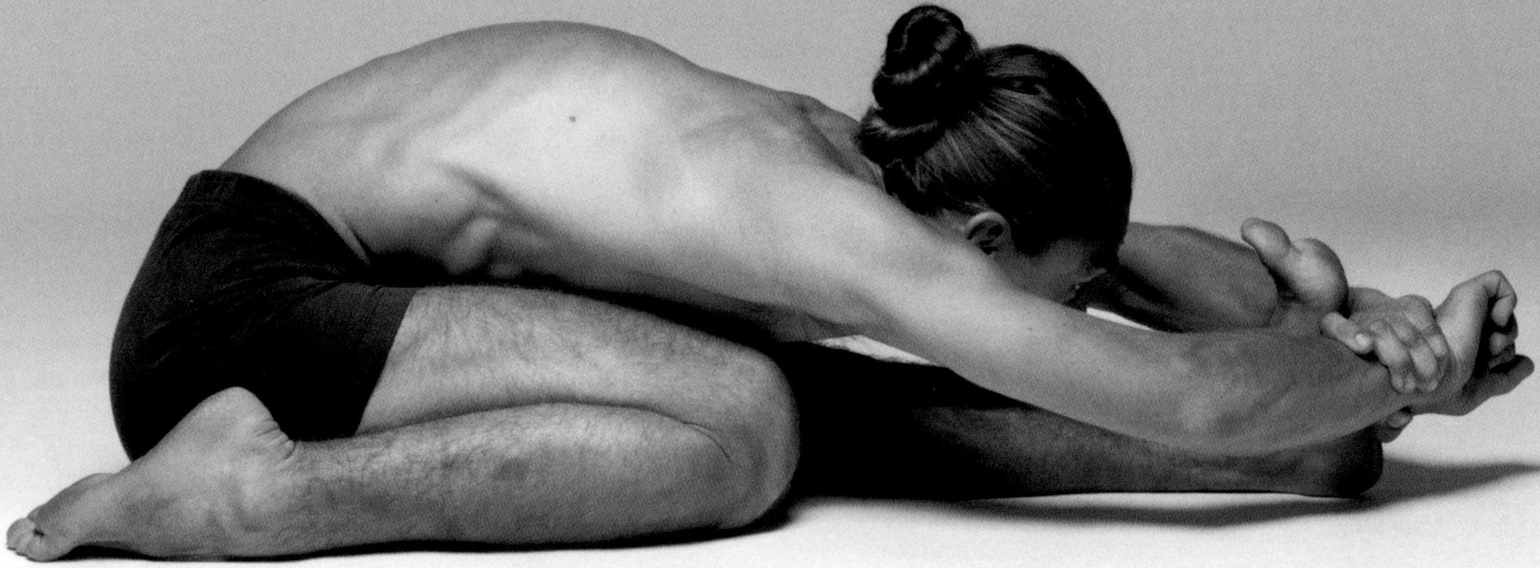

Tiryaṅ-mukhaikapāda-paścima-tānāsana
[one foot facing horizontally back forward bend pose]

22 vinyāsas

Tiryaṅ – horizontal, bent backwards, stretched back; *mukha* – face; *eka* – one; *pāda* – foot; *paścima* – western, backside; *ut* – deep, strong, intense; *tāna* – stretch, extend, lengthen; *āsana* – seat, posture

Tiryaṅ-mukhaikapāda-paścima-tānāsana is done right after the 20th vinyāsa of Ardha-baddha-padma-paścima-tānāsana.

7 Sapta
Inhale and jump through to sitting, as described in the earlier seated āsanas. Bend the right leg back beside the right hip so that the top of the right foot and toes are on the floor and touching the right hip. A second option is to inhale and jump directly into the position, by bending the right shin back and keeping the left leg straight while you jump. Once seated with the right leg back, straighten the left leg and bring the knees together. Continue the inhalation as you reach forwards with both hands to bind the wrist around the left foot. Straighten the spine, press both hips evenly down into the floor, open the chest and lift the head up. Straighten the arms and pull back slightly on the left foot to deepen the stretch. Engage the bandhas to expand the back and chest and to keep the hips grounded. Gaze at the tip of the nose.

8 Aṣṭau
Exhale, keep holding the bandhas and fold forwards over the left leg, placing the chin down to the shin. Press the left knee down and keep the body straight. This is the state of the āsana on the right side. Breathe deeply five times. Gaze at the left big toe.

9 Nava
Inhale, and while still holding the left foot, open the chest, straighten the spine and arms and lift the head up. Hold this position for an exhalation as well. Gaze at the tip of the nose.

10 Daśa
Begin inhaling and release the hands, bringing the right leg forwards and crossing the ankles in the air. Continue on with the jump-back, as described in the 11th vinyāsa in Paścima-tānāsana. Another technique is to inhale, place the palms on the floor beside the hips and leave the right leg where it is. As you continue with the inhalation, lift the whole body up off the floor by pressing the palms down, straightening the arms and engaging the bandhas. Lift the hips up high enough so the left leg can pass through the arms without touching the floor. Gaze at the tip of the nose.

Vinyāsa 11 is the same as the 12th vinyāsa in Paścima-tānāsana.

Repeat vinyāsas 7–11 on the left side, counting them as vinyāsas 14–18.

Vinyāsas 12 and 13 are the same as the 5th and 6th vinyāsas in Sūrya-namaskāra A.

Vinyāsa 15 is the state of the āsana on the left side. Breathe deeply five times.

Vinyāsas 19 and 20 are the same as the 5th and 6th vinyāsas in Sūrya-namaskāra A. After vinyāsa 20, go directly to the next āsana, the 7th vinyāsa in Jānu-śīrṣāsana A.

Beginners: It can take some time to do this āsana proficiently, with the knees together and the hips down.
- Bring the knees together as much as possible, and try to keep both sitting bones down.
- Lean the body slightly inwards, towards the bent knee, keeping the body straight.

Note 1:
According to Pattabhi Jois, this āsana is called Tiryaṅ-mukha-ekapāda paścima-tānāsana (tiryaṅg – horizontal). It is commonly pronounced as Tiryaṅ-mukhaikapāda-paścima-tānāsana, whereas some other traditions go by Triangmukha ekapāda paścima-tānāsana (triang – three limbs).

Note 2:
There are two breaths in the 9th and 16th vinyāsas.

Vinyāsa	Prāṇa (breath)	Āsana (posture)	Dṛṣṭi (gazing point)	Bandha (muscle lock)
Samasthitiḥ		stand straight		
Vinyāsas 1–6 according to Sūrya-namaskāra A				
7 Sapta	in	jump through to sit, bend right leg beside the hip, stretch out, head up		
8 Aṣṭau	out	bend forwards		
state of the āsana on the right side, hold for 5 deep breaths				
9 Nava	in & out	stretch out, head up, hold the pose		
10 Daśa	in	hands to floor, lift up		
11 Ekadaśa	out	catvāri position		
12 Dvādaśa	in	upward-facing dog		
13 Trayodaśa	out	downward-facing dog		
14 Caturdaśa	in	jump through to sit, bend left leg beside hip, stretch spine, head up		
15 Pañcadaśa	out	bend forwards		
state of the āsana on the left side; hold for 5 deep breaths				
16 Ṣoḍaśa	in & out	stretch out, head up, hold the pose		
17 Saptadaśa	in	hands to floor, lift up		
18 Aṣṭadaśa	out	catvāri position		
19 Ekoṇa-viṃśatiḥ	in	upward-facing dog		
20 Viṃśatiḥ	out	downward-facing dog		
21 Eka-viṃśatiḥ	in	jump forwards, stretch spine, head up		
22 Dva-viṃśatiḥ	out	bend forwards		
Samasthitiḥ	in	come up, stand straight		

Jānu-śīrṣāsana A

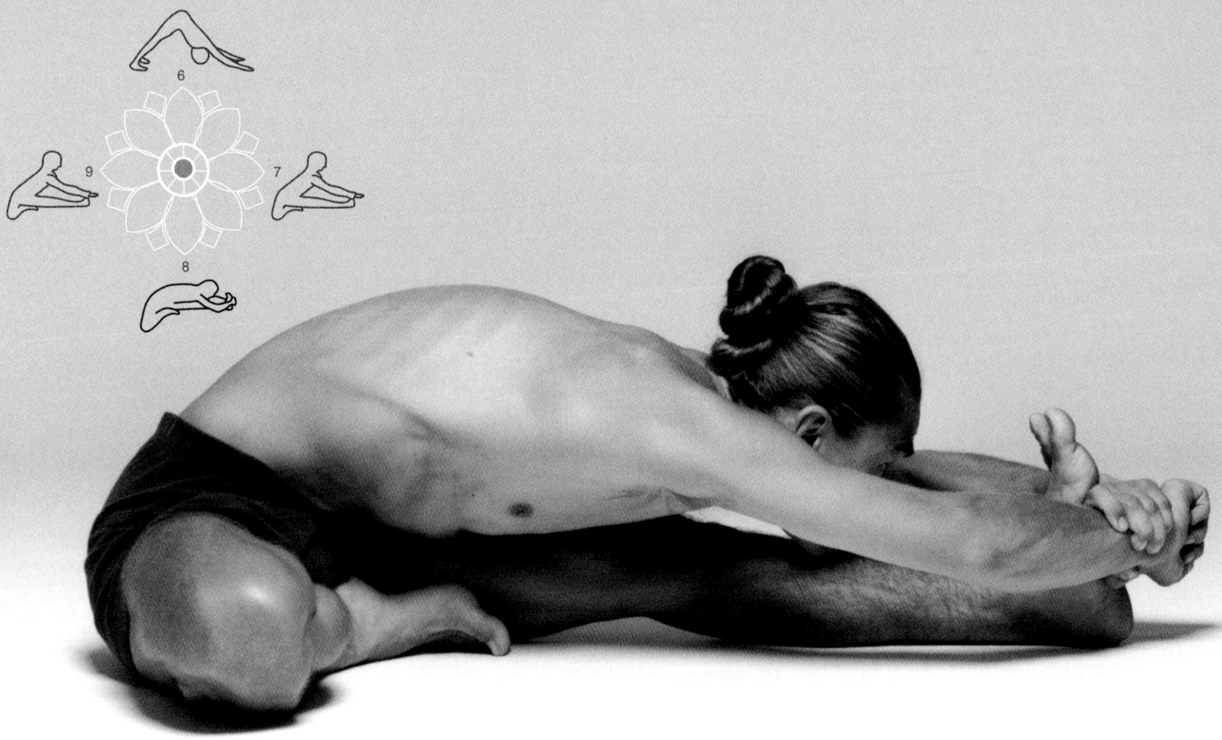

Jānu-śīrṣāsana B

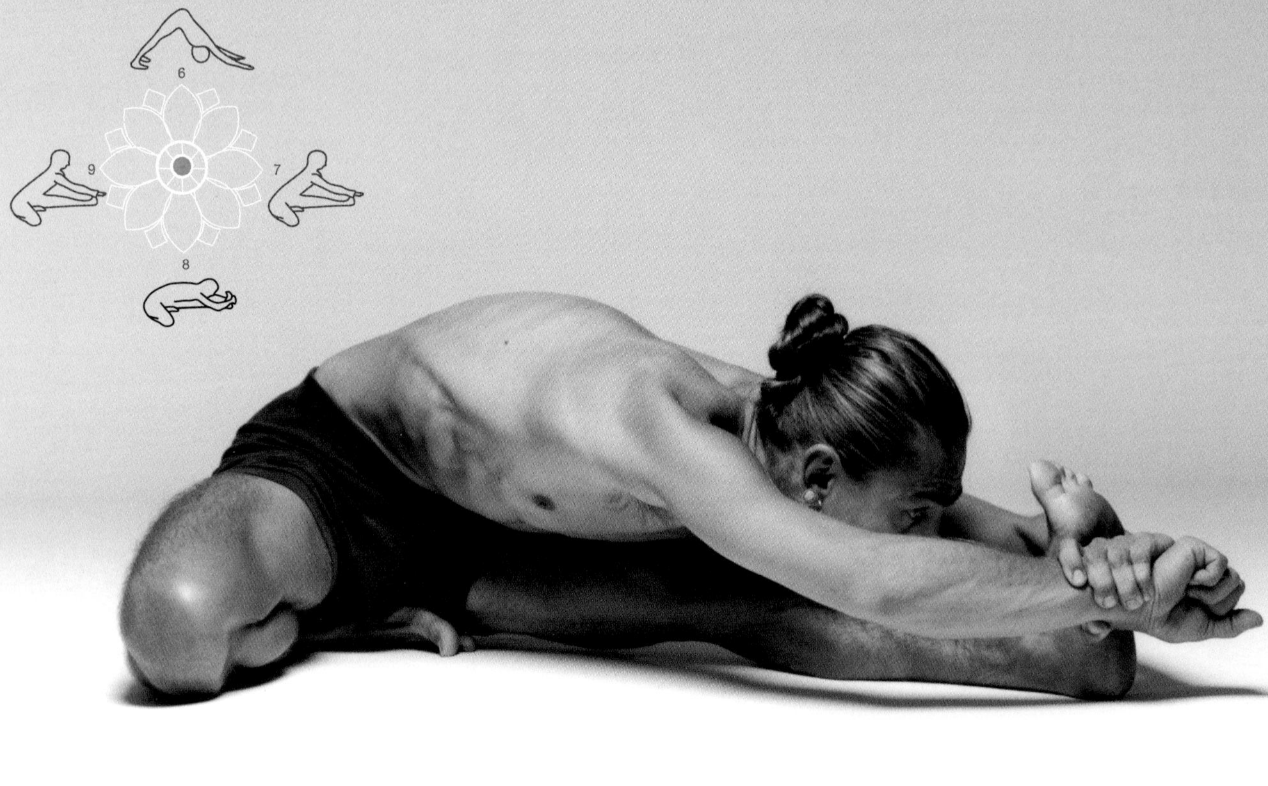

Jānu-śīrṣāsana C

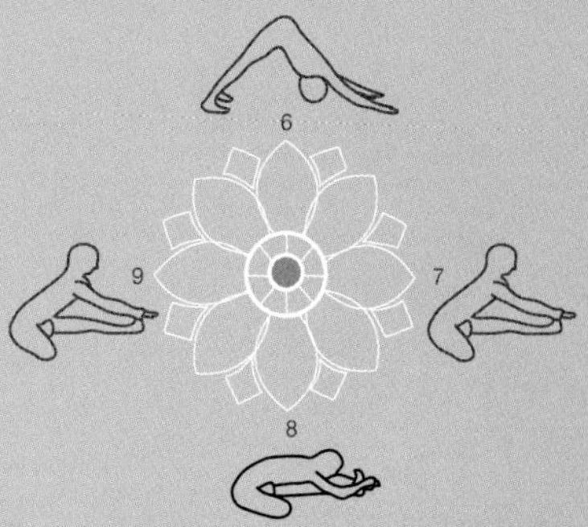

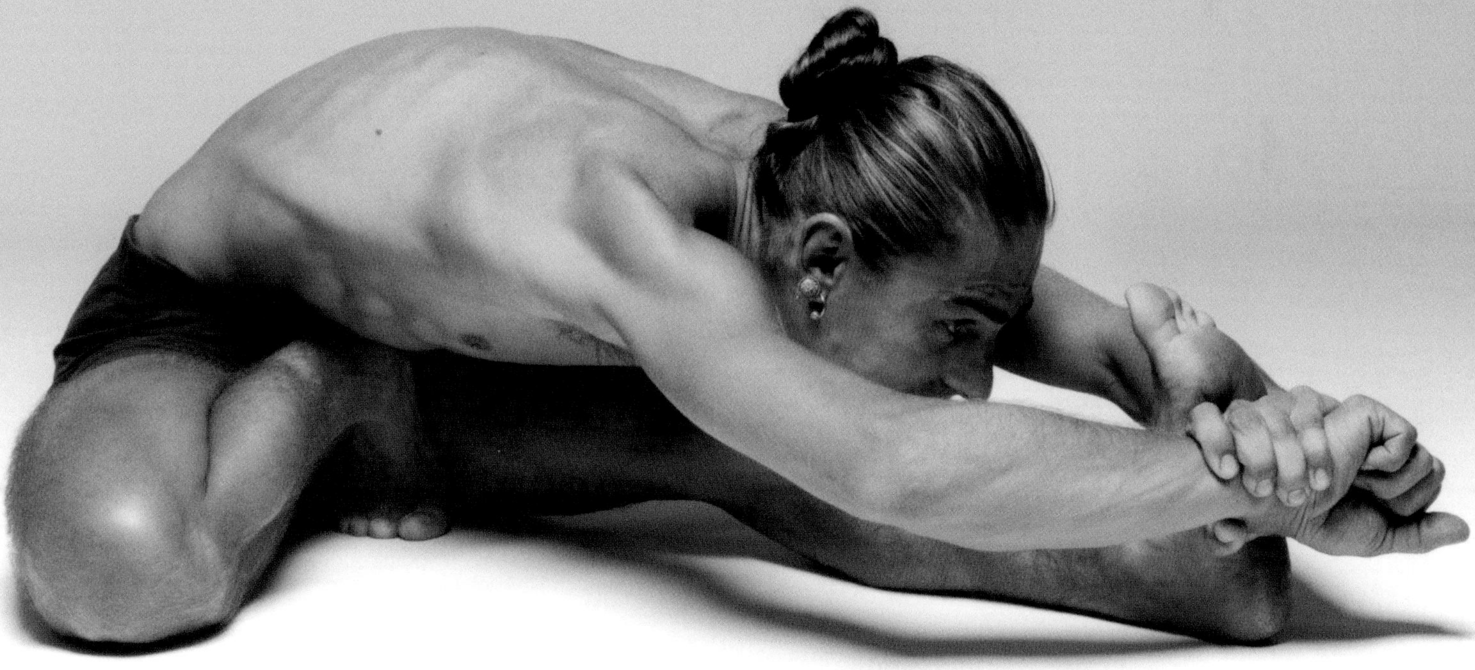

Jānu-śīrṣāsana A, B & C [head-to-knee pose]

22 vinyāsas

Jānu – knee; *śīrṣa* – head; *āsana* – seat, posture

Jānu-śīrṣāsana A follows the 20th vinyāsa in *Tiryaṅ-mukhaikapāda-paścima-tānāsana*.

7 Sapta
Inhale and jump through to sitting, without touching the feet to the floor. Gaze at the tip of the nose.

Jānu-śīrṣāsana A: Straighten the left leg forwards and bend the right knee, bringing the right foot in towards the groin. Male practitioners can place the sole of the foot on the inner thigh and the heel of the foot at the middle of the perineum (between the testicles and anus). Female practitioners can place the sole of the foot on the inner thigh and the heel at the groin. In the forward-bending position of this āsana, the heel presses on and stimulates the śīvani- and vīrya-nāḍīs (see p. 181). Once you have established the appropriate foot position, bend the right knee 90 degrees out to the side.

Jānu-śīrṣāsana B: Straighten your left leg forwards, bend the right knee 85 degrees out to the side and place the sole of the foot under the hips. Flex the right foot and move the hips onto the heel, so that you are essentially sitting on the anus (mūla-bandha). Mūla-bandha is fullly engaged here and pushing down onto the heel. Keep the right toes pointing forwards alongside the left leg; avoid turning them towards the side of the mat.

Jānu-śīrṣāsana C: Straighten the left leg forwards. Take hold of the right foot with both hands and, as you bring the foot in towards the left inner thigh, rotate it outwards so that the ball of the foot and toes root into the floor and the whole foot arches deeply. The arch of the right foot comes in towards the inner left thigh and the heel turns up and in towards the navel. When you bend forwards, the heel will press into the lower abdomen, stimulating vīrya-nāḍī in women (see p. 179). Press the ball of the foot into the floor and relax within the hip joint to open the knee out to a 45-degree angle and eventually touch the knee to the floor.

Keep inhaling as you place the foot into the correct position. Reach forwards with both hands and bind the wrist beyond the foot. Open the chest, lengthen the spine, lift the head up and gaze at the tip of the nose.

8 Aṣṭau
Exhale, fold slowly over the left leg and take the chin to the shin. Press the right knee down into the floor to stretch and open the hips. Lift uddīyana-bandha so there is space for the chest and stomach to fold forwards. Mūla-bandha keeps the hips down and grounded in the āsana. This is the state of the āsana. Breathe five times, gazing at the big toe.

9 Nava
Begin with an inhalation, open the chest, straighten the spine and lift the head up. Straighten the arms and pull back slightly on the left foot. Engage the bandhas to support the expansion in the back and chest as well as to keep the hips down. Hold this position and exhale here. Gaze at the tip of the nose.

10 Daśa
Inhale, place the hands on either side of the hips, cross the ankles in the air and jump back according to the description in the 11th vinyāsa of Paścima-tānāsana. Gaze at the tip of the nose.

11 Ekādaśa
Exhale, straighten the legs behind you and land in Catvāri position. Gaze at the tip of the nose.

Vinyāsas 12 and 13 are the same as the 5th and 6th vinyāsas in Sūrya-namaskāra A.

Repeat vinyāsas 7–11 on the left side, counting them as vinyāsas 14–18.

Vinyāsa 15 is the state of the āsana on the left side. Breathe deeply five times.

Vinyāsas 19 and 20 are the same as the 5th and 6th vinyāsas in Sūrya-namaskāra A.

After the 20th vinyāsa in Jānu-śīrṣāsana A, follow with the 7th vinyāsa in Jānu-śīrṣāsana B. Repeat this sequence again to transition from Jānu-śīrṣāsana B into Jānu-śīrṣāsana C. After the 20th vinyāsa in Jānu-śīrṣāsana C, begin with the 7th vinyāsa in Marīcy-āsana A.

Beginners: Jānu-śīrṣāsana B and C require much practice.

- If you cannot bring your chin to the shin at first, start by bringing the head to the knee and gazing at the tip of the nose.
- In B: Try to place the heel as close onto the anus as possible, keeping the foot flexed and toes pointing forwards as much as you can.
- In C: Turn the foot to face up as much as possible, eventually bringing the heel into the abdomen while you bend forwards. Try to press all toes into the floor, relax the hips and gently work the knee towards the floor.

Note:
There are two breaths in the 9th and 16th vinyāsas.

Vinyāsa	Prāṇa (breath)	Āsana (posture)	Dṛṣṭi (gazing point)	Bandha (muscle lock)
Samasthitiḥ		stand straight		
Vinyāsas 1–6 according to Sūrya-namaskāra A				
7 Sapta	in	jump through, place right foot, lift head		
8 Aṣṭau	out	bend forwards		
state of the āsana on the right side, hold for 5 deep breaths				
9 Nava	in & out	stretch out, head up, hold the pose		
10 Daśa	in	hands to floor, lift up		
11 Ekādaśa	out	catvāri position		
12 Dvādaśa	in	upward-facing dog		
13 Trayodaśa	out	downward-facing dog		
14 Caturdaśa	in	jump through, place left foot, head up		
15 Pañcadaśa	out	bend forwards		
state of the āsana on the left side in A, B & C, hold for 5 deep breaths				
16 Ṣoḍaśa	in & out	stretch out, head up, hold the pose		
17 Saptadaśa	in	hands to floor, lift up		
18 Aṣṭadaśa	out	catvāri position		
19 Ekona-viṃśatiḥ	in	upward-facing dog		
20 Viṃśatiḥ	out	downward-facing dog		
21 Ekaviṃśatiḥ	in	jump forward, head up		
22 Dvaviṃśatiḥ	out	bend forward		
Samasthitiḥ	in	come up, stand straight		

Note:
There are two breaths in the 9th and 16th vinyāsas.

Vinyāsa	Prāṇa (breath)	Āsana (posture)	Dṛṣṭi (gazing point)	Bandha (muscle lock)
Samasthitiḥ		stand straight		
Vinyāsas 1–6 according to Sūrya-namaskāra A				
7 Sapta	in	jump through, bend the right leg, head up		
8 Aṣṭau	out	bend forward, chin to shin		
state of the āsana on the right side, hold for 5 deep breaths				
9 Nava	in & out	stretch out, head up, hold the pose		
10 Daśa	in	hands to the floor, lift up		
11 Ekadaśa	out	catvāri position		
12 Dvādaśa	in	upward-facing dog		
13 Trayodaśa	out	downward-facing dog		
14 Caturdaśa	in	jump through, bend the left leg, head up		
15 Pañcadaśa	out	bend forward, chin to shin		
state of the āsana on the left side, hold for 5 deep breaths				
16 Ṣoḍaśa	in & out	stretch out, head up, hold the pose		
17 Saptadaśa	in	hands to floor, lift up		
18 Aṣṭadaśa	out	catvāri position		
19 Ekona-viṁśatiḥ	in	upward-facing dog		
20 Viṁśatiḥ	out	downward-facing dog		
21 Ekaviṁśatiḥ	in	jump forwards, head up		
22 Dvaviṁśatiḥ	out	bend forwards		
Samasthitiḥ	in	come up, stand straight		

Marīcy-āsana A [Sage Marīci's pose]

22 vinyāsas

Marīci – Sage Marīci; *āsana* – seat, posture

Marīcy-āsana A follows the 20th vinyāsa in Jānu-śīrṣāsana C.

7 Sapta
Inhale, jump through to sitting. Bend the right leg and place the right foot close to the right hip, with the knee up towards the ceiling. The heel should touch the buttock, and the outer edge of the foot should be in line with the outer edge of the right hip. The toes are pointed forwards. Another way to get into the āsana is to jump directly into the position, by bending the right knee as you jump through and landing with the right foot in place. Continue to inhale as you fold forwards and rotate the right arm, placing the armpit onto the shin. Wrap the arm around the knee and take the forearm and hand to the lower back. Bring the left hand up to meet the right and bind the left wrist with the right hand. Make a soft fist with the left hand. The left foot stays flexed. Open the chest, straighten the spine and lift the head up. Keep the right hip down as much as possible although it doesn't necessarily have to touch the floor. Gaze at the tip of the nose.

8 Aṣṭau
Exhale, fold forwards over the left leg and place the chin to the shin. Keep the shoulders in line with each other and over the left knee as evenly as possible. The hands will be relaxed around the back. Mūla-bandha keeps the hips down and works to ground the āsana. Uḍḍīyana-bandha gives the strength for the forward bend. This is the state of the āsana. Breathe five times and gaze at the left big toe.

9 Nava
Inhale, maintain the bound-hand position, lift the head up and elongate the upper body. Keep the bandhas engaged and stay here for an exhalation. Gaze at the tip of the nose.

10 Daśa
Inhale and release the hands and leg. Bring the right leg forwards and cross the ankles in the air. Jump back according to the description from the 11th vinyāsa in Paścima-tānāsana. Another option is to release the hands and bring the left hand to the floor beside the hip. Leave the right arm as it is in front of the right shin, and place the hand to the outside of the right foot. Both legs remain as they were in the 8th and 9th vinyāsas. Continue inhaling as you press the armpit into the right shin firmly to stabilize the lift. Hold the bandhas, stretch through the shoulders and straighten the arms. Lift the body using the strength of the arms and with the help of the right shin. Bend the left knee and bring it through the arms, lifting the hips up high.

Vinyāsa 11 is the same as the 12th vinyāsa in Paścima-tānāsana.

Vinyāsas 12 and 13 are the same as the 5th and 6th vinyāsas in Sūrya-namaskāra A.

Repeat vinyāsas 7–11 on the left side, but count them as vinyāsas 14–18.

Vinyāsa 15 is the state of the āsana on the left side. Breathe deeply five times.

Vinyāsas 19 and 20 are the same as the 5th and 6th vinyāsas in Sūrya-namaskāra A. After vinyāsa 20, go directly to the next āsana, the 7th vinyāsa in Marīcy-āsana B.

Beginners: To perform this āsana exactly, according to the description above, requires much practice.
- Bring your heel into the buttock as much as possible, with the knee upright and the foot pointing forwards.
- Instead of bringing the armpit to the shin on the 7th vinyāsa, bring the upper arm to the shin and wrap the arm from there.
- If you cannot reach the wrists to bind, take hold of the fingers instead or grasp a towel between the hands.
- Start by bringing the head to the knee and gaze at the nose tip.

Marīcy-āsana A

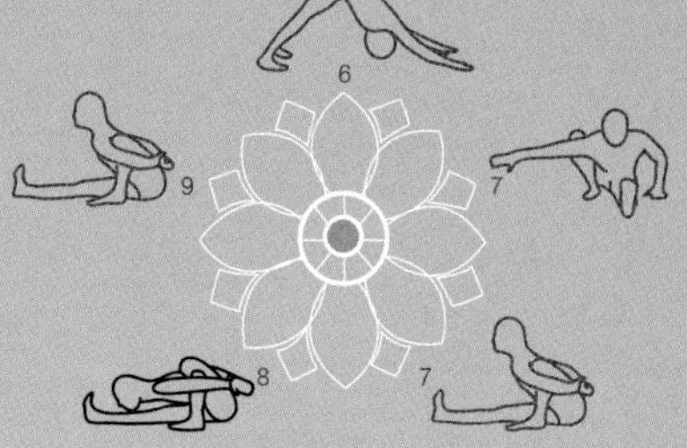

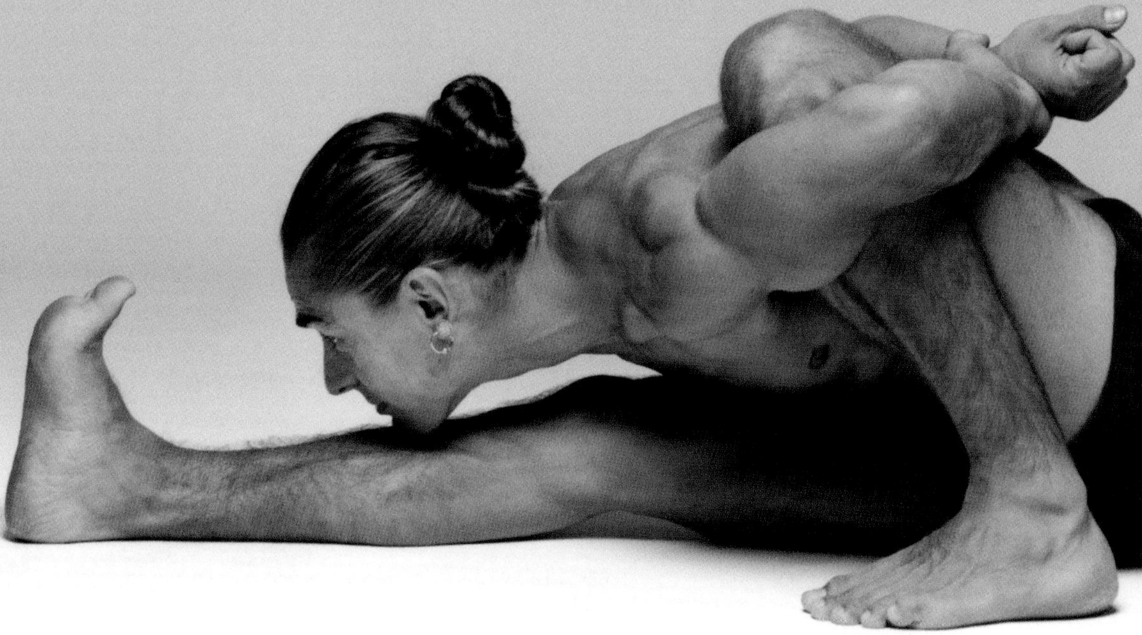

Note:
There are two breaths in the 9th and 16th vinyāsas.

Vinyāsa	Prāṇa (breath)	Āsana (posture)	Dṛṣṭi (gazing point)	Bandha (muscle lock)
Samasthitiḥ		stand straight		
Vinyāsas 1–6 according to Sūrya-namaskāra A				
7 Sapta	in	jump through to sit down, half-lotus with left leg, bend right leg, head up		
8 Aṣṭau	out	fold forward, chin to floor		
state of the āsana on the right side; hold for 5 deep breaths				
9 Nava	in & out	stretch out, head up, hold the pose		
10 Daśa	in	hands to the floor, lift up		
11 Ekādaśa	out	catvāri position		
12 Dvādaśa	in	upward-facing dog		
13 Trayodaśa	out	downward-facing dog		
14 Caturdaśa	in	jump through to sit down, make half-lotus with right leg, bend left leg,head up		
15 Pañcadaśa	out	fold forwards, chin to floor		
state of the āsana on the left side; hold for 5 deep breaths				
16 Ṣoḍaśa	in & out	stretch out, head up, hold the pose		
17 Saptadaśa	in	hands to floor, lift up		
18 Aṣṭadaśa	out	catvāri position		
19 Ekoṇa-viṁśatiḥ	in	upward-facing dog		
20 Viṁśatiḥ	out	downward-facing dog		
21 Ekaviṁśatiḥ	in	jump forwards, stretch spine, head up		
22 Dvaviṁśatiḥ	out	bend forwards		
Samasthitiḥ	in	come up, stand straight		

Marīcy-āsana B [Sage Marīci's pose]

22 vinyāsas

Marīci – Sage Marīci; *āsana* – seat, posture

Marīcy-āsana B is done right after the 20th vinyāsa in Marīcy-āsana A.

7 Sapta
Inhale, jump through to sitting. Continue to inhale as you bring your left foot into half-lotus, as in the 7th vinyāsa of Ardha-baddha-padma-paścima-tānāsana. Relax the left hip joint, and lower the knee down, 45 degrees out to the side. Bend the right knee and place the foot on the floor with the heel in towards the right buttock. This is the same leg position as in Marīcy-āsana A. Continue with the inhalation, and place the right armpit on the shin, just below the right knee. Take the arm around the knee and behind the lower back. Bring the left hand up to meet the right and bind the left wrist with the right hand, as you did in Marīcy-āsana A. Make a soft fist with the left hand. Open the chest, straighten the spine and lift the head up. Hold the hands in close to the back, press the hips into the floor, and engage the bandhas. Gaze at the tip of the nose.

8 Aṣṭau
Exhale and slowly bend forwards, bringing the head down in between the left knee and the right foot. Press the chin to the floor and relax the back of the neck. Keep the shoulders in line with each other, as you draw the right hip closer to the floor. In order to move further into the pose, use the strength in your hips, both the bandhas and the legs. Engage uddīyana-bandha, creating space for the left heel to massage the abdomen, liver and navel energy center (maṇipura cakra). Mūla-bandha keeps the hips grounded and works to stabilize the āsana. This is the state of the āsana. Breathe five times and gaze at the tip of the nose.

9 Nava
Inhale, maintain the bound-hand position, lift the head up and straighten the upper body. Keep the bandhas engaged, and stay here for an exhalation. Gaze at the tip of the nose.

10 Daśa
Inhale and release the hands and left leg. Bring the legs forwards and cross the ankles in the air. Jump back following the description from the 11th vinyāsa in Paścima-tānāsana. Another technique is to release the bind and place the left hand on the floor by the left thigh. Let the right armpit rest on the shin and place the hand on the floor. Keep the right knee and left leg in the position from the 8th vinyāsa. Continue inhaling and press the armpit firmly into the shin to stabilize the lift; hold the bandhas, stretch through the shoulders, and straighten the arms. Rest your body weight onto the arms and shin, and lift the legs through the arms, bringing the hips up high. A third option is to release the bind and bring the hands to the floor on either side of the hips. Continue with the inhalation as you engage the bandhas, straighten the arms and lift the body up off the floor, with the legs in the same position as in the state of the āsana.

Vinyāsa 11 is the same as the 12th vinyāsa in Paścima-tānāsana.

Vinyāsas 12 and 13 are the same as the 5th and 6th vinyāsas in Sūrya-namaskāra A.

Repeat vinyāsas 7–11 on the left side, counting them as vinyāsas 14–18.

Vinyāsa 15 is the state of the āsana on the left side. Breathe deeply five times.

Vinyāsas 19 and 20 are the same as the 5th and 6th vinyāsas in Sūrya-namaskāra A. After vinyāsa 20, go directly to the next āsana, the 7th vinyāsa in Marīcy-āsana C.

Beginners: It requires much practice to perform this āsana according to the description above.

- Try to bring the leg as far into half-lotus as your range of motion allows, with the foot along the inner thigh and groin.
- Bring your heel into the buttock as much as possible, with the knee upright and the foot pointing forwards.
- Instead of placing the armpit on the shin, bring the upper arm onto the shin and wrap the arm from there. If at first you need to place the hands on the ground for balance, do so, and work towards reaching the arms around later on.

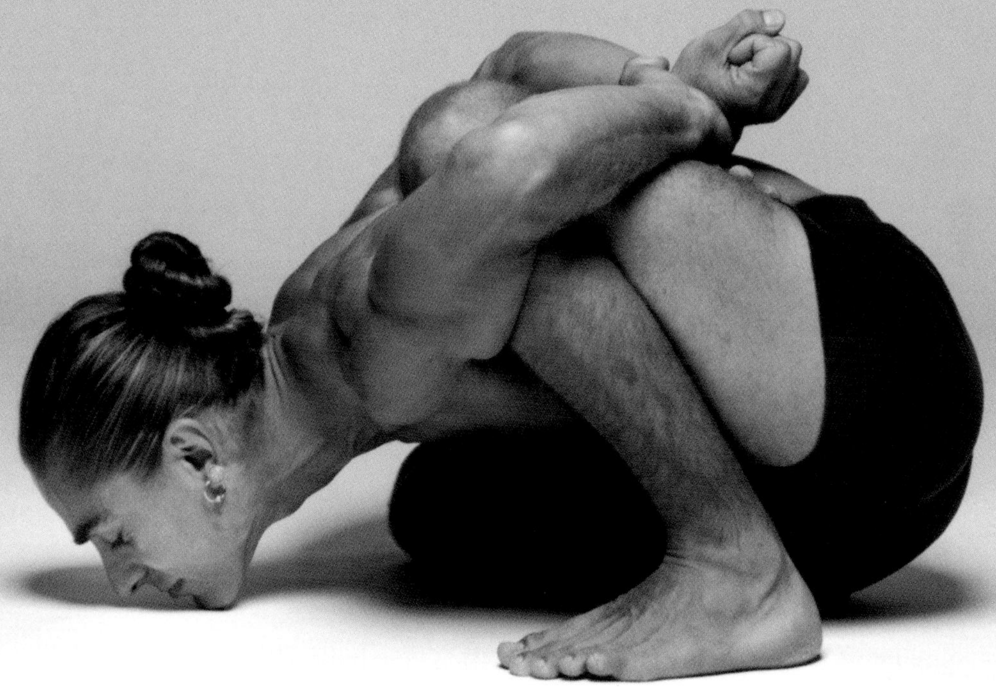

- If you cannot bind the wrists, take hold of the fingers instead or use a small towel between the hands.
- Bend forwards by first reaching the head towards the floor. When the forehead touches the floor, start to extend the chin forwards.
- Avoid using force to open the leg in lotus or to press the knee to the floor.
- Remember to keep relaxing deeply in the hip joint, opening the lotus pose with deep breathing.
- Do not create your own variations of this āsana, simply try to perform it as correctly as possible.

Marīcy-āsana C

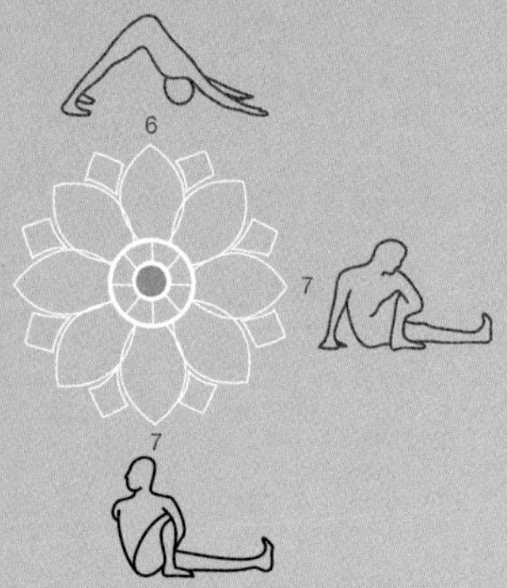

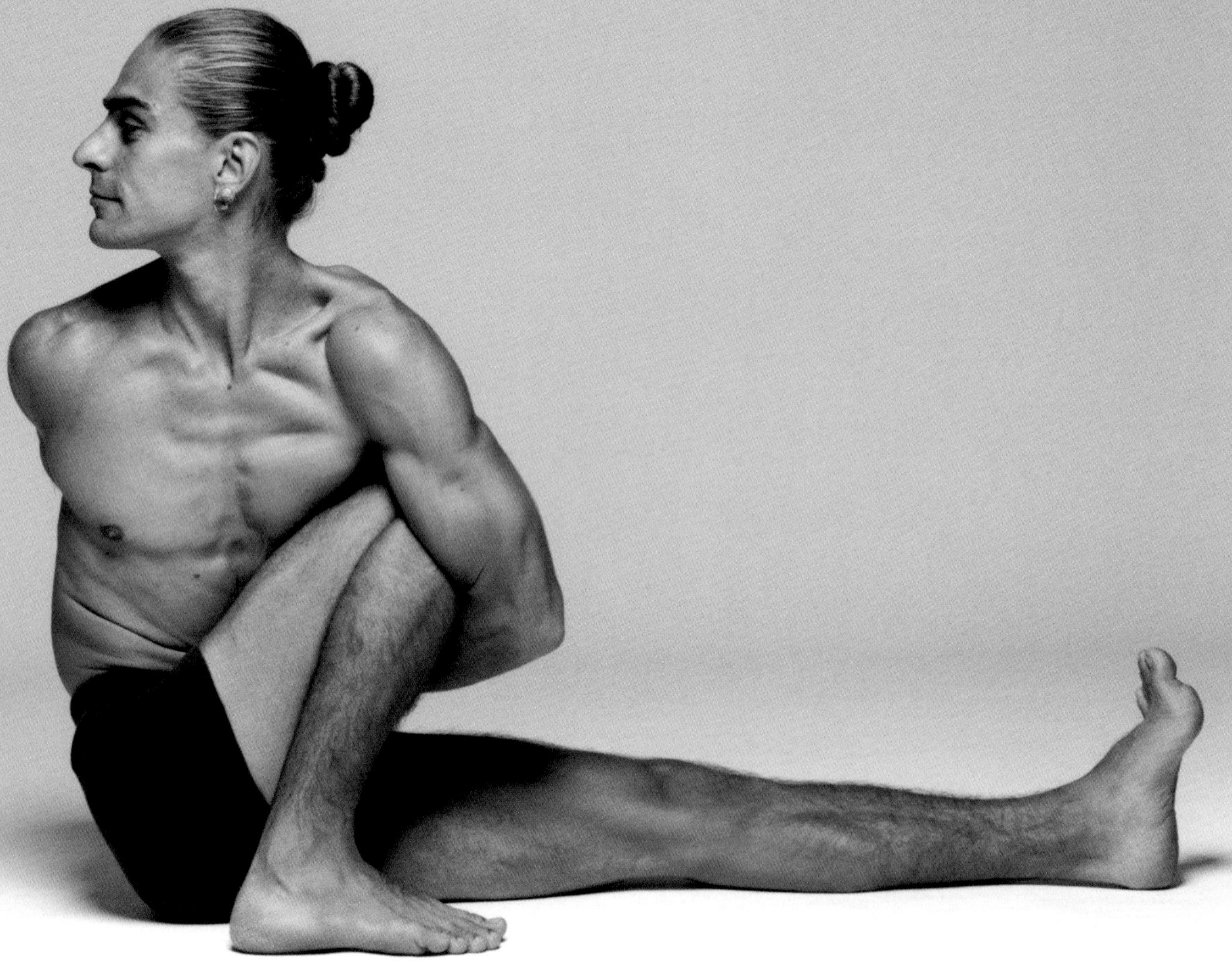

Marīcy-āsana C [Sage Marīci's pose]

18 vinyāsas

Marīci – Sage Marīci; *āsana* – seat, posture

Marīcy-āsana C comes after the 20th vinyāsa in *Marīcy-āsana B*.

7 Sapta
Inhale and jump through to sitting. Bend the right leg and place the right foot close to the right hip, as in Marīcy-āsana A. Another way is to jump directly into the position by bending the right knee as you jump through and land with the right foot in place. Continue to inhale as you twist the entire upper body towards the right. Bring the left arm and armpit around the right thigh and below the right knee. Internally rotate the left arm to twist it around, taking the hand towards the back as you wrap the right arm around to meet the left arm. Bind the left wrist with the right hand and make a soft fist with the left hand. The right knee stays facing up with the right foot firmly planted on the ground. The left leg remains straight, with the foot flexed. Open the chest, straighten the spine, expand the collarbones, and lengthen the back of the neck. Press the left hip into the floor. This is the state of the āsana. Breathe deeply five times. Gaze to the right side.

8 Aṣṭau
Slowly inhale and release the twist. Bring the legs forwards and cross the ankles in the air. Jump back according to the description from the 11th vinyāsa in Paścima-tānāsana A. Notice that after the fifth exhalation in the state of the pose, there is no extra breath (inhalation or exhalation) or opening. With the next inhalation (next vinyāsa), release the hands, set them on the floor beside the hips, and lift the body up.
The second option is to release the twist and bring the left hand to the floor beside the hip. Bring the right arm in front of the right shin, and place the hand outside the right foot, keeping the left leg straight. Continue with the inhalation as you press the armpit firmly onto the shin and stabilize the lift. Hold the bandhas, stretch through the shoulders and straighten the arms. Lift the body up with the strength of the arms and the help of the shin. Bend the left knee and bring it through the arms with the hips lifted high. Gaze at the tip of the nose.

Vinyāsa 9 is the same as the 12th vinyāsa in Paścima-tānāsana.

Vinyāsas 10 and 11 are the same as the 5th and 6th vinyāsas in Sūrya-namaskāra A.

Repeat vinyāsas 7–9 on the left side, counting them as vinyāsas 12–14.

Vinyāsa 12 is the state of the āsana on the left side. Breathe deeply five times.

Vinyāsas 15 and 16 are the same as the 5th and 6th vinyāsas in Sūrya-namaskāra A. After vinyāsa 16, go directly to the next āsana, the 7th vinyāsa in Marīcy-āsana D.

Beginners: The deep twist in Marīcy-āsana C requires practice.
- It can often take several breaths to come into the state of the 7th vinyāsa. Breathe calmly to set the pose, but try to limit the number of extra breaths you take.
- If you cannot bind the wrists, take hold of the fingers instead or use a small towel between the hands.
- If you cannot bind the hands with the towel, try to keep the hands off the floor and twist the body and head. This will develop the strength and flexibility needed to deepen the āsana.

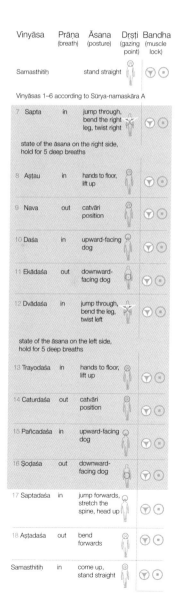

Vinyāsa	Prāṇa (breath)	Āsana (posture)	Dṛṣṭi (gazing point)	Bandha (muscle lock)
Samasthitiḥ		stand straight		
Vinyāsas 1–6 according to Sūrya-namaskāra A				
7 Sapta	in	jump through, bend the right leg, twist right		
state of the āsana on the right side, hold for 5 deep breaths				
8 Aṣṭau	in	hands to floor, lift up		
9 Nava	out	catvāri position		
10 Daśa	in	upward-facing dog		
11 Ekādaśa	out	downward-facing dog		
12 Dvādaśa	in	jump through, bend the leg, twist left		
state of the āsana on the left side, hold for 5 deep breaths				
13 Trayodaśa	in	hands to floor, lift up		
14 Caturdaśa	out	catvāri position		
15 Pañcadaśa	in	upward-facing dog		
16 Ṣoḍaśa	out	downward-facing dog		
17 Saptadaśa	in	jump forwards, stretch the spine, head up		
18 Aṣṭadaśa	out	bend forwards		
Samasthitiḥ	in	come up, stand straight		

Marīcy-āsana D

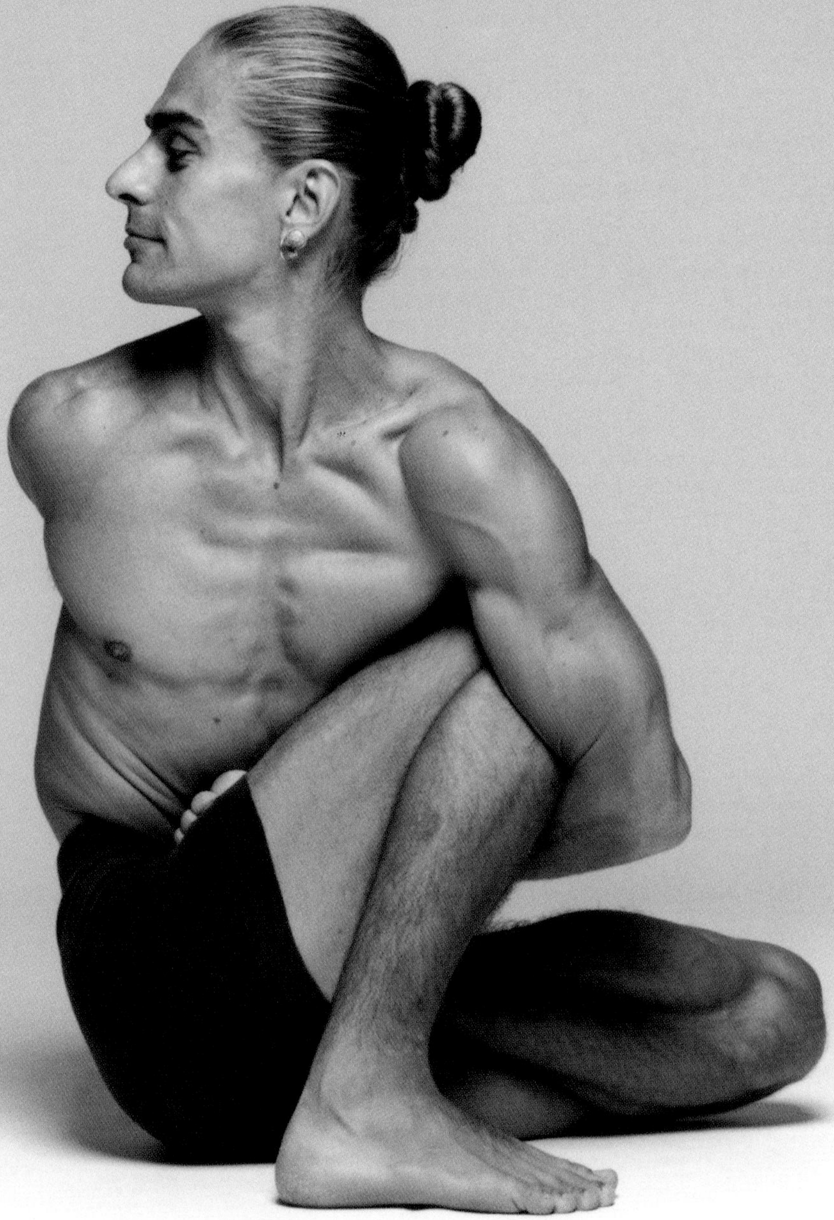

Marīcy-āsana D *[Sage Marīci's pose]*

18 vinyāsaa

Marīci – Sage Marīci; *āsana* – seat, posture

Marīcy-āsana D is done after the 16th vinyāsa in Marīcy-āsana C.

7 Sapta
Inhale and jump through to sitting. Continue inhaling as you bring the left foot up into the right groin, as in Marīcy-āsana B. In this āsana, however, the knee is lowered onto the floor and faces the front of the mat, whereas in Marīcy-āsana B the knee is 45 degrees out to the side. Bend the right knee, and place the foot on the floor with the heel next to the right buttock. The outer edge of the foot is in line with the outer edge of the hip, and the toes point towards the front of the mat. Keep inhaling as you twist the upper body to the right. Bring the left arm and armpit around the right thigh and below the right knee. Internally rotate the left arm to twist it around and bring the hand towards the back, while wrapping the right arm around the back as well. Bind the left wrist and make a soft fist with the left hand. The right knee faces the ceiling rather than tilting to the left, while the right foot stays grounded into the floor.
Twist the body to the right, open the chest, straighten the spine and lengthen the back of the neck. Keep the left knee on the floor (this is an important detail to remember) and press the right hip towards the floor. This is the state of the āsana. Breathe deeply five times and gaze towards the right side.

8 Aṣṭau
Slowly inhale and release the twist. The transition (and breathing) are the same as in Marīcy-āsana C. Use one of the three jump-back techniques described in Marīcy-āsana B.

Vinyāsa 9 is the same as the 12th vinyāsa in Paścima-tānāsana.

Vinyāsas 10 and 11 are the same as the 5th and 6th vinyāsas in Sūrya-namaskāra A.

Repeat vinyāsas 7–9 on the left side, counting them as vinyāsas 12–14.

Vinyāsa 12 is the state of the āsana on the left side. Breathe deeply five times.

Vinyāsas 15 and 16 are the same as the 5th and 6th vinyāsas in Sūrya-namaskāra A. After vinyāsa 16, go directly to the next āsana, the 7th vinyāsa in Navāsana.

Beginners: The deep twist in Marīcy-āsana D comes with practice. See the notes for both Marīcy-āsana B and C.

Vinyāsa	Prāṇa (breath)	Āsana (posture)	Dṛṣṭi (gazing point)	Bandha (muscle lock)
Samasthitiḥ		stand straight		
Vinyāsas 1–6 according to Sūrya-namaskāra A				
7 Sapta	in	jump through, left leg into half-lotus, twist right		
state of the āsana on the right side, hold for 5 deep breaths				
8 Aṣṭau	in	hands to floor, lift up		
9 Nava	out	catvāri position		
10 Daśa	in	upward-facing dog		
11 Ekādaśa	out	downward-facing dog		
12 Dvādaśa	in	jump through, right leg into half-lotus, twist left		
state of the āsana on the left side, hold for 5 deep breaths				
13 Trayodaśa	in	hands to floor, lift up		
14 Caturdaśa	out	catvāri position		
15 Pañcadaśa	in	upward-facing dog		
16 Ṣoḍaśa	out	downward-facing dog		
17 Saptadaśa	in	jump forwards, stretch spine, head up		
18 Aṣṭadaśa	out	bend forwards		
Samasthitiḥ	in	come up, stand straight		

Navāsana [boat pose]

13 vinyāsas

Nava – boat; *āsana* – seat, posture

Navāsana follows the 16th vinyāsa in Marīcy-āsana D.

Note:
Repeat the state of the āsana (the 7th vinyāsa) five times, holding for five breaths each time.

7 Sapta
Slowly inhale and jump directly into Navāsana without touching the feet to the floor. Balance the body, straighten the spine and legs and bring the (pointed) feet up to eye-level. Extend the arms out in front of you by the knees or ankles with the palms facing in. Engage mūla-bandha to support the hips and strengthen the upwards energy in the body. Engage uddīyana-bandha to lengthen the spine and to help keep the chest lifted. Keep the face and shoulders relaxed. This is the state of the āsana. Breathe deeply five times. Gaze at the toes.

8 Aṣṭau
Inhale, place the hands on the floor on either side of the hips, cross the ankles, keep the feet lifted up off the floor and draw the knees in towards the chest. Continue inhaling as you press the hands into the floor, lengthen through the shoulders, straighten the arms and lift the hips off the floor. Exhale, place the hips back down between the arms. On the next inhalation, straighten the legs back into the state of the āsana. Repeat this sequence five times, holding the state of the pose (the 7th vinyāsa) for five breaths each time. After the last exhalation on the fifth and final round of Navāsana, inhale, place the hands on the floor on either side of the hips, cross the ankles with the legs in the air and draw the knees in towards the chest. Continue the inhalation as you lift the hips up off the floor and bring the legs back between the arms. Gaze at the tip of the nose.

Vinyāsa 9 is the same as the 12th vinyāsa in Paścima-tānāsana.

Vinyāsas 10 and 11 are the same as the 5th and 6th vinyāsas in Sūrya-namaskāra A. After the 11th vinyāsa, go directly to the next āsana, the 7th vinyāsa in Bhuja-pīḍāsana.

Beginners: Navāsana, done five times in a row with straight legs, requires strength and practice.

- Keep the legs straight for as long as possible.
- Lift the body up, or just slightly off the floor, even if for a brief moment, in between repetitions.
- Work simultaneously to keep the back straight and the chest lifted.
- If you run out of breath before you get into Navāsana, breathe in and out again. Avoid holding the breath.

Vinyāsa	Prāṇa (breath)	Āsana (posture)	Dṛṣṭi (gazing point)	Bandha (muscle lock)
Samasthitiḥ		stand straight		
Vinyāsas 1–6 according to Sūrya-namaskāra A				
7 Sapta	in	jump into Navasana		
state of the āsana; hold for 5 deep breaths				
8 Aṣṭau	in	hands to floor, lift up		
exhale, hips down, inhale, come back into vinyasa 7; repeat 5 times				
9 Nava	out	catvāri position		
10 Daśa	in	upward-facing dog		
11 Ekādaśa	out	downward-facing dog		
12 Dvādaśa	in	jump forwards, stretch spine, head up		
13 Trayodaśa	out	fold forwards		
Samasthitiḥ	in	come up, stand straight		

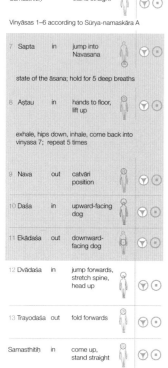

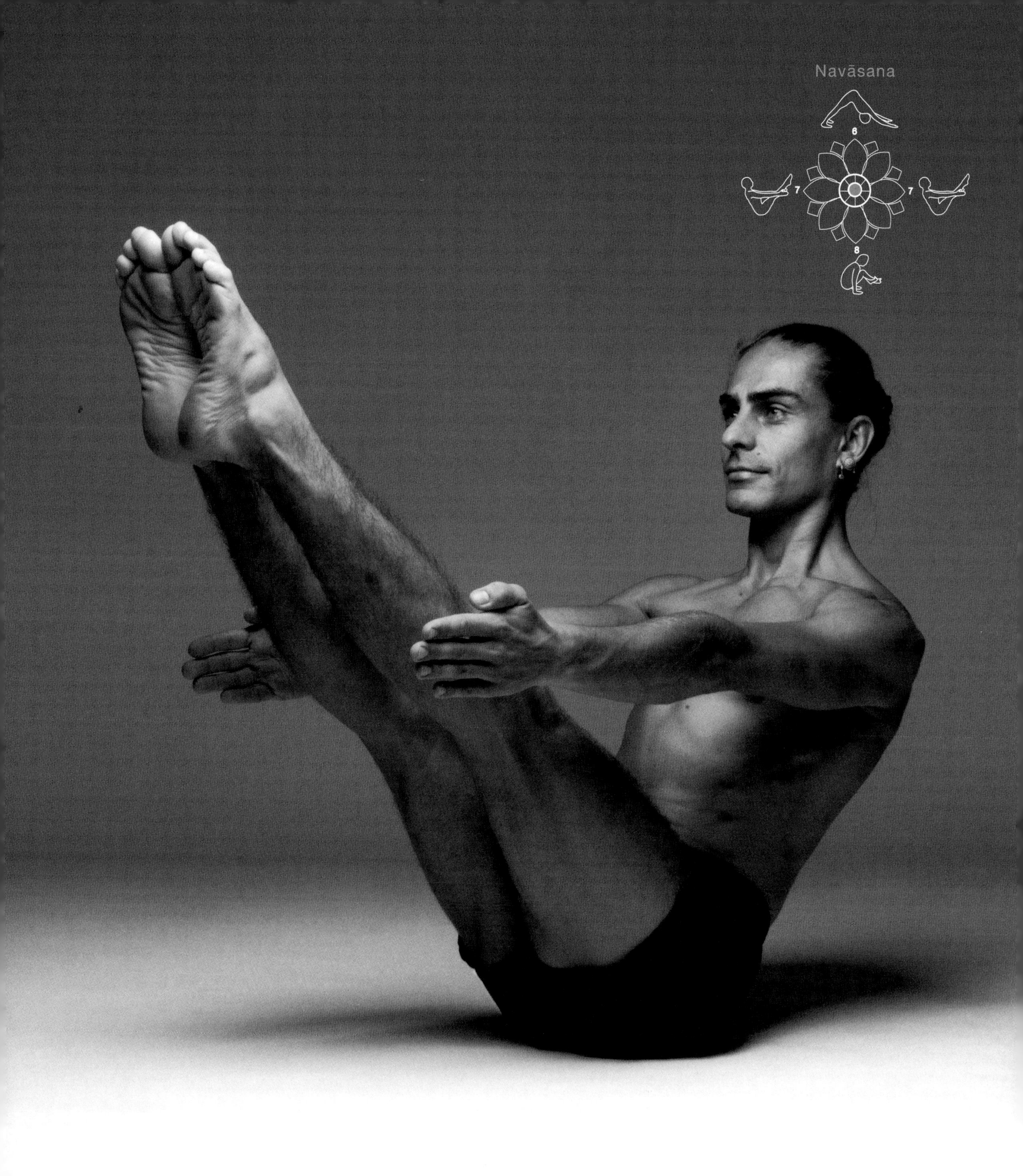
Navāsana
6
7
7
8

Bhuja-pīḍāsana [arm pressure pose]

15 vinyāsas

Note 1:
There are two breaths in the 9th vinyāsa.

Note 2:
There is no Tittibhāsana position in the 9th or 10th vinyāsa.

Bhuja – arm; *pīḍā* – pressure, pressing; *āsana* – seat, posture

7 Sapta
Inhale, bend the elbows and knees, and jump so that the legs (i.e. hamstrings) land onto the upper arms. This action requires the strength of the arms. Keeping the elbows bent will make it easier to balance. Once you are balanced, cross your ankles, right over left, and straighten the arms, keeping the feet in the air throughout. Straighten the back and gaze at the nose-tip with the head up.

8 Aṣṭau
Exhale, draw in the bandhas, lift the hips and bring yourself slowly forwards. Point the feet and shift them between the arms, keeping them off the ground. Bend the elbows until the chin touches the floor. Support your body with the arms so that the chin does not carry much weight. Keep lifting the feet up, between and behind the hands. This is the state of the āsana. Hold for five deep breaths and gaze at the tip of the nose.

9 Nava
Inhale, press the hands into the floor, engage the bandhas and slowly come back up to the position in the 7th vinyāsa. Straighten the back and arms, lift the head and lengthen the back of the neck. Keep the feet lifted throughout the āsana. Exhale here and hold this position. Gaze at the tip of the nose.

10 Daśa
Inhale, uncross the feet, maintain strength in the arms and keep the bandhas engaged. Lift the hips upwards, as you bend the knees and take the feet and shins behind you, bringing the knees onto the upper arms. Let the knees slide into position next to the armpits. Bring the feet together and keep them pointed. This is Bakāsana position and is held briefly, only until the end of the inhalation. Gaze at the tip of the nose.

11 Ekādaśa
Exhale, and lift or jump the legs back through the air to land into Catvāri position. Gaze at the tip of the nose.

Vinyāsas 12 and 13 are the same as the 5th and 6th vinyāsas in Sūrya-namaskāra A. After vinyāsa 13, go directly to the next āsana, the 7th vinyāsa in Kūrmāsana.

Beginners: It can be quite challenging to perform this āsana exactly as described above.

- When you first attempt the 7th vinyāsa, jump and set the feet besides the hands. You can take a few steps to bring the feet further forwards in front of the fingertips. Bend the elbows out to the side, and sit onto the upper arms. Find the balance and keep the bandhas strong to stay supported. Try to bring the feet together in the air, or slowly walk them together along the floor. Try to cross the right foot over the left and work towards lifting the legs up.
- In the 8th vinyāsa, bend the elbows and bring the feet onto the floor between the arms. Bend the elbows some more and slowly place the crown of the head onto the floor. Gradually work towards placing the forehead, and eventually the chin, to the floor. Try to lift the feet up off the floor and bring them in between and behind the arms.
- In the 9th vinyāsa, place the feet on the floor between the hands. Bring the head up next and finally lift the feet back up in front of the body.
- In the 10th vinyāsa, instead of taking both legs back into Bakāsana simultaneously, you can take them back one at the time. If you can't keep the hips up high enough to bring the legs onto the upper arms, lower the feet onto the floor and position them behind the arms. Then place the knees onto the upper arms and take Bakāsana position. Try to keep the legs up as much as possible, developing the strength needed for this transition.
- In the 11th vinyāsa, begin by touching the feet to the floor and hopping back into Catvāri position.

Vinyāsa	Prāṇa (breath)	Āsana (posture)	Dṛṣṭi (gazing point)	Bandha (muscle lock)
Samasthitiḥ		stand straight		
Vinyāsas 1–6 according to Sūrya-namaskāra A				
7 Sapta	in	jump over the arms, cross the legs, head up		
8 Aṣṭau	out	chin to floor		
state of the āsana; hold for 5 deep breaths				
9 Nava	in & out	come up, head straight, hold the pose		
10 Daśa	in	legs into Bakāsana		
11 Ekādaśa	out	catvāri position		
12 Dvādaśa	in	upward-facing dog		
13 Trayodaśa	out	downward-facing dog		
14 Caturdaśa	in	jump forwards, stretch the spine, head up		
15 Pañcadaśa	out	bend forwards		
Samasthitiḥ	in	come up, stand straight		

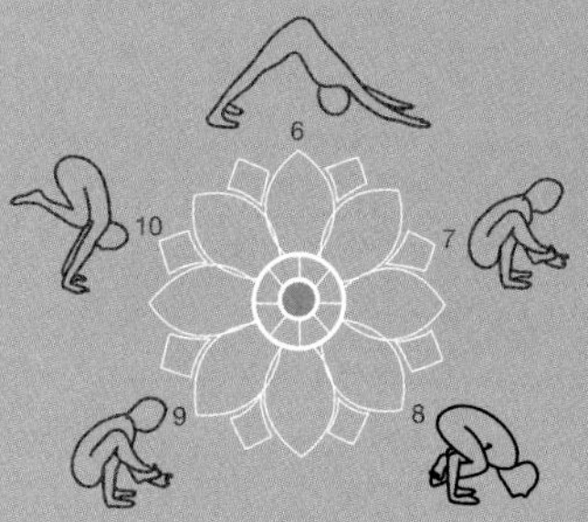
6
7
8
9
10

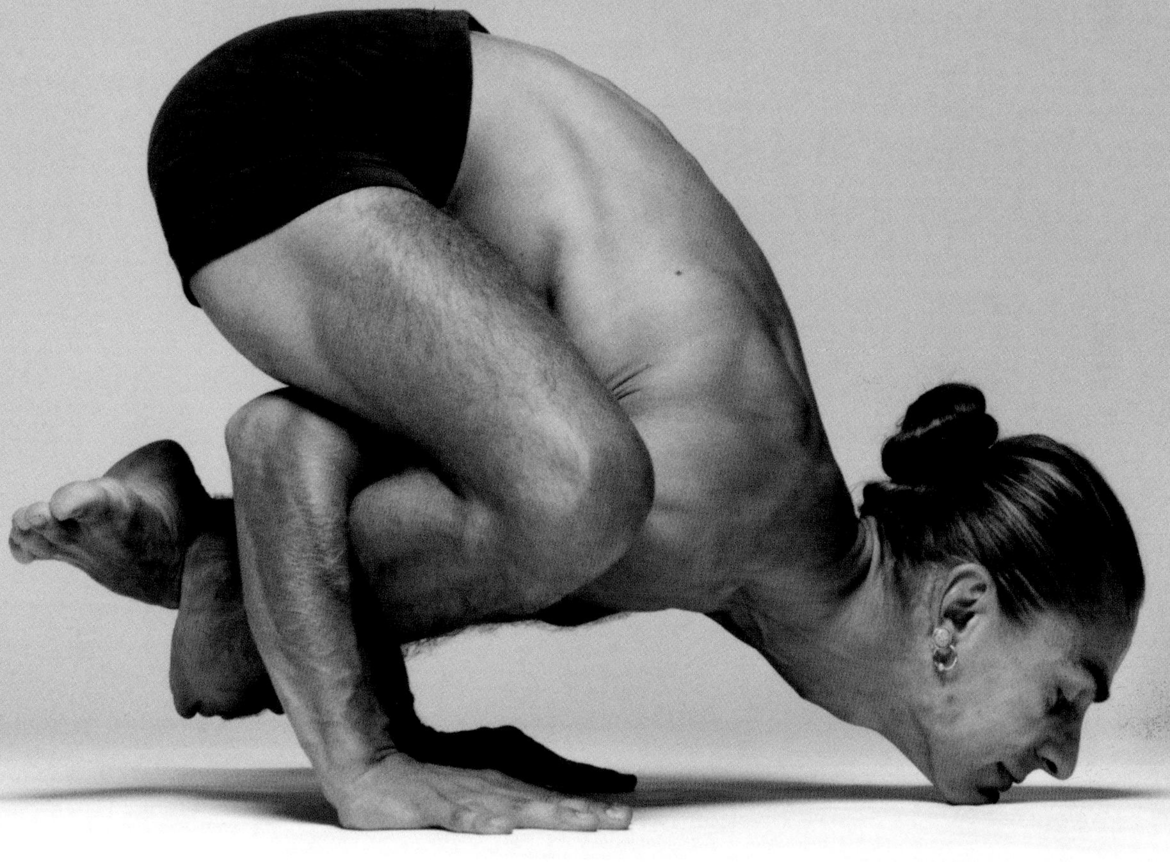

Kūrmāsana & supta-kūrmāsana

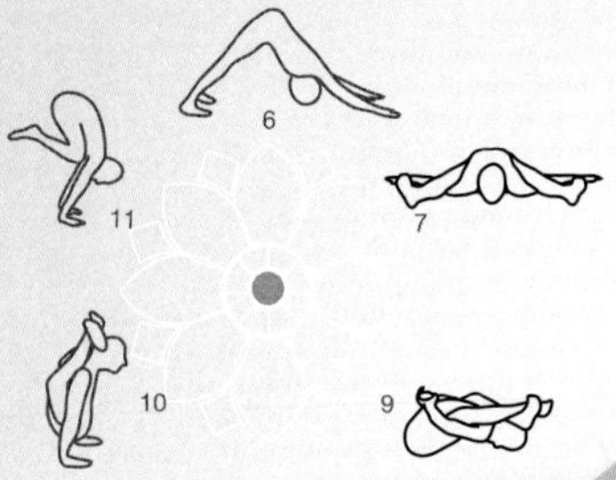

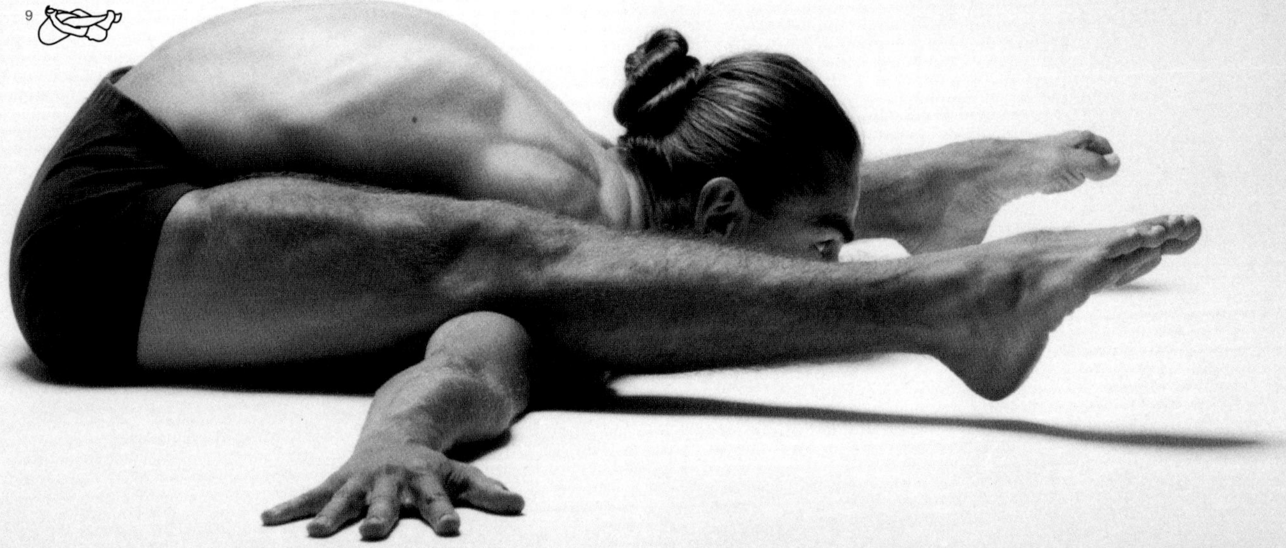

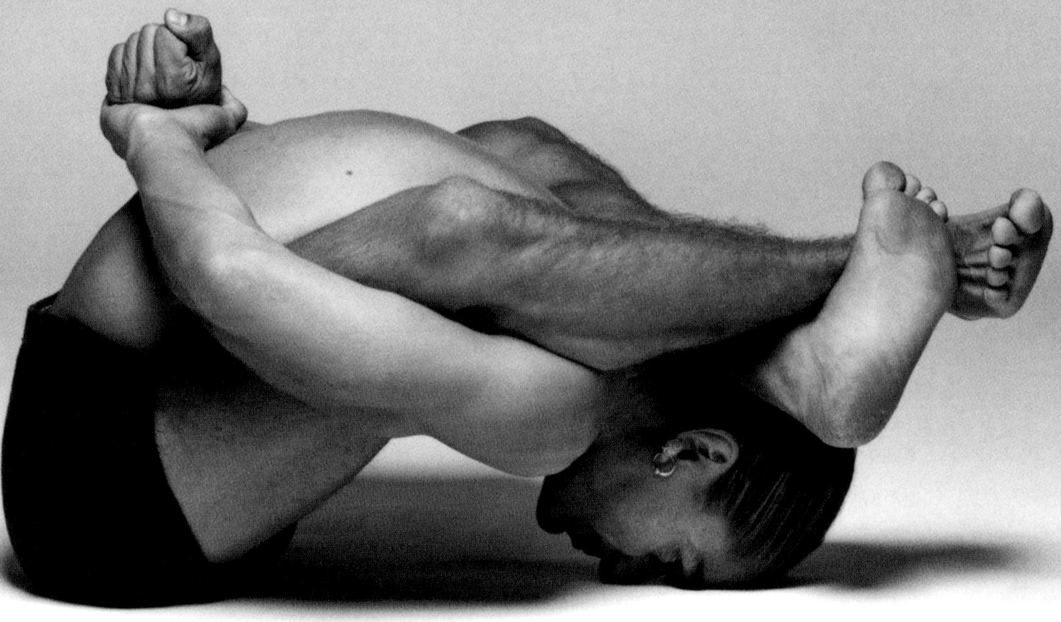

Kūrmāsana & supta-kūrmāsana [tortoise and sleeping tortoise pose]

16 vinyāsas

Kūrmā – tortoise, turtle; *supta* – reclining, sleeping; *āsana* – seat, posture

Kūrmāsana is done directly after the 13th vinyāsa in Bhuja-pīḍāsana.

7 Sapta
Inhale, and jump onto the upper arms as in the 7th vinyāsa in Bhuja-pīḍāsana, but without crossing the legs. Keep inhaling as you bend the elbows deeper and place the whole body on the floor. Straighten the arms directly out to the sides, palms down, and bring the shoulders in and under the knees. Straighten out the legs, keeping them approximately mat-width apart. Press the shoulders and chest into the floor, and the backs of the knees into the shoulders while stretching through the legs. As a result of straightening the legs, the heels may lift off the floor, but this is an optional detail. Point the feet and slide the chin forwards along the floor. This is the state of Kūrmāsana. Stay here for five breaths. Gaze in between the eyebrows.

8 Aṣṭau
Exhale, take the hands towards the lower back and bind the wrist, making a soft fist with the free hand. The gaze stays in between the eyebrows.
Note: Advanced students and/or those with uneven body proportions (e.g. a long torso and shorter legs) can sit up here and do Dvi-pāda-śīrṣāsana. Afterwards, lower the body down into the 9th vinyāsa in Supta-kūrmāsana and point the feet (see the following vinyāsa description below).

9 Nava
Inhale, bend the knees, bring the feet together and cross the right foot over the left. Bring the head in between the legs and the forehead on the floor. If the feet do not remain crossed easily, flex the feet. If you feel stable in the pose, point the toes.This is the state of Supta-kūrmāsana. Stay here for five breaths and gaze in between the eyebrows.

10 Daśa
Inhale, release the bind and place the hands on the floor, beside the hips. Keep the feet crossed behind the head, engage the bandhas, and lift the body up by pressing the palms into the floor. If the legs are not behind the head entirely, keep them crossed in front of the head while you lift the legs and body up and try to take the feet further behind the head. Stretch the spine and the back of the neck. Straighten the arms, open the chest and draw the shoulders back. Exhale and hold the position. Gaze at the tip of the nose with the head forwards.

11 Ekādaśa
Inhale, release the legs, lean forwards slightly into the palms, engage the bandhas and lift the hips up high. Follow the instructions from the 10th vinyāsa of Bhuja-pīḍāsana.

12 Dvādaśa
Exhale, jump back, following the 11th vinyāsa in Bhuja-pīḍāsana and land in Catvāri.

Vinyāsas 13 and 14 are the same as the 5th and 6th vinyāsas in Sūrya-namaskāra A. After vinyāsa 14, go directly to the next āsana, the 7th vinyāsa in Garbha-piṇḍāsana.

Beginners: Kūrmāsana and Supta-kūrmāsana are two of the most challenging āsanas in the primary series. It requires consistent practice to do them fully.

- In the 7th vinyāsa (Kūrmāsana), jump the feet outside the hands and set the feet in front of the fingertips. Bend the elbows out to the side, and sit with the hamstrings on the upper arms. Keep bending the elbows and come to sit on the floor. Take the shoulders under the knee joints as much as possible, and stretch the arms out to the sides with the feet forwards. Relax the back of the neck, and bring the head towards the floor. Place the feet about mat-width apart, with the feet pointed. Glide the heels forwards as far as possible, straightening the legs as much as you can.
- In the 8th vinyāsa (Supta-kūrmāsana), first bend the knees slightly to help bring the shoulders under. This creates more space for the arms to reach further behind you and helps with the hand bind. If you cannot reach the wrist, bind the fingers or use a small towel between the hands.
- In the 9th vinyāsa, if you cannot cross the feet, leave them next to each other and breathe five times.

Note 1:
There are two breaths in the 10th vinyāsa.

Note 2:
There is a second option for dṛṣṭi (the tip of the nose) in the 7th, 8th and 9th vinyāsas.

Vinyāsa	Prāṇa (breath)	Āsana (posture)	Dṛṣṭi (gazing point)	Bandha (muscle lock)
Samasthitiḥ		stand straight		
Vinyāsas 1–6 according to Sūrya-namaskāra A				
7 Sapta	in	jump over the arms, sit back, straighten the legs and arms		
state of Kūrmāsana; hold for 5 deep breaths				
8 Aṣṭa	out	hands bind behind back		
9 Nava	in	cross the feet		
state of Supta-kūrmāsana; hold for 5 deep breaths				
10 Daśa	in & out	lift up, keep feet behind neck, hold the pose		
11 Ekādaśa	in	legs into Bakāsana		
12 Dvādaśa	out	catvāri position		
13 Trayodaśa	in	upward-facing dog		
14 Caturdaśa	out	downward-facing dog		
15 Pañcadaśa	in	jump forwards, stretch the spine, head up		
16 Ṣoḍaśa	out	bend forwards		
Samasthitiḥ	in	come up, stand straight		

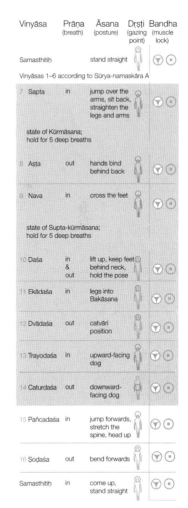

Garbha-piṇḍāsana

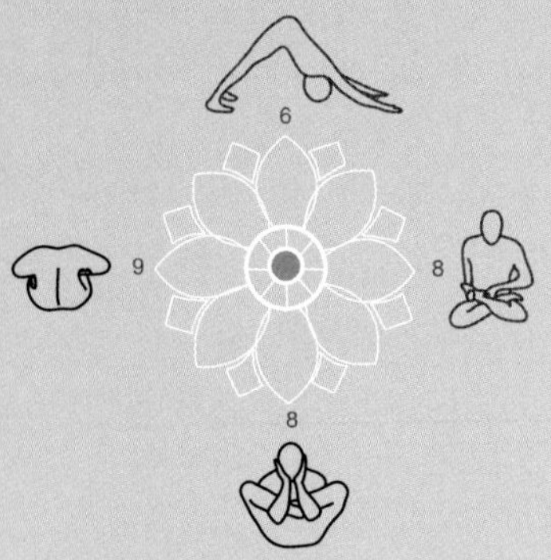

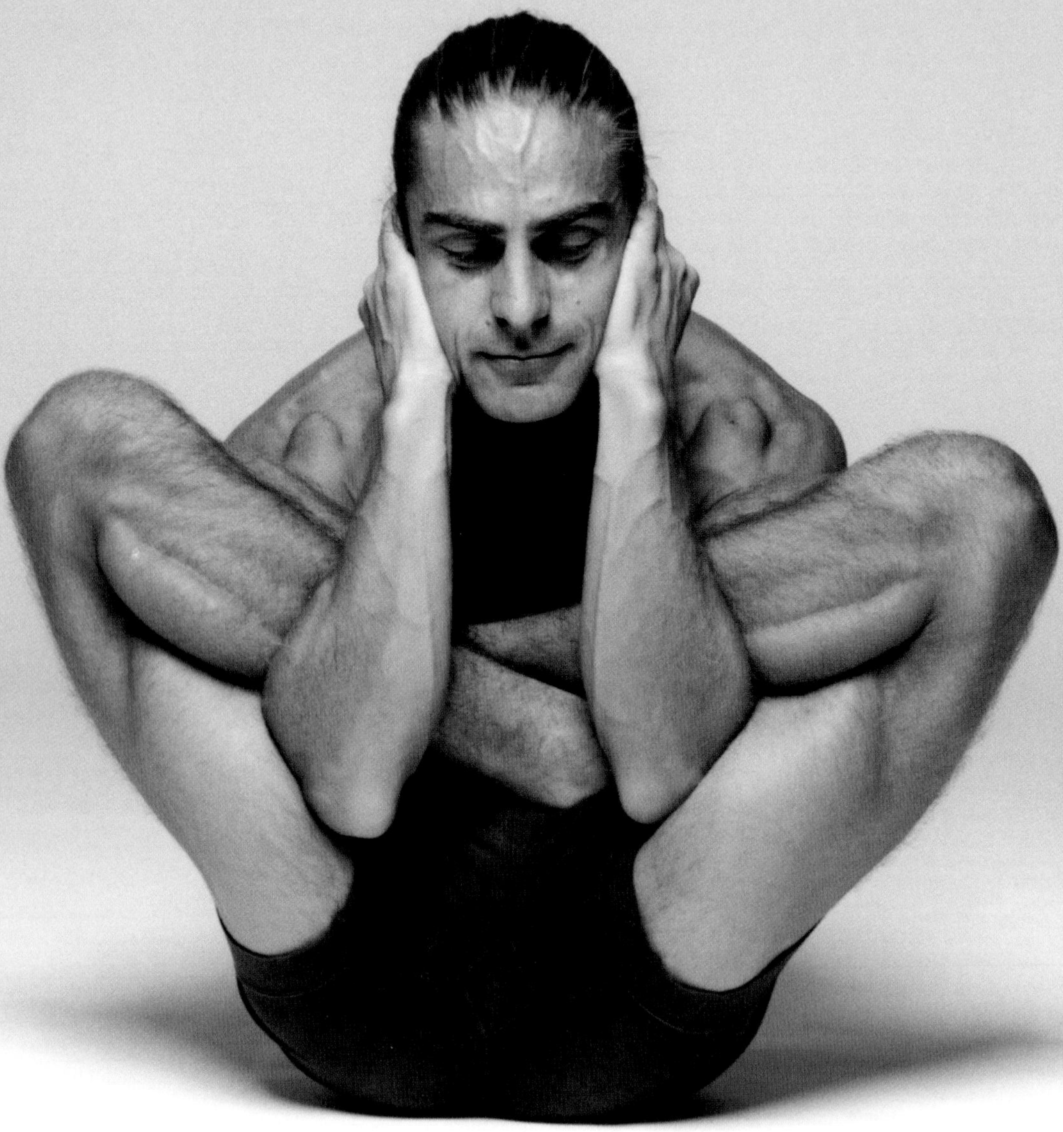

Garbha-piṇḍāsana [embryo in womb pose]

15 vinyāsas

Garbha – womb; *piṇḍa* – embryo, fetus; *āsana* – seat, posture

Garbha-piṇḍāsana comes after the 14th vinyāsa in Supta kūrmāsana.

Note:
Garbha-piṇḍāsana is combined with the next āsana, Kukkuṭāsana.

7 Sapta
Inhale and jump through to sitting. Straighten the legs and gaze at the tip of the nose.

8 Aṣṭau
Exhale, bring the right foot up and into the left groin (into half-lotus). Relax the right hip and take the knee out to a 45-degree angle. Lift the left foot and bring it in towards the right groin, on top of the right calf or lower leg, deeply releasing through the left hip. The left heel is pointing towards the right side of the navel. This is Padmāsana (lotus pose). Keep exhaling as you bring the legs up and into the chest.
Take hold of the right shin with the left hand and slide the right arm in between the right calf and right hamstring. Push the arm all the way through, so that you can bend your elbow on the other side of your thigh. Do the same with the left arm, sliding it deeply in between the left calf and left hamstring so that you can bend the elbow on the outer side of the thigh. Balance on the sitting-bones, take both hands up towards the head and cup the palms over the ears. Straighten the spine and the back of the neck and open the chest. Engage the bandhas and press the heels into the both sides of the navel. This is the state of the āsana. Breathe here five times. Gaze at the tip of the nose.

9 Nava
Exhale, round the back, bring the chin into the chest and place the hands onto the crown of the head. Lean back and roll through the spine on the first exhalation, keeping your spine and back of the neck rounded. Roll forwards to come back up to sitting on the next inhalation, keeping the hands and palms on the crown of the head. Roll clockwise, five to nine times, forwards (on an inhalation) and backwards (on an exhalation) along the spinal column. Coordinate the rolling movement and the breath so that you take the five breath minimum. Use the strength of the bandhas to control both the fall-back and lift-up movements. Gaze at the tip of the nose throughout.

10 Daśa
After the last exhalation and fall-back in the 9th vinyāsa, begin to inhale and, with the support of the bandhas, transfer the weight from the shoulders and come up directly into the next āsana: Kukkuṭāsana. Roll forwards with some speed and momentum, shifting your palms from the crown of the head and placing them on the floor with the fingers facing forwards. The whole body is lifted and balanced on top of the palms. This roll-up counts as the 10th vinyāsa in Garbha-piṇḍāsana and the balanced arm-lift position is the 8th vinyāsa in Kukkuṭāsana.

Beginners: This āsana requires much practice. Sliding the arms in between the calves and hamstrings, in particular, can be difficult in the beginning. Over time, this action relieves tension in the calves, making them more pliable.

- If the hips and knees are still too tight to come into lotus, cross the legs, take hold of the shins and draw the legs up to the chest.
- Coming into lotus and sliding the arms through can require more than one breath. Cross the legs into lotus and use as many breaths as you need to bring the arms through the lotus pose.
- Always place the right leg into lotus first, followed by the left, even if it feels as though it would be easier to switch legs.
- To help slide the arms through, you can moisten the arms and legs with plain/soapy water or oil.
- In the 8th vinyāsa, bring the hands up as close as possible to the head, aiming first at placing the palms onto the chin, then higher up towards the ears as the āsana progresses.
- When you roll along the spine, remain balanced along the spine with a rounded back. If you fall over to one side, keep the hands where they are and try to come up using the strength of the bandhas. This will develop the muscles you need in order to keep the balance as you roll.
- If you feel the bones of the spine digging into the floor, create an extra layer by folding your mat over or placing a cotton mat or towel over the yoga mat before starting Garbha-piṇḍāsana.

Vinyāsa	Prāṇa (breath)	Āsana (posture)	Dṛṣṭi (gazing point)	Bandha (muscle lock)
Samasthitiḥ		stand straight		
Vinyāsas 1–6 according to Sūrya-namaskāra A				
7 Sapta	in	jump through, legs out straight		
8 Aṣṭau	out	lotus pose, arms through, hands to ears		
state of the āsana, breathe five times				
9 Nava	out & in	roll around, exhale back, inhale up 5–9 times		
10 Daśa	in	come up, release arms, hands to floor, lift up		
11 Ekādaśa	out	catvāri position		
12 Dvādaśa	in	upward-facing dog		
13 Trayodaśa	out	downward-facing dog		
14 Caturdaśa	in	jump forward, stretch spine, head up		
15 Pañcadaśa	out	bend forwards		
Samasthitiḥ	in	stand straight		

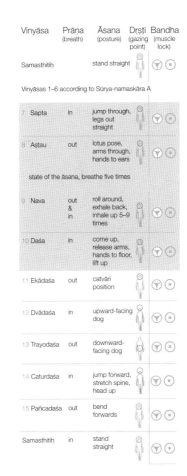

Kukkuṭāsana [rooster pose]

14 vinyāsas

Note 1:
Kukkuṭāsana is done in combination with the preceding āsana, Garbha-piṇḍāsana.

Note 2:
At the end of the 8th vinyāsa, you can also release the body with the last exhalation.

Vinyāsa	Prāṇa (breath)	Āsana (posture)	Dṛṣṭi (gazing point)	Bandha (muscle lock)
Samasthitiḥ		stand straight		
Vinyāsas 1–6 according to Sūrya-namaskāra A				
7 Sapta	in	jump through, straight legs		
8 Aṣṭau	out & in	lotus position, arms through, lift up		
state of the āsana; hold for 5 deep breaths				
9 Nava	in	lower down, take out arms, lift up		
10 Daśa	out	catvāri position		
11 Ekādaśa	in	upward-facing dog		
12 Dvādaśa	out	downward-facing dog		
13 Trayodaśa	in	jump forwards, stretch the spine, head up		
14 Chaturdaśa	out	bend forwards		
Samasthitiḥ	in	come up, stand straight		

Kukkuṭa – rooster; *āsana* – seat, posture

Kukkuṭāsana is done directly after the 10th vinyāsa in Garbha-piṇḍāsana.

8 Aṣṭau
After rolling forwards with an inhalation in Garbha-piṇḍāsana's 10th vinyāsa and balancing on the arms, continue lifting the legs up on the arms. Stabilize the body and hold the legs up high, preventing the knees from sliding down and touching the floor. Straighten the arms, and/or lengthen through the shoulders and back of the neck. Open the chest and lengthen the spine. Press the heels into both sides of the navel, massaging the abdomen. Release mūla-bandha. This is the state of the āsana. Stay here for five breaths and gaze at the tip of the nose.

Note: According to *Yoga Mala*, one does nauli here, one technique of the purification actions known as kriyās, which is done by creating wave-like motions in the stomach. This should be learned directly from a guru or an experienced teacher. Performing nauli with full force is not recommended for women, as it can damage the womb.

9 Nava
Inhale, release the body down to the floor and remove the hands, placing them on the floor beside the thighs (in practice, it is easier to release the body with the last exhalation of the 8th vinyāsa, but this is how Pattabhi Jois often counted the vinyāsa. In *Yoga Mala* this breath is an exhalation and is counted as part of the 8th vinyasa). Strengthen the arms, press the palms into the floor, and lift the body up off the floor with the legs still in lotus. Strongly engage mūla-bandha to help with the lift and uddīyana-bandha to support the chest and back. Lift the hips high to bring the legs through the arms into Padmāsana. Gaze at the tip of the nose.

10 Daśa
When the legs have passed through the arms, begin to exhale and release the lotus pose in the air. Straighten the legs out and land back in Catvāri. Gaze at the tip of the nose.

Vinyāsas 11 and 12 are the same as the 5th and 6th vinyāsas in Sūrya-namaskāra A. After the 12th vinyāsa, go directly to the next āsana, the 7th vinyāsa in Baddha-koṇāsana.

Beginners:
- If the hips and legs are too tight for lotus pose in the 8th vinyāsa, keep the legs crossed, place the hands on the floor and lift the hips (the feet can stay on the floor).
- If the legs do not stay in the air throughout the jump-back in the 9th vinyāsa, try to keep them lifted as long as you can. Undo the lotus pose, touch the feet to the floor and jump back, straightening the legs in the air on your way back to Catvāri. If the legs are not in lotus pose, jump back as in the 12th vinyāsa of Paścima-tānāsana.

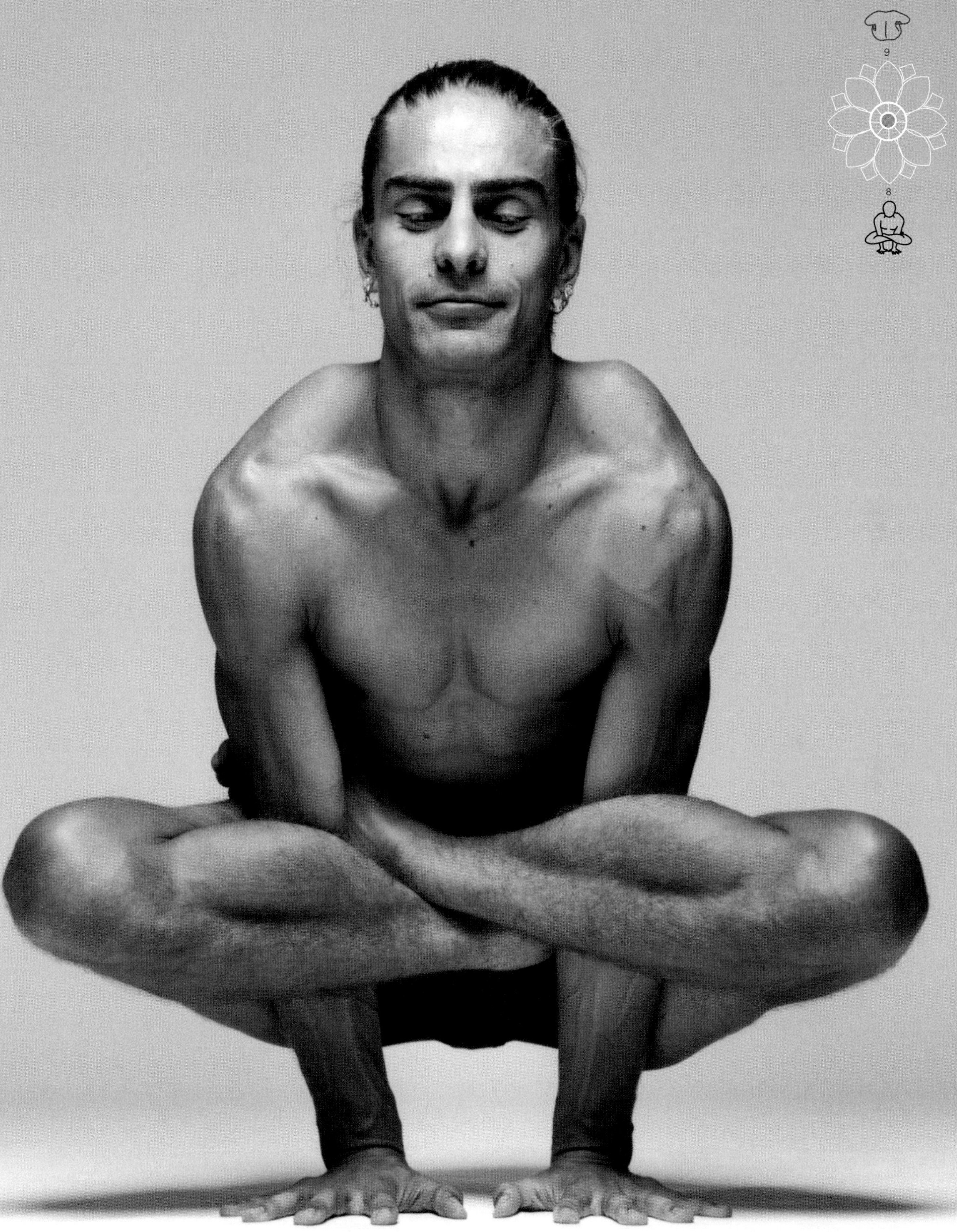
9
8

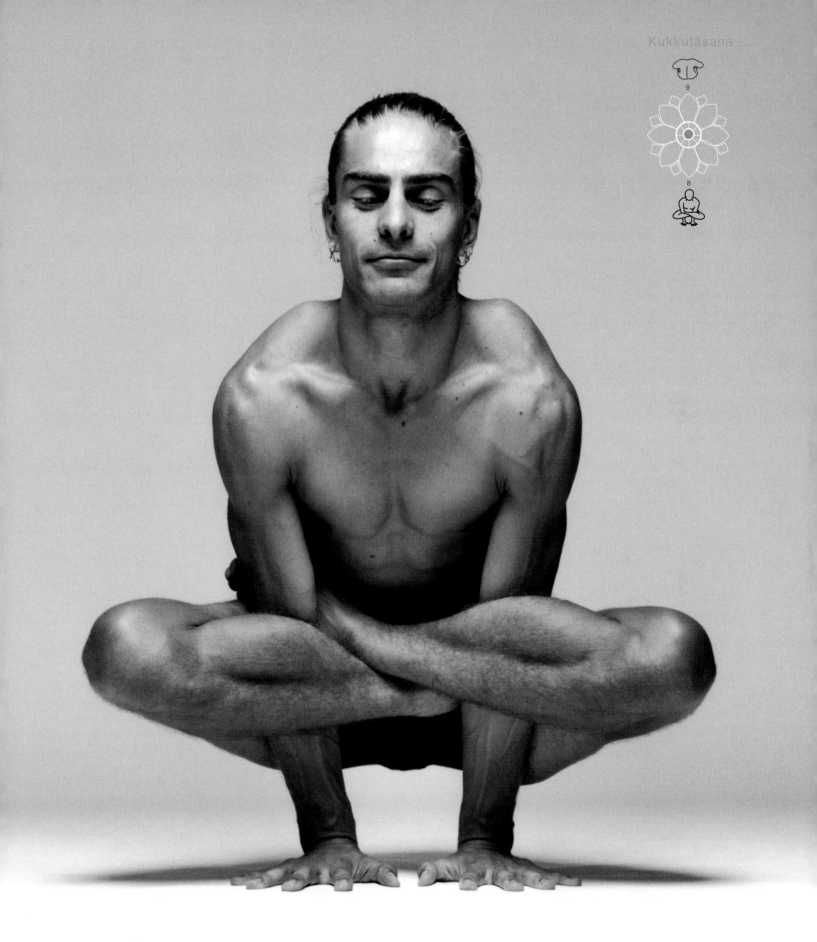

Baddha-koṇāsana

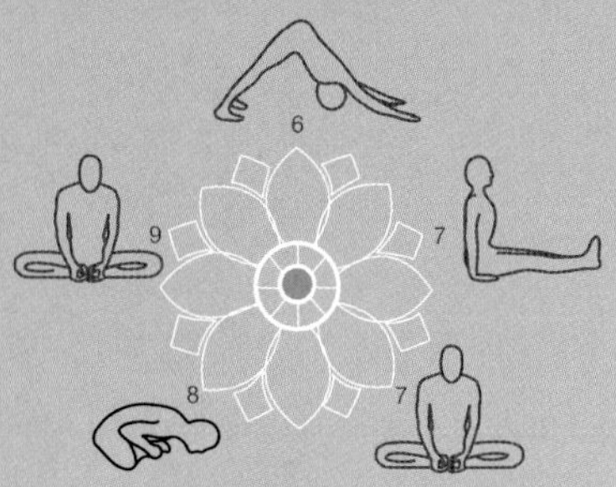

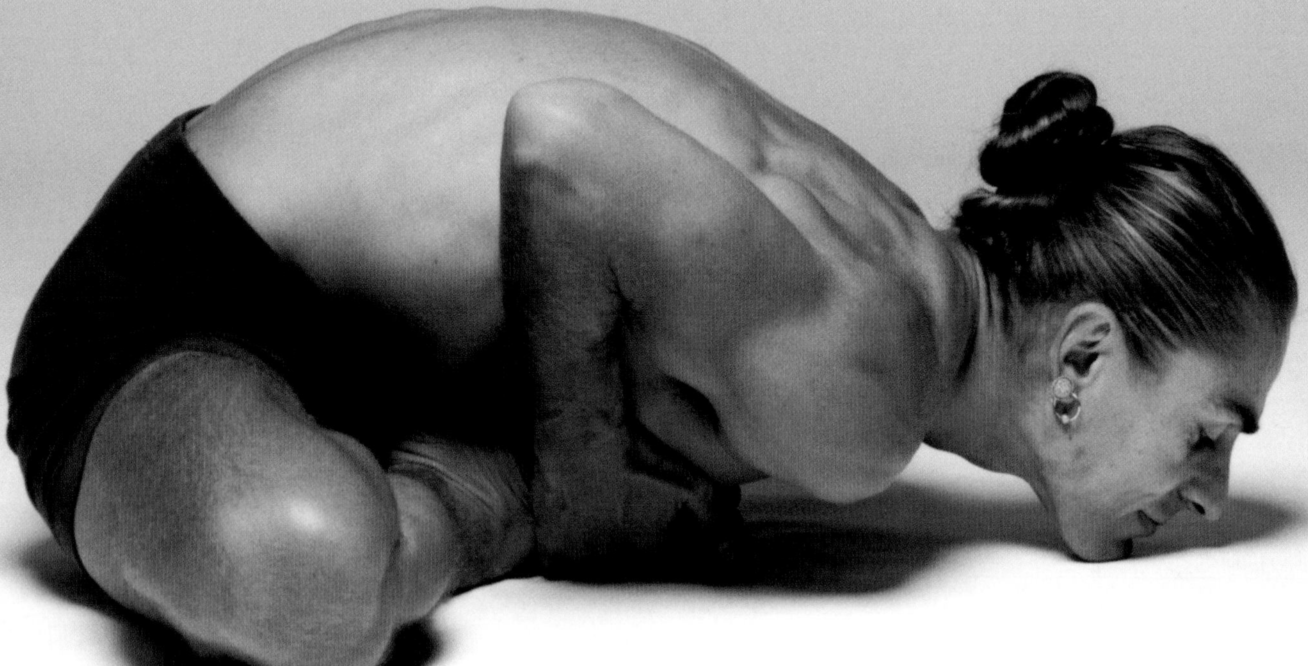

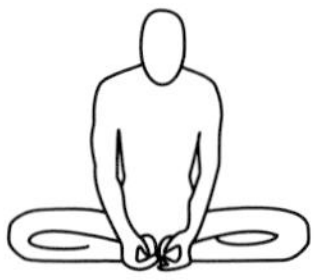

The 7th vinyāsa in
Baddha-koṇāsana

Baddha-koṇāsana *[bound angle pose]*

15 vinyāsas

Baddha – bound; *koṇa* – angle; *āsana* – seat, posture

Baddha-koṇāsana comes after the 12th vinyāsa in Kukkuṭāsana.

7 Sapta
Inhale and jump through to sitting. Bend the knees, draw the feet in towards the groin and lower the knees out to the sides. Take hold of the soles of the feet. Lean back slightly to pull the feet as close into the groin as possible. Straighten the back and open the feet. The soles of the feet open evenly, at a 90-degree angle, similar to a half-open book. Do not turn up the entire sole of the foot as the heels are then no longer able to be brought into śīvani-nāḍī (in the middle of the perineum muscle). The ability to open the hips up decreases as well if the soles of the feet are turned up too much. The outside edges stay pressed together, and the heels and balls of the feet do not overlap. Relax both hip joints deeply, pressing the knees into the floor with the help of the thigh muscles. Keep inhaling, lengthen the back, open the chest and lower the chin slightly. Engaging mūla-bandha will help open the hips, and engaging uddīyana-bandha will help expand the upper body. Gaze at the tip of the nose.

8 Aṣṭau
Exhale, extend through the spine and chest, fold forwards over the soles of the feet and place the chin on the floor. Keep pulling the heels in towards the groin as much as possible. Uddīyana-bandha helps keep the spine straight while mūla-bandha keeps the hips grounded and provides therapeutic benefits for the rectum. This is the state of the āsana. Breathe deeply five times. Relax the back of the neck and gaze at the tip of the nose.
From here, move into Baddha-koṇāsana B.
Inhale, come up briefly, as if to move into the state of the 7th vinyāsa. Then, round the back deeply and tilt the head down. Exhale, bring the crown of the head onto the toes or into the soles of the feet. Press the knees down to the floor and take five deep breaths. Gaze at the tip of the nose.
Note: Baddha-koṇāsana B is combined with Baddha-koṇāsana A. Pattabhi Jois didn't usually count a vinyāsa number for Baddha-koṇansana B. Instead, he instructed us to, "Inhale, straighten up (after the last exhalation in Baddha-koṇāsana A), exhale head down to Baddha-koṇāsana B." If you want to use the vinyāsa number for Baddha-koṇāsana B, it is also considered as the 8th vinyāsa.

9 Nava
Inhale, roll the back up and into the state of the 7th vinyāsa. Hold here and exhale slowly. Direct the gaze to the tip of the nose.

10 Daśa
Inhale and bring the hands to the floor on either side of the hips. Cross the ankles in the air and lift the knees into the chest. Continue with the inhalation and, engaging the bandhas and using the strength of the arms, lift the whole body up off the floor. Lift the hips up high, so the legs can begin to move back in between the arms. Gaze at the tip of the nose.

Vinyāsa 11 is the same as the 12th vinyāsa in Paścima-tānāsana.

Vinyāsas 12 and 13 are the same as the 5th and 6th vinyāsas in Sūrya-namaskāra A. After vinyāsa 13, move to the next āsana, the 7th vinyāsa in Upaviṣṭa-koṇāsana.

Beginners:
- Opening the feet out 90 degrees in the 8th vinyāsa will automatically guide the knees towards the floor, making the forward bend easier.
- If the knees do not touch the floor, use the elbows to press them down lightly as you bend forwards.
- First bring the crown of the head to the floor; over time, as you begin to open up in the pose, take the forehead, and eventually the chin, to the floor.
- It is beneficial to sit for five to ten breaths in the 9th vinyāsa instead of two breaths, to release the hips even further.

Note 1:
There are two āsanas in the 8th vinyāsa, Baddha-koṇāsana A & B.

Note 2:
There are two breaths in the 9th vinyāsa.

Vinyāsa	Prāṇa (breath)	Āsana (posture)	Dṛṣṭi (gazing point)	Bandha (muscle lock)
Samasthitiḥ		stand straight		
Vinyāsas 1–6 according to Sūrya-namaskāra A				
7 Sapta	in	jump through to sitting, feet together		
8 Aṣṭau	out	head to floor		
state of the Baddha-konāsna A; hold for 5 deep breaths				
	in	come up		
	out	round the back, head to toes		
state of the Baddha-konāasna B; hold for 5 deep breaths				
9 Nava	in & out	come up, hold the pose		
10 Daśa	in	hands to floor, lift up		
11 Ekādaśa	out	catvāri position		
12 Dvādaśa	in	upward-facing dog		
13 Trayodaśa	out	downward-facing dog		
14 Caturdaśa	in	jump forwards, stretch spine, head up		
15 Pañcadaśa	out	bend forwards		
Samasthitiḥ		come up, stand straight		

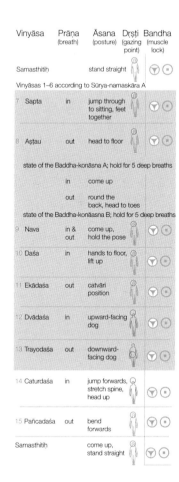

Upaviṣṭa-koṇāsana *[seated angle pose]*

15 vinyāsas

Note 1:
The gaze can also be at the tip of the nose in the 8th vinyāsa.

Note 2:
There are three breaths in the 9th vinyāsa.

Vinyāsa	Prāṇa (breath)	Āsana (posture)	Dṛṣṭi (gazing point)	Bandha (muscle lock)
Samasthitiḥ		stand straight		
Vinyāsas 1–6 according to Sūrya-namaskāra A				
7 Sapta	in	jump to sitting, open the legs, hold the feet, head up		
8 Aṣṭau	out	head to floor		
first state of the āsana; hold for 5 deep breaths				
9 Nava	in & out & in	stretch out, head up, hold the pose, lift up to balance		
second state of the asana; hold for 5 deep breaths				
10 Daśa	in	hands to floor, lift up		
11 Ekādaśa	out	catvāri position		
12 Dvādaśa	in	upward-facing dog		
13 Trayodaśa	out	downward-facing dog		
14 Caturdaśa	in	jump forwards, stretch spine, head up		
15 Pañcadaśa	out	bend forwards		
Samasthitiḥ	in	come up, stand straight		

Upaviṣṭa – seated, sitting; *koṇa* – angle; *āsana* – seat, posture

Upaviṣṭa-koṇāsana comes after the 13th vinyāsa in Baddha-koṇāsana.

7 Sapta
Inhale and jump through to sitting, keeping the feet lifted. Separate the legs as widely as possible while still being able to take hold of the outside edges of the feet. Flex the feet, straighten the arms, pull back slightly on the feet and open the chest. Lift the head and gaze at the tip of the nose.

8 Aṣṭau
Exhale, strongly engage uḍḍīyana-bandha to expand the chest and back as you lift mūla-bandha to ground the hips. Fold the upper body forwards, in between the legs, lowering the chin and chest onto the floor. Keep stretching the legs with the thighs engaged and the toes pointing up. This is the first state of the āsana. Stay here for five breaths and gaze in between the eyebrows.

9 Nava
Inhale, come back up to the position of the 7th vinyāsa (head up, back and arms straight), gazing at the tip of the nose. Exhale and hold the pose.
Inhale and while keeping a firm grip on the feet, lift the whole body up to balance on the sitting-bones. You can come up with bent knees or straight legs. Straighten the legs completely once you are balanced. This is the same position as in the 8th vinyāsa, except that now your legs and body are angled up to the ceiling. Point the feet and tilt the head back. Elongate the spine upwards, expand the chest, and engage the bandhas to help with the balance. Do not separate the legs any wider than they were in the first state of the āsana. This is the second state of the āsana. Stay here for five breaths and gaze upwards.

Note: The second position in Upaviṣṭa-koṇāsana is part of the āsana. It could be called Upaviṣṭa-koṇāsana B, but it never had its own name. The vinyāsa number (9th) is also the same as in the first position, even though Pattabhi Jois didn't usually count the number during led class. Often, the transition between the first and second position has been counted as the 10th vinyāsa, which would change this āsana's final vinyāsa number to 16. This was not what Pattabhi Jois wanted to do.

Vinyāsas 10 and 11 are the same as the 10th and 11th vinyāsas in Baddha-koṇāsana.

Vinyāsas 12 and 13 are the same as the 5th and 6th vinyāsas in Sūrya-namaskāra A. After vinyāsa 13, move to the next āsana, the 7th vinyāsa in Supta-koṇāsana.

Beginners:

- First bring the forehead to the floor in the 8th vinyāsa. As you begin to release into the pose over time, move the chin, shoulders, and eventually the chest onto the floor.
- When you lift the legs up in the second part of the pose, the feet can be held throughout. A second option is to release the feet, lift the legs up and then take hold of the feet once you are balanced on the sitting-bones.

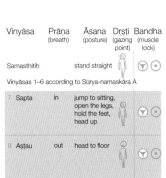

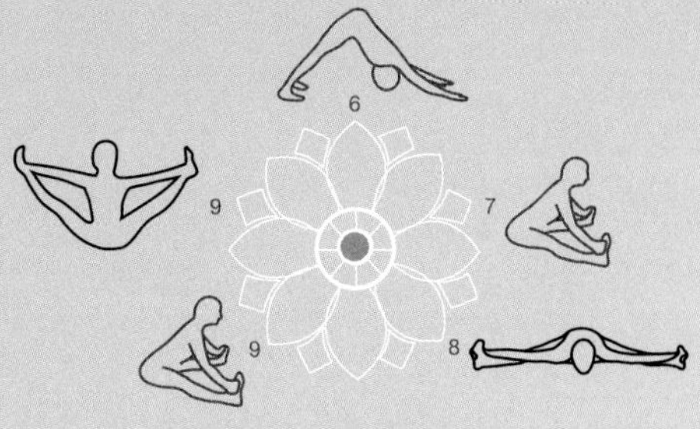

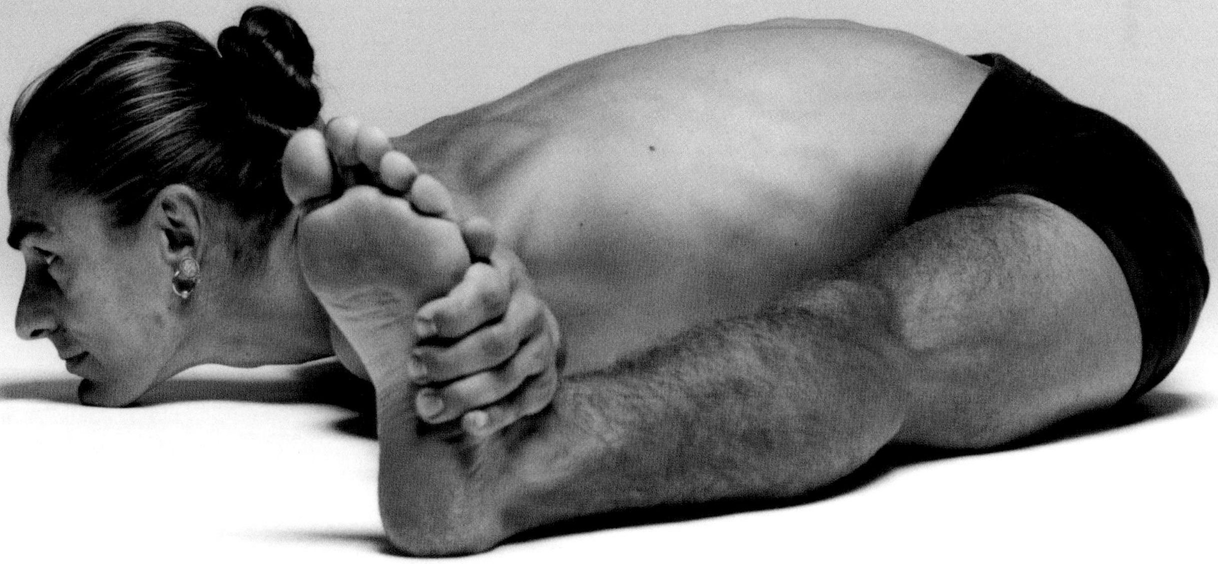

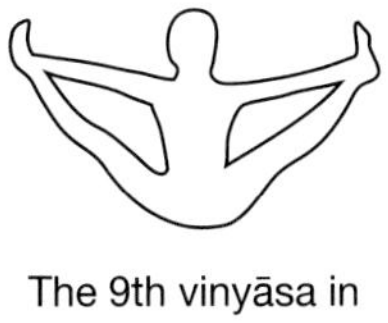

The 9th vinyāsa in
Upaviṣṭa-koṇāsana

Supta-koṇāsana

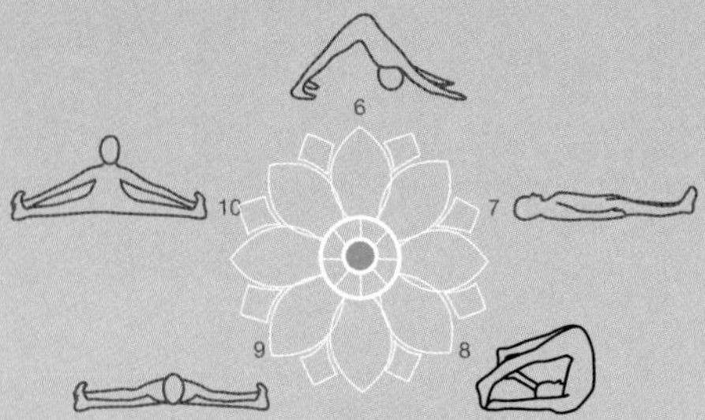

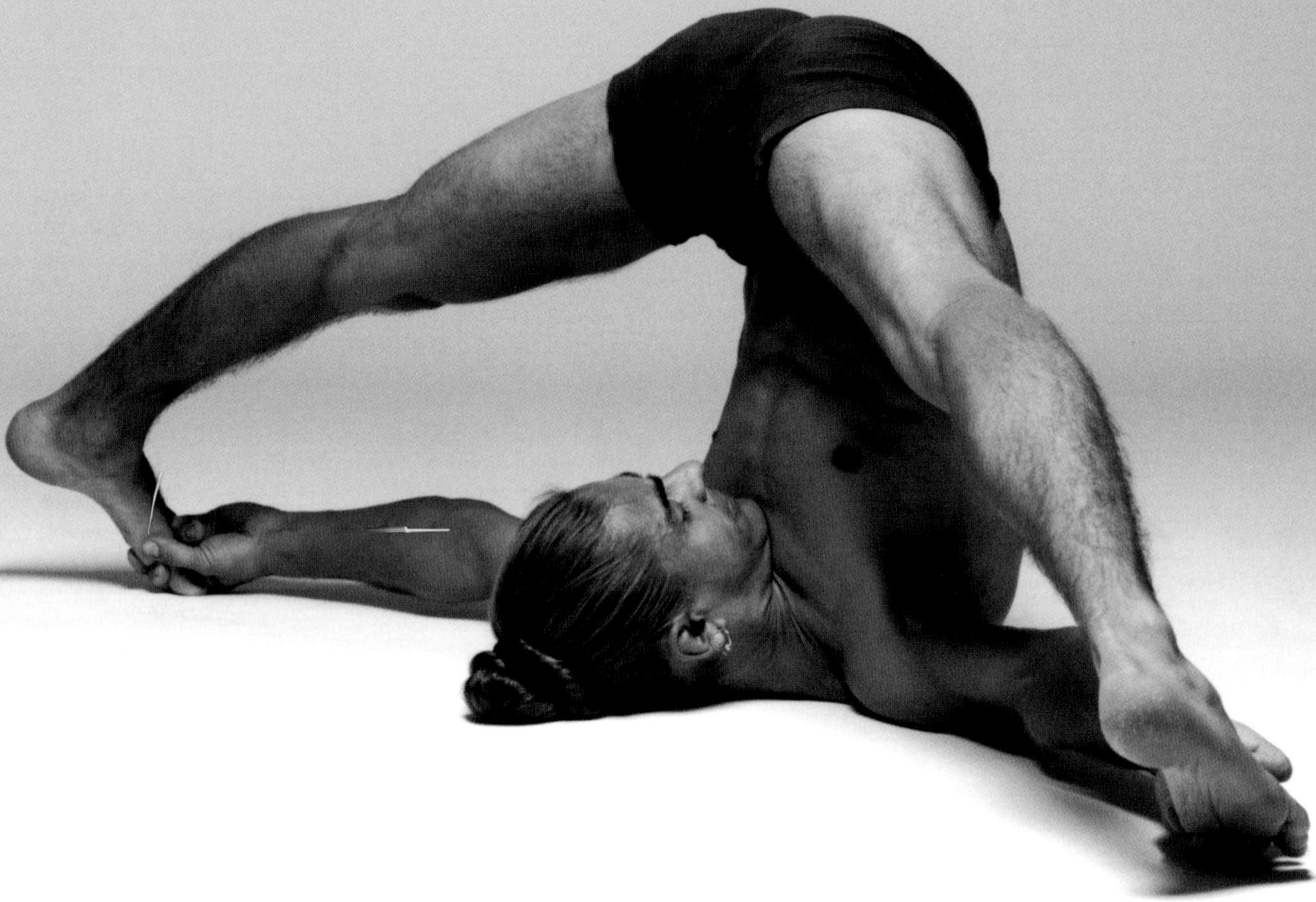

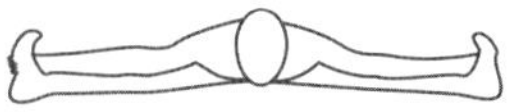

The 9th vinyāsa in Supta-koṇāsana

Supta-koṇāsana [sleeping angle pose]

16 vinyāsas

Supta – reclining, sleeping, lying down; *koṇa* – angle; *āsana* – seat, posture

Supta-koṇāsana comes after the 13th vinyāsa in Upaviṣṭa-koṇāsana.

7 Sapta
Inhale, jump through to sitting. Continue with the inhalation, engage uddīyana-bandha, roll down the back and come to lie down with straight legs. Press the palms into the floor, by the thighs, expand the chest and lengthen the spine along the mat. Gaze at the tip of the nose and exhale here.

8 Aṣṭau
Inhale, press the palms down, engage the bandhas, and lift the hips up off the floor, taking the legs up and over the body. Lower the legs to the floor, and spread them apart, taking hold of the big toes with the first two fingers and thumb. The arms are straight and the weight of the body rests on the shoulders. The chin moves in towards the collarbones, and the stomach pulls lightly inward. Do not hold uddīyana-bandha here, as it can restrict blood circulation. Keep the feet flexed with the heels pointing straight up. This is the state of the āsana. Stay here for five deep breaths and gaze at the tip of the nose.

9 Nava
Inhale, lean the body slightly back, keep a firm grip on the big toes with straight arms, and push the feet off the floor, rolling forwards on a rounded spine. To gain some momentum, nudge the back and the back of the head just before they leave the floor. With the help of the bandhas, the strength of the upper body and the rhythm of the breathing, come up to balance on the sitting-bones for the remainder of the inhalation. This balance is a transition; do not stay here for any additional breaths. Instead, slowly fall forwards and down on the next exhalation. Flex the feet and pull the toes enough towards you that the calves touch the ground first, followed by the heels. Straighten the spine and, in the deep forward bend, open the chest and push the chin and chest onto the floor. Engage the thighs and keep flexing the feet to stretch the calves, hamstrings and hips. Gaze in between the eyebrows.

10 Daśa
Inhale, straighten the arms, pulling back slightly on the feet; open the chest, straighten the back, and lift the head. Stay here for an exhalation. Gaze at the tip of the nose.

Vinyāsas 11 and 12 are the same as the 10th and 11th vinyāsas in Baddha-koṇāsana.

Vinyāsas 13 and 14 are the same as the 5th and 6th vinyāsas in Sūrya-namaskāra A. After vinyāsa 14, move into the next āsana, the 7th vinyāsa in Supta-pādāṅguṣṭhāsana.

Beginners: Rolling up and down with control requires practice.
- Separate the legs only as wide as you can while still being able to hold the big toes.
- Keep the spine rounded by pressing the chin into the chest as you roll up.
- Pulling firmly on the big toes will help get the calves onto the floor before the heels.
- When you bend forwards at the end of the āsana, begin by bringing the forehead to the floor. As you gain flexibility, move the chin and chest onto the floor.

Note 1:
There are two breaths in the 7th, 9th and 10th vinyāsas.

Note 2:
The second option for the dṛṣṭi in the 9th vinyāsa is the tip of the nose.

Vinyāsa	Prāṇa (breath)	Āsana (posture)	Dṛṣṭi (gazing point)	Bandha (muscle lock)
Samasthitiḥ		stand straight		
Vinyāsas 1–6 according to Sūrya-namaskāra A				
7 Sapta	in & out	jump to sitting, lie on the back, hold position		
8 Aṣṭau	in	legs back and wide, take hold of toes		— —
state of the āsana; hold for 5 deep breaths				
9 Nava	in & out	roll up, hold toes, come up, bend forward		
10 Daśa	in & out	stretch out, head up, hold the pose		
11 Ekādaśa	in	hands to floor, lift up		
12 Dvādaśa	out	catvāri position		
13 Trayodaśa	in	upward-facing dog		
14 Caturdaśa	out	downward-facing dog		
15 Pañcadaśa	in	jump forwards, stretch spine, head up		
16 Ṣoḍaśa	out	bend forwards		
Samasthitiḥ	in	come up, stand straight		

Note 1:
There are two breaths in the 7th and 24th vinyāsas.

Note 2:
Supta-pādāṅguṣṭhāsana has two parts. It is combined with Supta-pārśva-sahita. The vinyāsas are counted according Supta-pārśva-sahita.

Vinyāsa	Prāṇa (breath)	Āsana (posture)	Dṛṣṭi (gazing point)	Bandha (muscle lock)
Samasthitiḥ		stand straight		
Vinyāsas 1–6 according to Sūrya-namaskāra A				
7 Sapta	in & out	jump through, lie down, hold the pose		
Right side				
8 Aṣṭau	in	left hand to thigh, right leg up, bind the big toe		
9 Nava	out	bring the chin to the shin		
state of Supta-pādāṅguṣṭhāsana; hold for 5 deep breaths				
10 Daśa	in	stretch out, head to floor		
11 Ekādaśa	out	leg to the right, look left		
state of Supta-pārśva-sahita; hold for 5 deep breaths				
12 Dvādaśa	in	leg back up		
13 Trayodaśa	out	chin to the shin		
14 Caturdaśa	in	head to floor, hold big toe		
15 Pañcadaśa	out	lower the leg and arm		
Left side				
16 Ṣoḍaśa	in	right hand to thigh, left leg up, bind the big toe		
17 Saptadaśa	out	bring the chin to the shin		
state of Supta-pādāṅguṣṭhāsana; hold for 5 deep breaths				
18 Aṣṭadaśa	in	stretch out, head to floor		
19 Ekoṇa-viṃśatiḥ	out	leg to the left, look right		
state of Supta-pārśva-sahita; hold for 5 deep breaths				
20 Viṃśatiḥ	in	leg back up		
21 Ekaviṃśatiḥ	out	chin to the shin		
22 Dvaviṃśatiḥ	in	head to floor, hold toe		

Supta-pādāṅguṣṭhāsana & Supta-pārśva-sahita

[sleeping big toe pose & following sleeping side pose]

28 vinyāsas

Supta – reclining, sleeping, lying down; *pāda* – leg; *aṅguṣṭha* – big toe; *āsana* – seat, posture; *pārśva* – side; *sahita* – fill in, together, to be with, to follow

Supta-pādāṅguṣṭhāsana comes after the 14th vinyāsa in Supta-koṇāsana.

7 Sapta
Inhale, jump through to sitting. Continue with the inhalation as you engage uddīyana-bandha and, with the legs straight together, roll the back slowly down to the floor. Press the palms into the floor next to the thighs, expand the chest and lengthen the whole body along the mat. Gaze at the tip of the nose and exhale here.

8 Aṣṭau
Inhale and place the left hand on the left thigh, keeping the hip and leg down. Lift the right arm directly overhead. Gaze for a moment at the right hand and lift the right leg up to take hold of the big toe with the first two fingers and thumb (keeping the head on the floor). Firmly hook the right big toe by pressing it slightly forwards and gaze at the big toe.

9 Nava
Exhale, and keeping a firm grip on the right big toe, engage the bandhas as you lift the upper body towards the right leg. Flex the right foot, touching the chin to the shin. The left leg stays actively engaged into the floor, with the foot pointed. This is the state of the āsana on the right side of Supta-pādāṅguṣṭhāsana. Breathe deeply five times. Gaze at the right big toe.

10 Daśa
Inhale, lower the head back to the floor, to the same position as the 8th vinyāsa, and gaze at the big toe.

11 Ekādaśa
Exhale and open the right leg out to the side, turning the head to look over the left shoulder. Lower the right leg so the foot and heel touch the floor. Keep both hips firmly on the floor by engaging the left thigh and mūla-bandha. Engage uddīyana-bandha to stretch the chest, press the back into the floor and strengthen the muscles of the upper body. Open the hips, keeping both legs and the right arm straight. Relax the shoulders and ground them onto the floor. This is the state of Supta-pārśva-sahita. Breathe deeply five times and gaze to the left side.

12 Dvādaśa
Inhale, bring the head and right leg back up to the center, as in the 8th vinyāsa. Use the same muscle control to lift the leg up as when you lowered it out to the side. Gaze at the big toe.

13 Trayodaśa
Exhale, keep a firm grip on the right big toe, engage the bandhas and bring the chin up to meet the right shin. The left leg stays firmly on the floor with the foot pointed. Gaze at the big toe.

14 Caturdaśa
Inhale, lower the back and head onto the floor while keeping hold of (and gazing at) the big toe.

15 Pañcadaśa
Exhale, release the big toe, and lower the right leg and arm straight down. This is the same position as in the 7th vinyāsa. Gaze at the tip of the nose.

Left side: Repeat vinyāsas 8–15 but on the left side, counting them as vinyāsas 16–23.

Vinyāsa 17 is the state of the left side of Supta-pādāṅguṣṭhāsana. Breathe deeply five times.

Vinyāsa 19 is the state of Supta-pārśva-sahita. Breathe deeply five times.

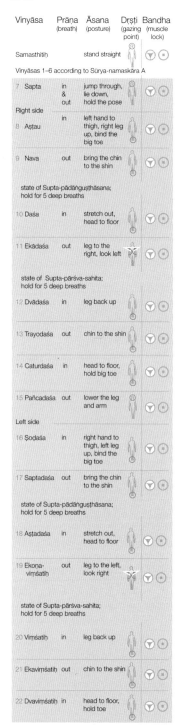

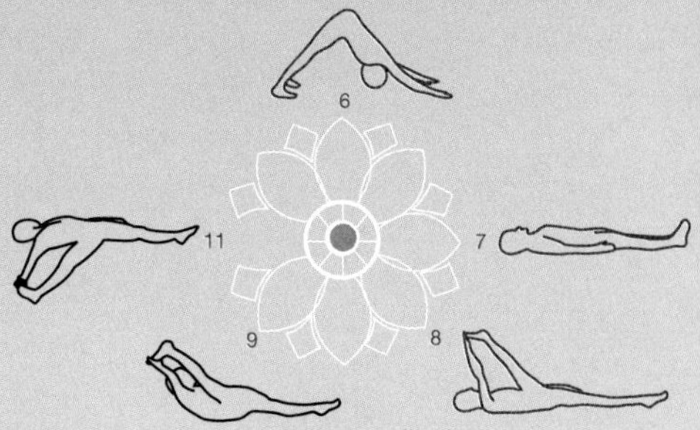

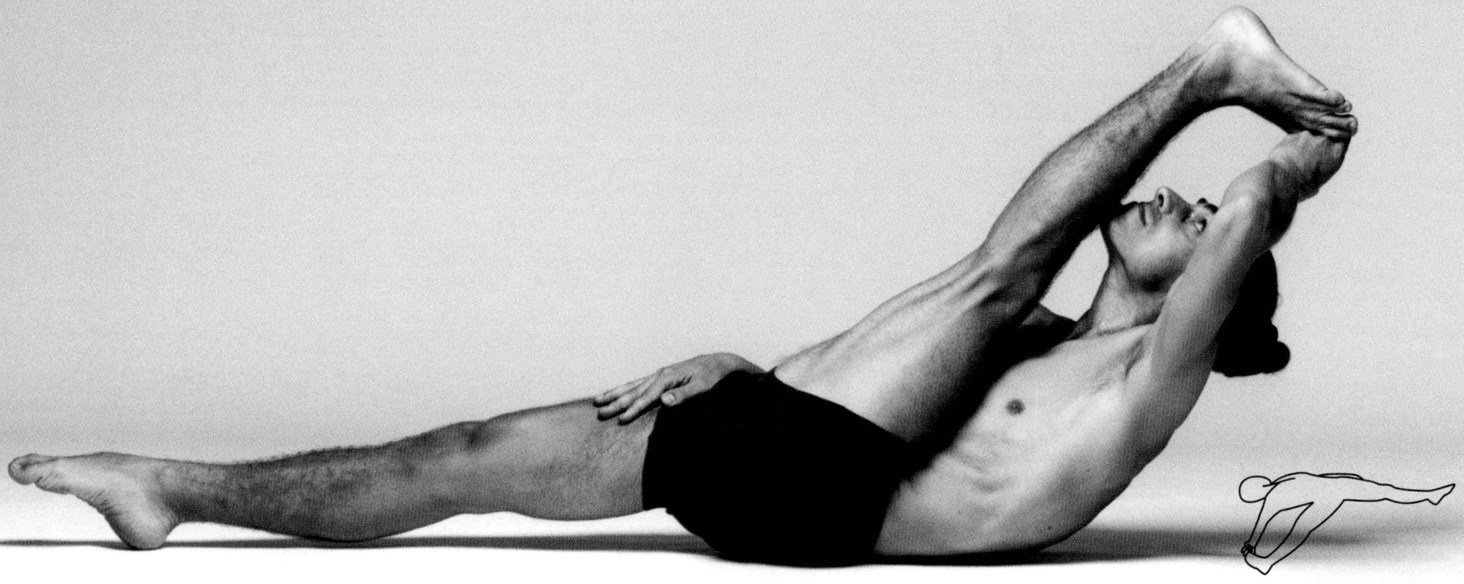

The 11th vinyāsa in Supta-pārśva-sahita

24 Caturviṃśatiḥ
Inhale, press the palms into the floor beside the thighs, and lift the legs up. Strongly engage uddīyana-bandha, bringing the legs up and over and touching the feet to the floor. Move the hands from the sides of the thighs to the ears, and press them into the floor. Push with the strength of the arms to roll over the spine, back of the neck and the head. If the legs are bent, straighten them behind you as you move through the roll. Take the weight of the body into the arms and lift the head up from the floor. Begin an exhalation as you continue the backwards-roll into Catvāri. This backwards-roll is called Cakrāsana (cakra - circle, wheel).

Vinyāsas 25 and 26 are the same as the 5th and 6th vinyāsas in Sūrya-namaskāra A. After vinyāsa 26, move to the next āsana, the 7th vinyāsa in Ubhaya-pādāṅguṣṭhāsana.

Beginners:
- Start by bringing the forehead towards the knee and looking at the tip of the nose in the 9th vinyāsa. Later on, touch the chin to the shin and look at the big toe.
- When you take the leg to the side in the 11th and 19th vinyāsas, try to keep the hips evenly on the floor. Avoid tilting to the side in order to get the leg further down.
- Try to do the backwards roll in the 24th vinyāsa in a straight line, with both palms on the floor.
- If you have back or neck problems, instead of doing Cakrāsana as described in the 24th vinyāsa, sit up, cross the legs and jump back, like in the 11th vinyāsa in Paścima-tānāsana.
- Those with back or neck problems should consult a doctor or an experienced teacher before attempting the backwards roll (Cakrāsana).

23 Trayo-viṃśati	out	lower the leg and arm		
24 Catur-viṃśati	in & out	cakrāsana, backwards roll, catvāri position		
25 Pañca-viṃśatiḥ	in	upward-facing dog		
26 Ṣoḍa-viṃśatiḥ	out	downward-facing dog		
27 Sapta-viṃśatiḥ	in	jump forwards, stretch spine, head up		
28 Aṣṭa-viṃśatiḥ	out	bend forwards		
Samasthitiḥ	in	come up, stand straight		

Note:
There are two breaths in the 7th and 8th vinyāsas.

Vinyāsa	Prāṇa (breath)	Āsana (posture)	Dṛṣṭi (gazing point)	Bandha (muscle lock)
Samasthitiḥ		stand straight		
Vinyāsas 1–6 according to Sūrya-namaskāra A				
7 Sapta	in & out	jump through, lie down, hold the pose		
8 Aṣṭau	in & out	take legs over the head grab big toes		
9 Nava	in	roll up, hold the position		
state of the āsana; hold for 5 deep breaths				
10 Daśa	in	hands to floor, lift up		
11 Ekādaśa	out	catvāri position		
12 Dvādaśa	in	upward-facing dog		
13 Trayodaśa	out	downward-facing dog		
14 Caturaśa	in	jump forwards, stretch spine, head up		
15 Pañcadaśa	out	bend forwards		
Samasthitiḥ	in	come up, stand straight		

Ubhaya-pādāṅguṣṭhāsana [both big toes pose]

15 vinyāsas

Ubhaya – both; *pāda* – foot; *aṅguṣṭha* – big toe; *āsana* – seat, posture

Ubhaya-pādāṅguṣṭhāsana comes after the 26th vinyāsa in Supta-pādāṅguṣṭhāsana.

7 Sapta
Inhale, jump through to sitting. Continuing with the inhalation, press the hands onto the floor by the thighs, and lie down, keeping the legs together. Gaze at the tip of the nose and exhale here.

8 Aṣṭau
Inhale, press the hands to the floor, engage the bandhas, and lift the legs, hips and back straight up off the floor. Lower the legs onto the floor behind you, keeping them straight together. Take hold of the big toes with the first two fingers and thumb. Stay here for a deep exhalation. Gaze at the tip of the nose.

9 Nava
Inhale, round the spine and keep a firm grip on the big toes with straight arms as you roll up to balance on the sitting bones. Use the bandhas, the strength of the upper body, and the rhythm of the breath to control the momentum and balance the body in an upright position. The muscles in the back of the neck, throat and torso are all activated in order to maintain balance. Straighten out the spine and broaden the chest. Draw the shoulders back and down. Keep a firm grip on the big toes, straighten the legs, point the feet and release the head back. This is the state of the āsana. Breathe here five times and gaze upwards.

Vinyāsas 10 and 11 are the same as the 10th and 11th vinyāsa in Baddha-koṇāsana.

Vinyāsas 12 and 13 are the same as the 5th and 6th vinyāsas in Sūrya-namaskāra A. After vinyāsa 13, move to the next āsana, the 7th vinyāsa in Ūrdhva-mukha-paścimottānāsana.

Beginners: Rolling up to balance in the state of the āsana requires some practice.
- The key to finding balance in this pose requires control of the bandhas and proper alignment of the spine and chest.
- Pointing the feet can be difficult at first. Do as much as you can while keeping the legs straight.
- Try to synchronize the movement with the breath as you roll over the spine. Keep the knees slightly bent if you need to.

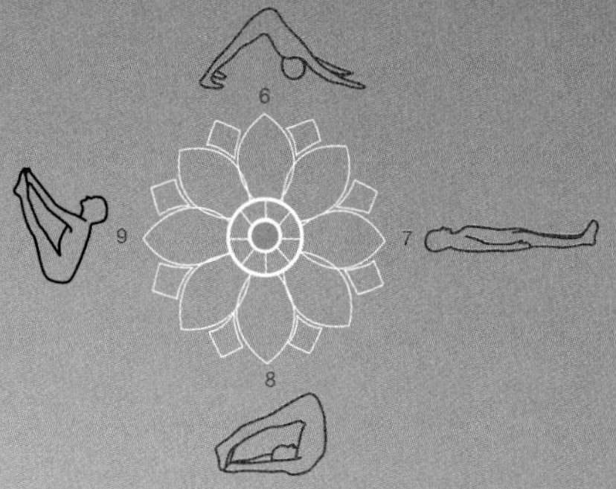

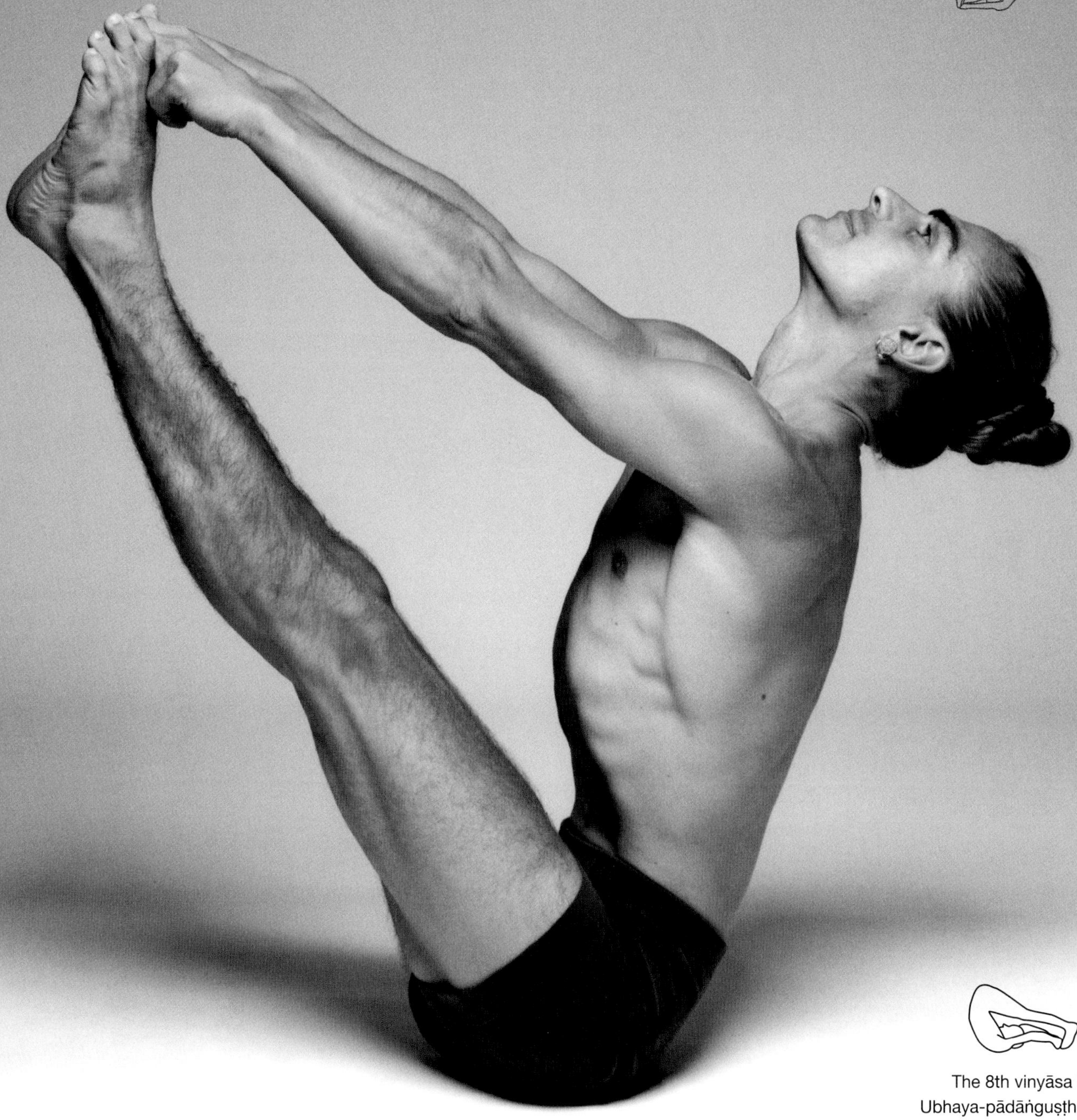

The 8th vinyāsa in
Ubhaya-pādāṅguṣṭhāsana

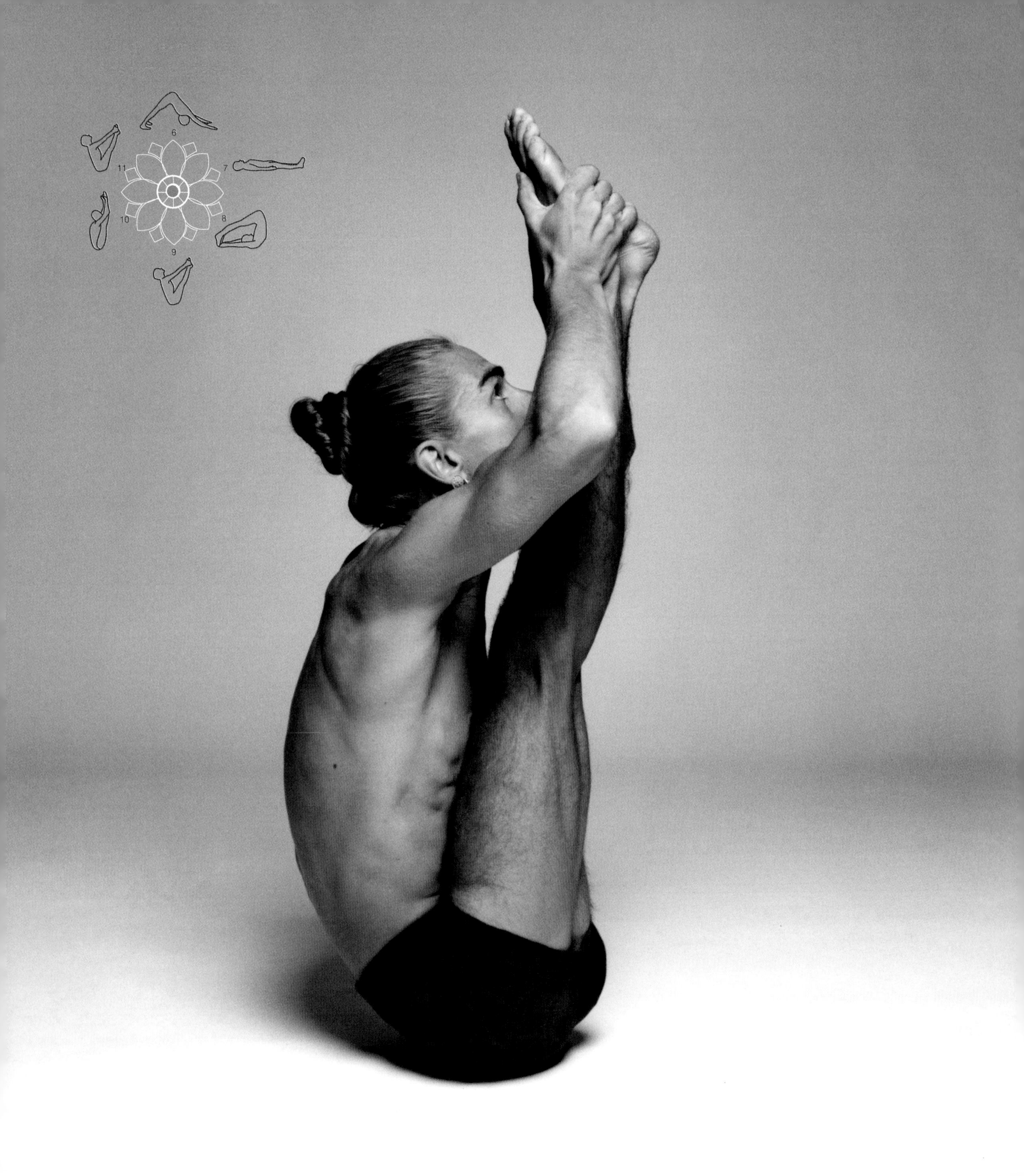
6
7
8
9
10
11

Ūrdhva-mukha-paścimottānāsana

[upward-facing forward stretch pose]

17 vinyāsas

Ūrdhva – upwards; *mukha* – facing, mouth; *paścima* – western, backside of the body, back; *ut* – deep, strong, intense; *tāna* – stretch, extend, lengthen; *āsana* – seat, posture

Ūrdhva-mukha-paścimottānāsana comes directly after the 13th vinyāsa in Ubhaya-pādāṅguṣṭhāsana.

Vinyāsas 7–9 are the same as vinyāsas 7–9 in Ubhaya-pādāṅguṣṭhāsana with the exception that, in this āsana, you take hold of the outside edge of the feet instead of the big toes. After rolling up, continue onto the 10th vinyāsa.

10 Daśa
Exhale, engage mūla-bandha so that the hips stay grounded. Hold uddīyana-bandha to straighten the spine, widen the chest and lengthen the entire body. Pull firmly on the feet to keep the balance and counter the upwards movement. Fold the chest forwards into the thighs, keeping the legs straight. Touch the chin to the shins, point the feet and hold the balance. This is the state of the āsana. Breathe deeply five times. Gaze up at the toes.

11 Ekādaśa
Inhale, stretch the arms and return to the position of the 9th vinyāsa. Hold the pose, release the head back, gaze upwards and and exhale deeply.

Vinyāsas 12 and 13 are the same as the 10th and 11th vinyāsas in Baddha-koṇāsana.

Vinyāsas 14 and 15 are the same as the 5th and 6th vinyāsas in Sūrya-namaskāra A. After vinyāsa 15, go directly to the next āsana, the 7th vinyāsa in Setu-bandhāsana.

Beginners: Holding the balance in this āsana with a straight body and straight legs requires a good deal of practice.

- Pointing the feet can be difficult at first. Do as much as you can while keeping the legs straight.
- First touch the nose or forehead to the knees and gaze at the tip of the nose. As you gain more flexibility and strength, bring the chin up to the shins and gaze at the toes.
- Try to synchronize the movement with the breath as you roll over the spine; if need be, keep the knees slightly bent in the 8th and 9th vinyāsas.

Note 1:
There are two breaths in the 7th, 8th and 11th vinyāsas.

Note 2:
According to Pattabhi Jois, Paścimottanāsana is written with the letter "o" in this āsana.

Vinyāsa	Prāṇa (breath)	Āsana (posture)	Dṛṣṭi (gazing point)	Bandha (muscle lock)
Samasthitiḥ		stand straight		
Vinyāsas 1–6 according to Sūrya-namaskāra A				
7 Sapta	in & out	jump through, lie down, hold the pose		
8 Aṣṭau	in & out	take legs over head, hold outside edge of feet		
9 Nava	in	roll up, look up		
10 Daśa	out	bring the chin to the shins, look to toes		
state of the āsana; hold for 8–10 deep breaths				
11 Ekādaśa	in & out	straighten arms, head up, hold the pose		
12 Dvādaśa	in	hands on the floor, lift up		
13 Trayodaśa	out	catvāri position		
14 Caturaśa	in	upward-facing dog		
15 Pañcadaśa	out	downward-facing dog		
16 Ṣoḍaśa	in	jump forwards, stretch spine, head up		
17 Saptadaśa	out	bend forwards		
Samasthitiḥ	in	come up, stand straight		

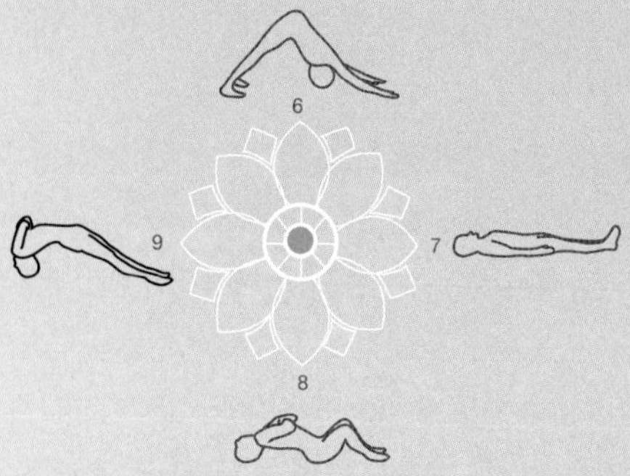

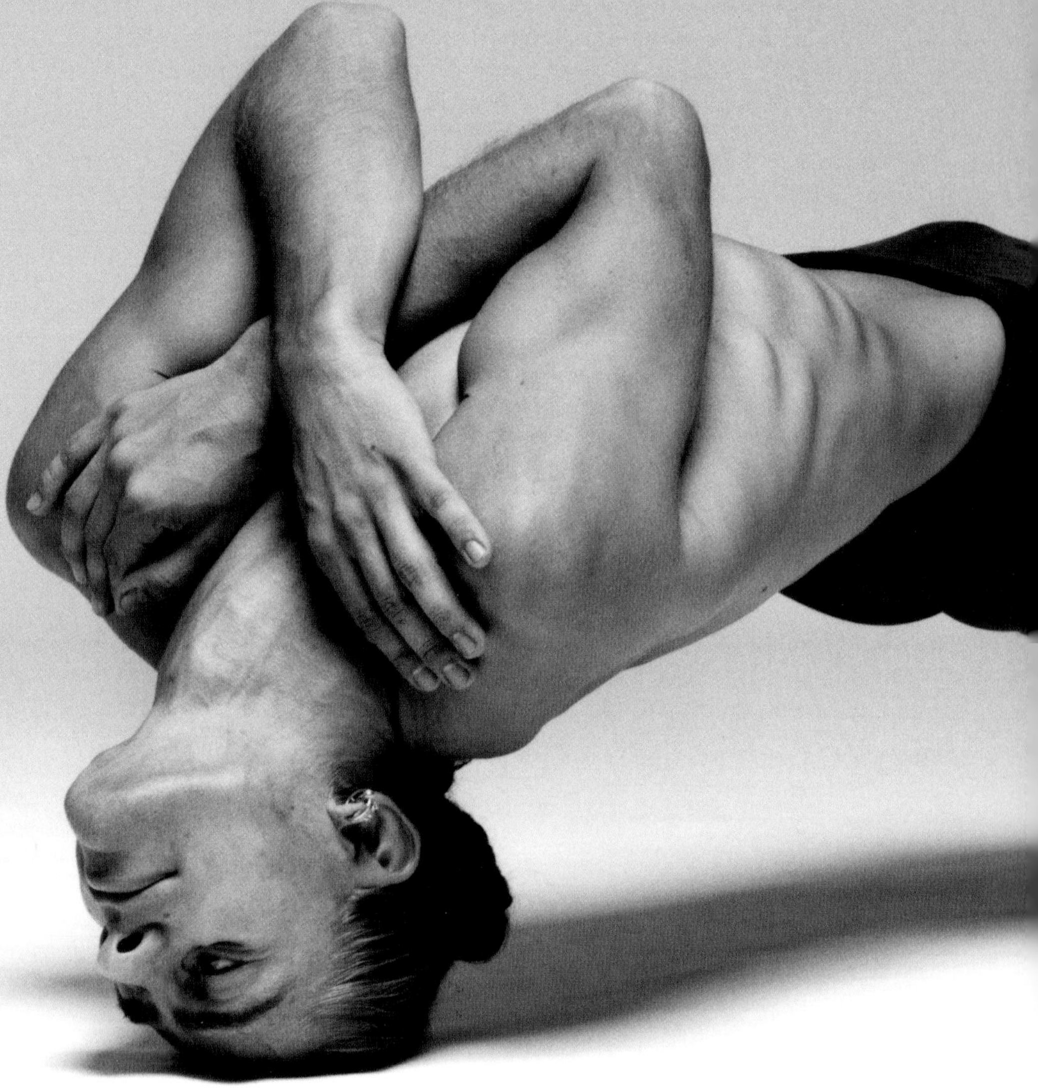

Vinyāsa	Prāṇa (breath)	Āsana (posture)	Dṛṣṭi (gazing point)	Bandha (muscle lock)
Samasthitiḥ		stand straight		
Vinyāsas 1–6 according to Sūrya-namaskāra A				
7 Sapta	in & out	jump through, lie down, hold the pose		
8 Aṣṭau	in & out	arrange the feet, chest, head and arms		
9 Nava	in	lift up to bridge		
state of the āsana; hold for 5 deep breaths				
10 Daśa	out	lie on the back		

Setu-bandhāsana *[sealed bridge pose]*

15 vinyāsas

Setu – bridge; *bandha* – bound, closed with a seal; *āsana* – seat, posture

Setu-bandhāsana comes after the 15th vinyāsa in Ūrdhva-mukha-paścimottānāsana.

7 Sapta
Inhale, jump through to sitting. On the same inhalation, slowly roll down onto the floor with the legs together. Press the palms into the floor by the thighs, expand the chest and lengthen the body along the mat. Gaze at the tip of the nose and exhale here.

8 Aṣṭau
Inhale, bend the knees and bring the heels together, making a diamond shape with the legs and a V shape with the feet. Press the outside edges of the feet into the floor, and keep the feet a good distance away from the groin. Exhale, press the elbows into the floor and lift the chest up so you can arch the back into a bridge. Lift and lean the head back slightly, placing the crown of the head on the floor. Place the arms across the chest, opposite palms over opposite shoulders, or hands under the armpits, creating a seal over the breastbone. Gaze at the tip of the nose.

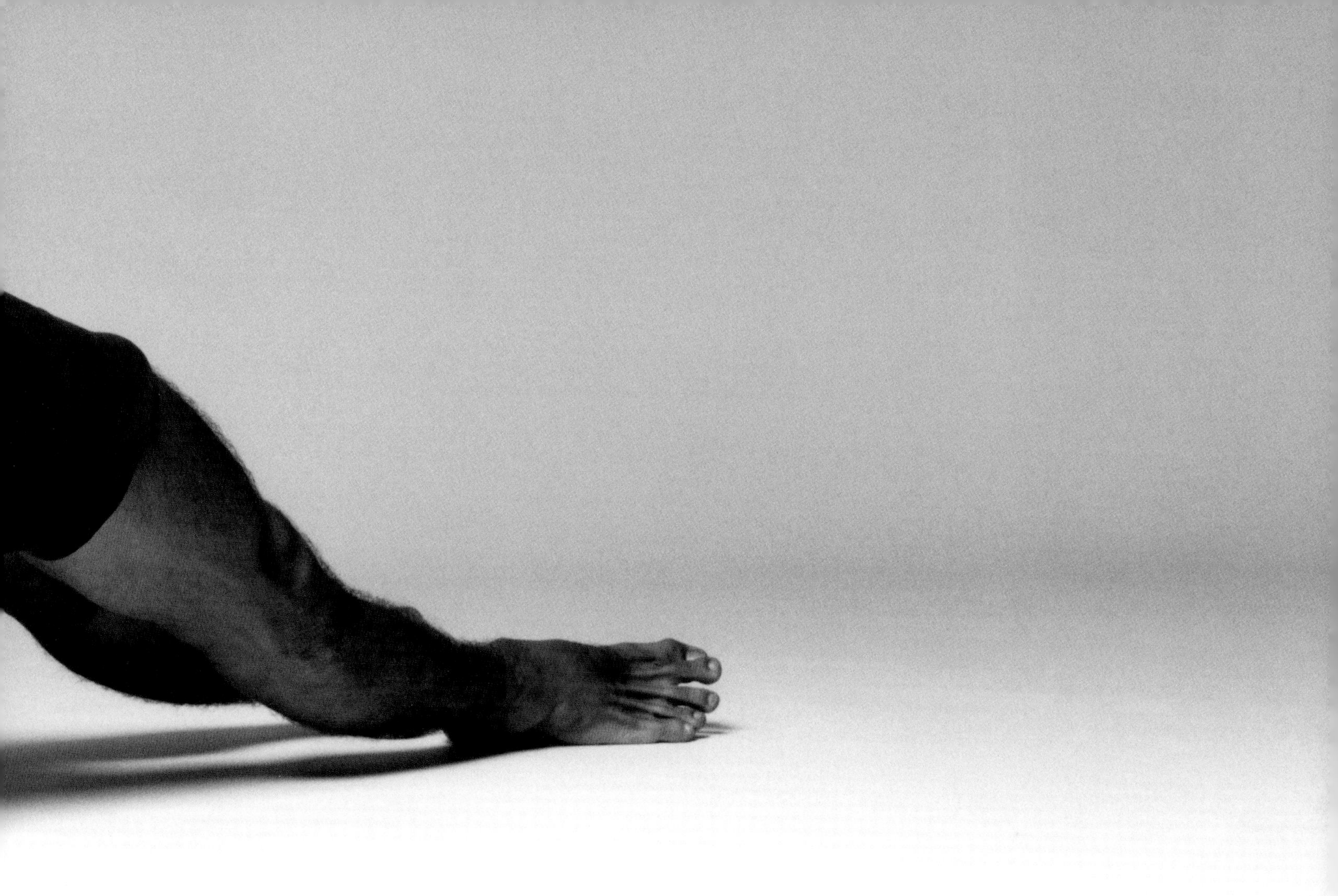

9 Nava
Inhale, lift the hips off the floor, open the chest upwards, and balance on the crown of the head and the outside edges of the feet. Do not push the soles of the feet into the floor. Straighten the legs completely, keep the heels together and strongly engage the bandhas to support the bridge. This is the state of the āsana. Breathe here five times and gaze at the tip of the nose.

10 Daśa
Exhale and lower the body slowly back to the mat by bending the knees and releasing the head down. Strong bandhas help in keeping the balance during this transition; the arms remain crossed over the chest. Keep the knees bent after rolling down, so that you can transition into Cakrāsana immediately.

11 Ekādaśa
Inhale and place the hands by the ears. Roll backwards through Cakrāsana as described in the 24th vinyāsa of Supta-pādāṅguṣṭhāsana.

Vinyāsas 12 and 13 are the same as the 5th and 6th vinyāsas in Sūrya-namaskāra A. After vinyāsa 13, go to the next āsana, the 7th vinyāsa in Ūrdhva-dhanur-āsana.

Beginners: Coming up and balancing on the crown of the head requires much practice and a strong, stable neck.
- In the beginning, you can take some of the weight off the neck by keeping the hands on the floor, with either bent elbows by the ears, or straight beside you by the hips.
- Straighten the legs as much as possible in the state of the āsana.
- Those with neck problems should consult a doctor or a competent teacher before trying either Setu-bandhāsana or Cakrāsana.

Note:
There are two breaths in the 7th, 8th and 11th vinyāsas.

11 Ekādaśa	in & out	cakrāsana, backwards roll, catvāri position
12 Dvādaśa	in	upward-facing dog
13 Trayodaśa	out	downward-facing dog
14 Caturaśa	in	jump forwards, stretch spine, head up
15 Pañcadaśa	out	bend forwards
Samasthitiḥ	in	come up, stand straight

Ūrdhva-dhanur-āsana [upward bow pose]

15 vinyāsas

Note 1:
Paścima-tānāsana C is combined with Ūrdhva-dhanur-āsana.

Note 2:
There are two breaths in the 7th, 8th and 11th vinyāsas.

Ūrdhva – upward; *dhanu* – bow (as in archery); *āsana* – seat, pose, posture

Ūrdhva-dhanur-āsana comes after the 13th vinyāsa in Setu-bandhāsana.

7 Sapta
Inhale and jump through to sitting. Continue with the inhalation as you roll down onto the floor, keeping the legs together. Press the palms into the floor by the thighs, expand the chest and lengthen the whole body along the mat. Gaze at the tip of the nose and exhale here.

8 Aṣṭau
Inhale, bend the knees and pull the heels in as close to the hips as possible, keeping the feet hip-width apart with the toes pointing forwards. Exhale, place the hands on the floor by the ears, palms down, fingers spread wide and the fingertips pointing towards the shoulders. Gaze at the tip of the nose.

9 Nava
Inhale, hold mūla- and uddīyana-bandha and press the hands and feet into the floor. Lift the body up into an arch, bridge or backbend, with the head between the shoulders. Straighten the arms, and engage the thighs to straighten the knees. Lift up through the chest, shoulders and hips, keeping the back relaxed. Mūla-bandha will keep the hips lifted, lighten the body and help relax the buttocks. Uddīyana-bandha supports the chest and opens the sternum up and into the arch. Lean the head back to release the shoulders and chest.
Note that while the spine is deeply arched in this backbend, the front side of the body (thighs, psoas, stomach and sternum) will also open up tremendously. In this way, the āsana requires that the flexibility of the back and spine, as well as that of the front side of the body, work complementary to each other. This is the state of the āsana. Breathe deeply five times and gaze at the tip of the nose.

10 Daśa
Exhale, bend the elbows and knees and lower the crown of the head, or the back, slowly to the floor. The soles of the feet and the palms should stay firmly in place. On the next inhalation, come back up to the state of the āsana, as described in the 9th vinyāsa. Repeat this vinyāsa three times, taking a minimum of five deep breathes each time. On the second and third attempt, try to walk the hands closer to the feet, bending the elbows to help bring the hands in, and straightening the arms again into the state of the āsana. After the third lift-up into the 9th vinyāsa, lie back down on the exhalation. Do not straighten the legs here but move straight into the 11th vinyāsa (Cakrāsana). Gaze at the tip of the nose.
Note: Advanced students can come up to standing from Ūrdhva-dhanur-āsana on an inhalation, and continue with further back-bending practice by themselves, or with the help of a teacher.

11 Ekādaśa
Inhale, lift the legs up and over the head into Cakrāsana (backwards-roll). Follow the instructions given in the 24th vinyāsa of Supta-pādāṅguṣṭhāsana (see p. 141).

Vinyāsas 12 and 13 are the same as the 5th and 6th vinyāsas in Sūrya-namaskāra A.

Do vinyāsas 7–14 of Paścima-tānāsana C directly after the 13th vinyāsa in Ūrdhva-dhanur-āsana, as a counter pose to the deep backbending. Breathe deeply ten times in the state of this āsana.

The 14th vinyāsa in Paścima-tānāsana C is the same as the 13th vinyāsa in Ūrdhva-dhanur-āsana (downward-facing dog). Continue on from here to the next āsana, the 7th vinyāsa in Salamba-sarvāṅgāsana.

Beginners: It takes some practice to straighten the arms and breathe calmly with a relaxed back in Ūrdhva-dhanur-āsana.

- First try to lift the head up off the floor, gazing at the tip of the nose, or, to make it easier, look in between the hands.
- Extend through the arms until they are completely straight.
- Relax the back in the state of the āsana and lengthen the breath. Breathe deeply and calmly.

Vinyāsa	Prāṇa (breath)	Āsana (posture)	Dṛṣṭi (gazing point)	Bandha (muscle lock)
Samasthitiḥ		stand straight		
Vinyāsas 1–6 according to Sūrya-namaskāra A				
7 Sapta	in & out	jump through, lie down, hold the pose		
8 Aṣṭau	in & out	prepare the hands and feet		
9 Nava	in	lift up to bow		
state of the āsana; hold for 5 deep breaths				
10 Daśa	out	head or back to floor		
back up to vinyāsas 9 on an inhale; repeat 3 times; hold for 5 deep breaths				
11 Ekādaśa	in & out	cakrāsana, backwards roll, catvāri position		
12 Dvādaśa	in	upward-facing dog		
13 Trayodaśa	out	downward-facing dog		
14 Chaturdaśa	in	jump forwards, stretch spine, head up		
15 Pañcadaśa	out	bend forwards		
Samasthitiḥ	in	come up, stand straight		

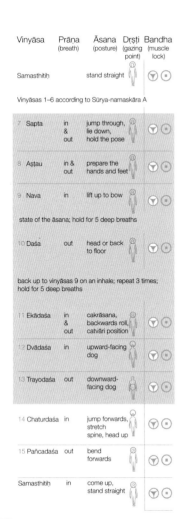

Ūrdhva-dhanur-āsana

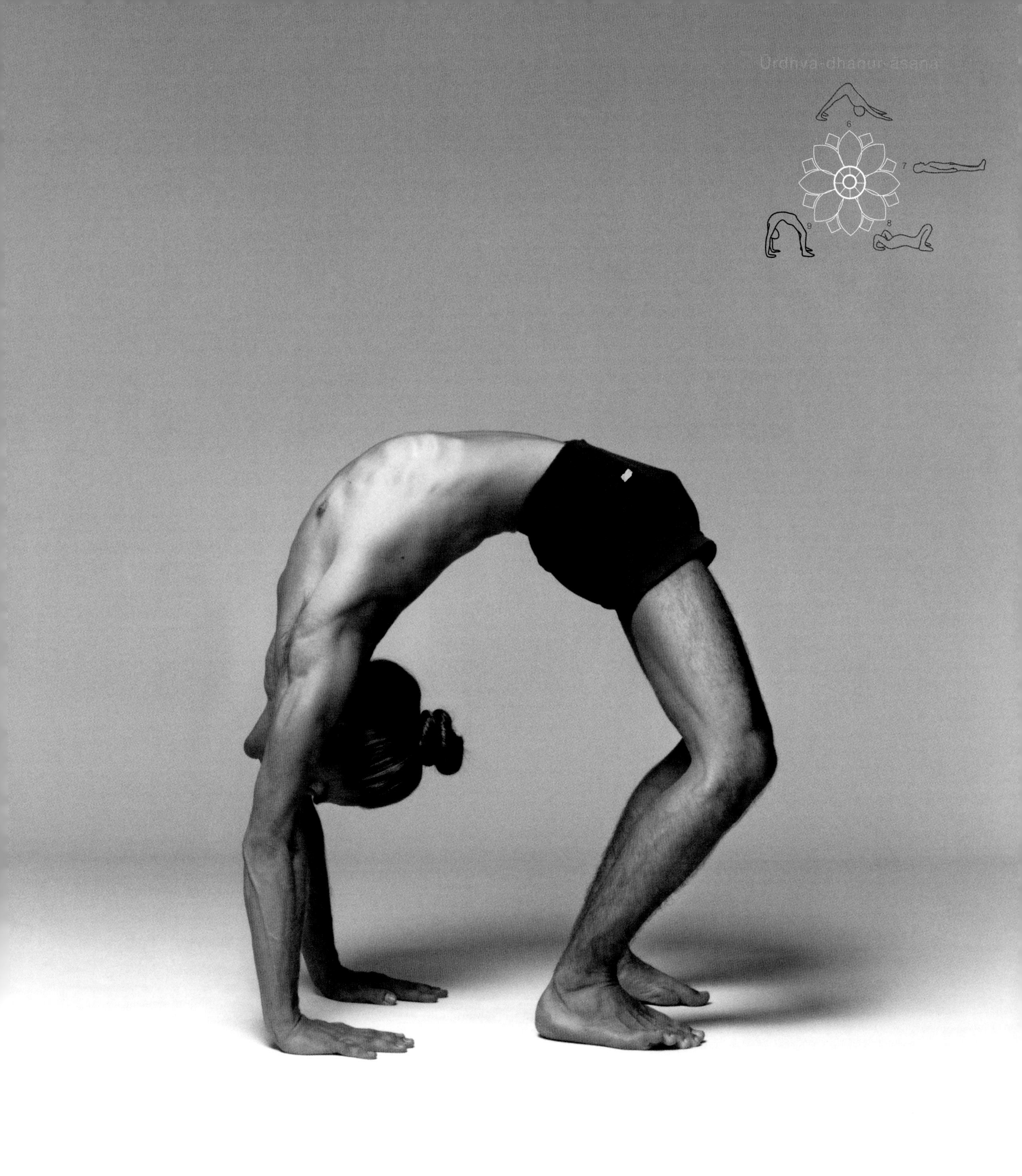

finishing āsanas

The practice ends with a series of primarily inverted postures (viparīta-karaṇi) which guide the energy upwards after the seated āsana sequence. The poses are held longer than in the standing or seated āsanas and are done at a slower pace with long, extended breathing. The finishing sequence can be divided into five parts, each with its own specific focus.

1. The first five āsanas are made up of the shoulderstand and its variations. Shoulderstanding strengthens and purifies the muscles and joints in the body. Shoulderstanding also warms the blood, so that it can flow easily throughout the upper body, nourishing, among others, the following systems in the body: the digestive organs, skin, lungs, heart, brain and cell reproduction.

   This āsana and its variations benefit the heart by slowing down the heart rate. Blood circulation and the quality of blood (and other bodily fluids) improves. The effect of gravity on the body is reversed when doing inversions, thus relieving pressure from the organs and tension in the muscles and nervous system. Furthermore, when the flow of blood is reversed, this relieves the build-up of fluid in the legs and aids proper circulation, while delivering restorative life-energy to the head. Illnesses such as dry cough, digestive problems, constipation, high-blood pressure and chronic hiccups can be cured.

   Moreover, the shoulderstanding sequence brings equlibrium to the the body's inner energy system. It works on the energy channels (nāḍīs), the energy centers (cakras), the blood vessels and nervous system (dhamani), the three doṣas (vāta, pitta, kapha), the metabolism (vaiśvānara) and the digestive fire (jāṭharāgni).

   The body's lower regions are purified, including but not limited to, the stomach, lower back, intestines, anus and sexual organs. The digestive and elimination systems also benefit from shoulderstanding. As these āsanas stimulate the throat and neck, the energy center located here, viśuddha-cakra, is purified and strengthened. The two lowest energy centers (mūlādhāra- and svādhiṣṭhāna-cakras) are also stimulated, which releases the three energy knots (granthi-traya – Brahmā, Viṣṇu and Rudra), so that prāṇa can flow without restriction through the suṣumnā-nāḍī.

   Shoulderstanding and headstanding generate amṛta-bindu (created in part through digestion), so that it can move up from the stomach to the brahma-randhra, or Brahmā's opening, located on the crown of the head. In this way, practising inversions, along with getting plenty of fresh air, leading a sattvic lifestyle and following the principles of brahmacarya, increases the amount of amṛta-bindu in the brahma-randhra.
2. Matsyāsana and Uttāna-pādāsana are counter-poses to the shoulderstanding āsanas.
3. Headstanding has similar effects as shoulderstanding, but works at a deeper level. When performed correctly, the head shouldn't press down too strongly, if at all, on the floor. This āsana activates the sahasrāra-cakra, or crown cakra. In order to get the full effects of headstand, it should be done consistently and held for a considerable amount of time. *Yoga Mala* recommends holding the headstand anywhere from a minimum of five minutes to as long as three hours.
4. Padmāsana and its variations: Baddha-padmāsana and Yoga-mudrā are strengthening and cleansing poses. They prepare the body for Padmāsana, which stabilizes the mind and breath. Padmāsana is ideal for meditation, chanting and prāṇāyama. According to ancient texts, through the purification process in the Padmāsana sequence, the body will be cleansed of impurities and the mind will be freed

from latent karmic impressions (samsara). Utplutiḥ strengthens the bandhas and arms, and prepares the practitioner for the relaxation pose that completes the practice.

5. The āsana series culminates with the relaxation pose, giving the practitioner time to recover while restoring energy to the body and mind. In addition, the relaxation pose allows the nervous system to process the effects of the deep purification that has taken place throughout the āsana sequence.

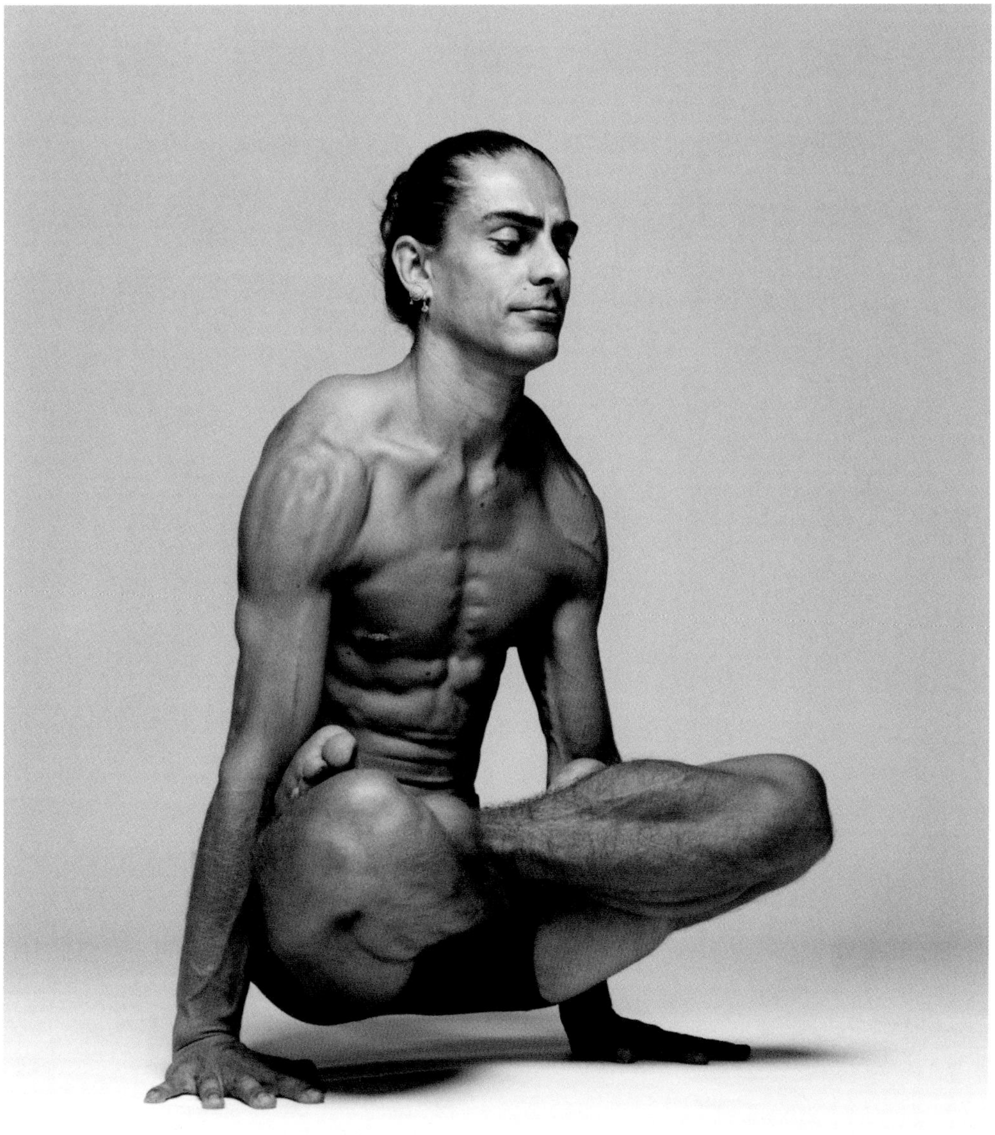

Utplutiḥ, the 9th vinyāsa in Padmāsana

Salamba-sarvangasana

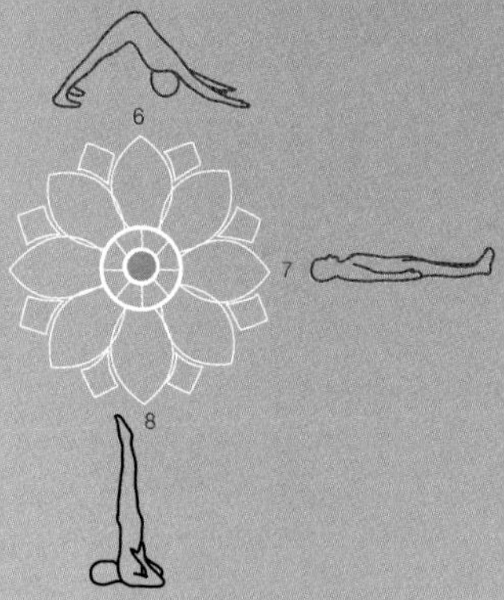

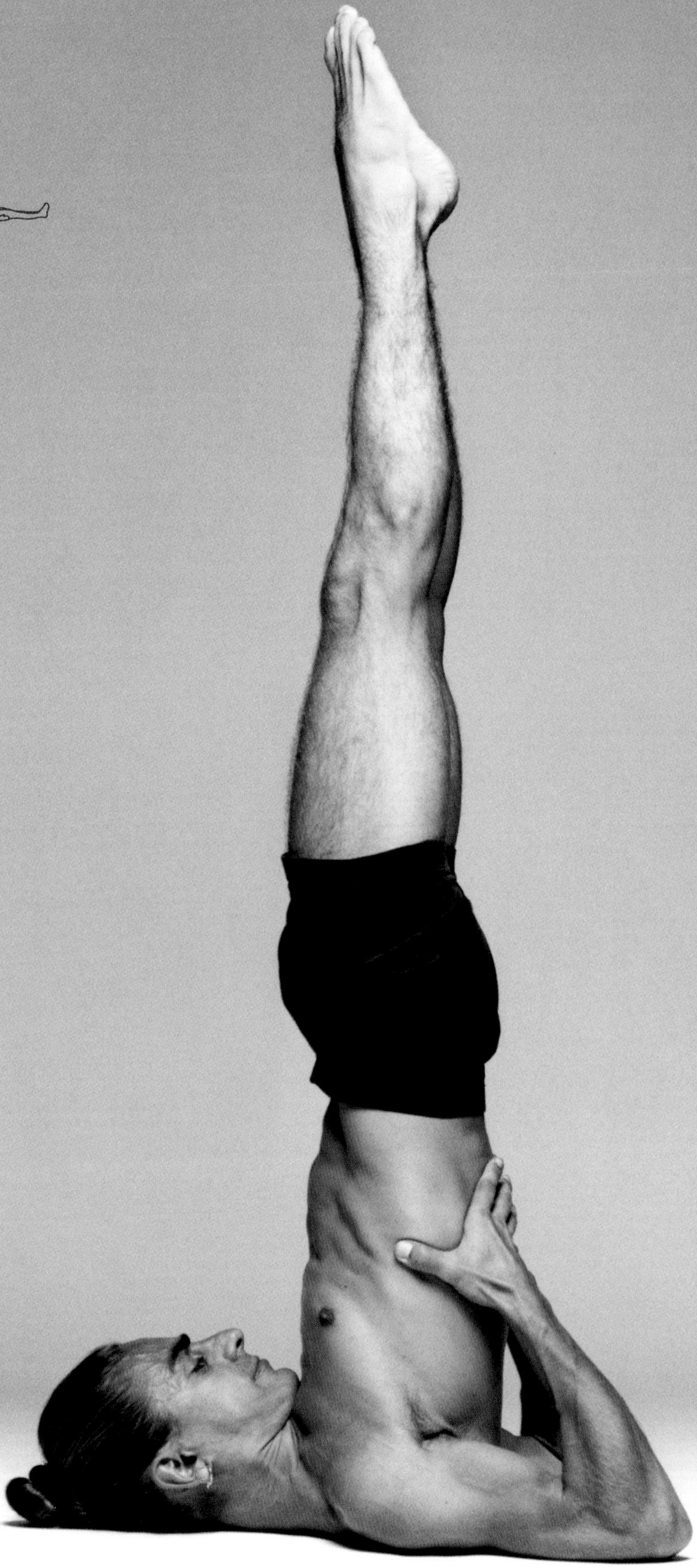

Salamba-sarvāṅgāsana [supported all-limbs pose; shoulderstand]

13 vinyāsas

Salamba – supported, with help; *sarva* – all, full; *aṅga* – limb; *āsana* – seat, posture

Salamba-sarvāṅgāsana follows the 13th vinyāsa in Ūrdhva-dhanur-āsana.

7 Sapta
Inhale, bend the knees and jump through to sitting. Continuing with the inhalation, slowly roll down onto the floor keeping the legs straight and together. Press the palms into the floor and expand the chest, lengthening the body along the mat. Start to slow the heartbeat down by increasing the length of the breath. Exhale once or stay for five deep breaths here. These five breaths are not part of the vinyāsa system but are added here often to calm down both mind and breath. Gaze at the tip of the nose.

8 Aṣṭau
Inhale, press the palms into the floor next to the thighs. Draw in the bandhas and lift the legs, hips and spine straight up, keeping the legs straight and together. Point the feet towards the ceiling. Bend the elbows and support the torso by placing the hands on either side of the spine. The fingers face up towards the hips and the thumbs are out to the sides. Draw the elbows in, shoulder-width apart, and move the shoulders closer together to support the body's straight alignment. Most of the weight is supported by the shoulders, so the neck should not be pressing uncomfortably into the floor. Only the shoulders, upper arms, elbows and back of the head touch the floor. Tuck the chin in between the collarbones and sternum. This is not jalandhara-bandha, even though the positions look similar. Engage mūla-bandha to support the hips and uddīyana-bandha to stretch the body. This is the state of the āsana. Breathe deeply for 10–25 breaths and gaze at the tip of the nose.

Note: In *Yoga Mala*, it is recommended to hold Salamba-sarvāṅgāsana for a minimum of five minutes and up to a maximum of three hours, and anywhere in between, to benefit fully from the healing aspects of this āsana.

After the last inhalation in the 8th vinyāsa, go directly to the next āsana, the 8th vinyāsa in Halāsana.

Beginners: It takes some practice to be able to stand on the shoulders with a completely straight spine.
- If you cannot bring your hips up on the arms, or if you have back problems, lift the legs, keeping the hips on the ground until the body becomes stronger and the tension has released.
- Lift the legs up slowly, support the back with the arms, and allow the body to get accustomed to the pose. You can then lower the hands towards the shoulder blades, draw the elbows in towards each other, lift the hips some more and straighten the spine.
- Draw the shoulders under the body as far as you can and avoid touching the back of the neck to the floor.
- Remember that all āsanas become easier and more fluid with time and practice.

Note 1:
There are one to five breaths in the 7th vinyāsa, and 10–25 breaths in the 8th vinyāsa.

Note 2:
The breathing in the finishing sequence is slower than in the standing and sitting poses.

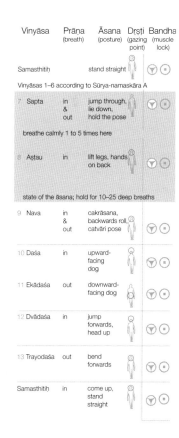

Vinyāsa	Prāṇa (breath)	Āsana (posture)	Dṛṣṭi (gazing point)	Bandha (muscle lock)
Samasthitiḥ		stand straight		
Vinyāsas 1–6 according to Sūrya-namaskāra A				
7 Sapta	in & out	jump through, lie down, hold the pose		
breathe calmly 1 to 5 times here				
8 Aṣṭau	in	lift legs, hands on back		
state of the āsana; hold for 10–25 deep breaths				
9 Nava	in & out	cakrāsana, backwards roll, catvāri pose		
10 Daśa	in	upward-facing dog		
11 Ekādaśa	out	downward-facing dog		
12 Dvādaśa	in	jump forwards, head up		
13 Trayodaśa	out	bend forwards		
Samasthitiḥ	in	come up, stand straight		

Vinyāsa	Prāṇa (breath)	Āsana (posture)	Dṛṣṭi (gazing point)	Bandha (muscle lock)
Samasthitiḥ		stand straight		
Vinyāsas 1–6 according to Sūrya-namaskāra A				
7 Sapta	in & out	jump through, lie down, hold the pose		
8 Aṣṭa	in & out	lift the legs up, lower them to the floor		
state of the āsana; hold for 8–10 deep breaths				
9 Nava	in & out	cakrāsana, backwards roll, catvāri pose		
10 Daśa	in	upward-facing dog		
11 Ekādaśa	out	downward-facing dog		
12 Dvādaśa	in	jump forwards, head up		
13 Trayodaśa	out	bend forwards		
Samasthitiḥ	in	come up, stand straight		

Halāsana [plow pose]

13 vinyāsas

Hala – plow; *āsana* – seat, posture

Halāsana comes directly after the 8th vinyāsa in Salamba-sarvāṅgāsana.

8 Aṣṭau
Exhale, bring the legs down behind the head. Keep the legs straight, point the feet and stretch through the toes. Lower the hands from the back and interlace the fingers, squeezing the palms together and pressing the arms straight out onto the floor. The shoulders and back of the head are on the floor. However, keep the back of the neck lifted up off the floor. Engage mūla-bandha to support and lift the hips, and to relax the buttocks. Engage uddīyana-bandha to open the back, and to straighten and lift the spine. This is the state of the āsana. Breathe deeply eight to ten times. Gaze at the tip of the nose.

After the last inhalation, go directly to the 8th vinyāsa in Karṇa-pīḍāsana.

Beginners: Refer back to shoulderstanding.

- Straighten the legs behind the head. If your legs do not touch down to the floor at first, breathe deeply and gradually let the legs sink lower.
- Try to interlace the fingers behind the back, straighten the arms and press the arms towards the floor.

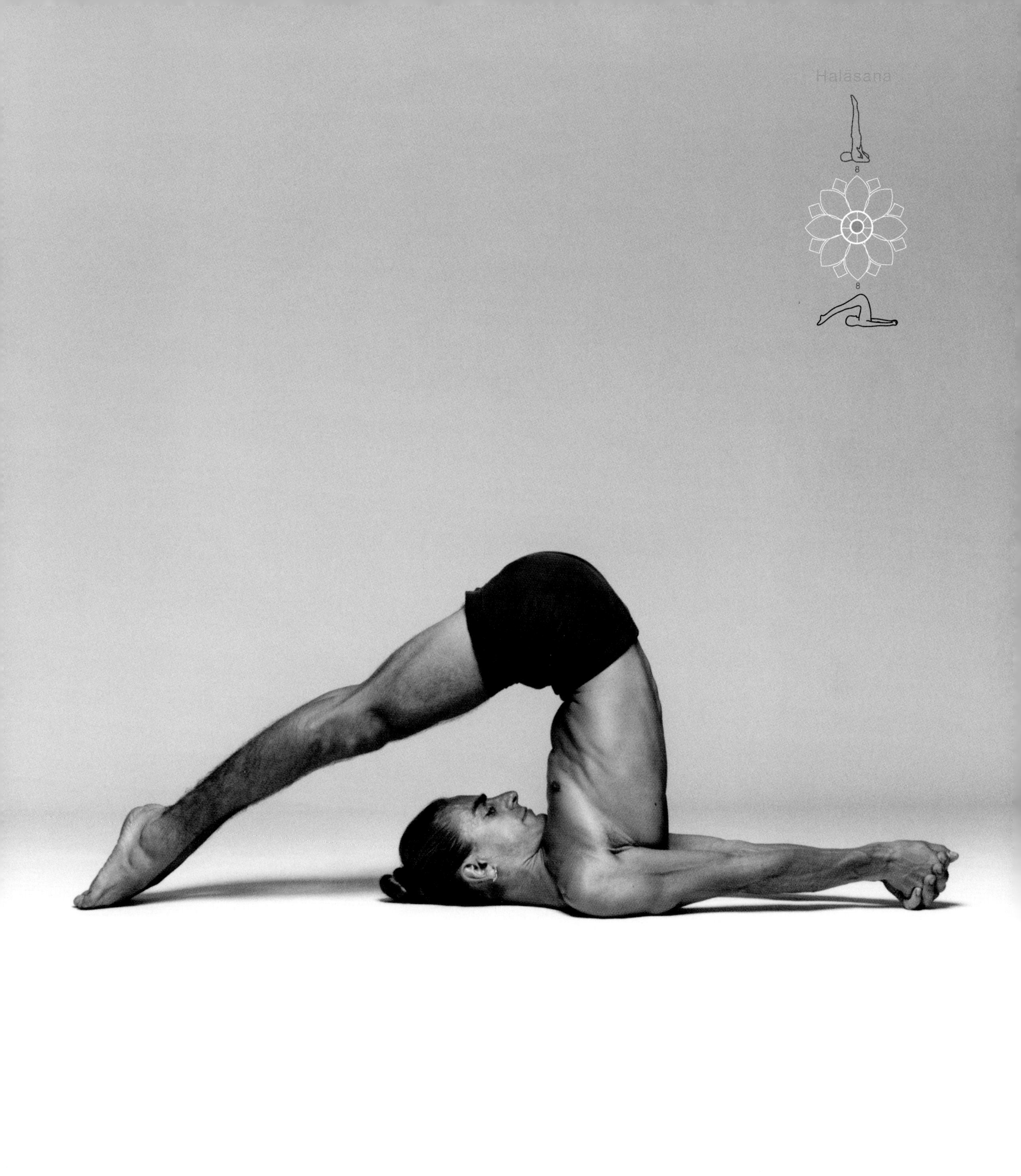
Halāsana
8
8

Karṇa-pīḍāsana

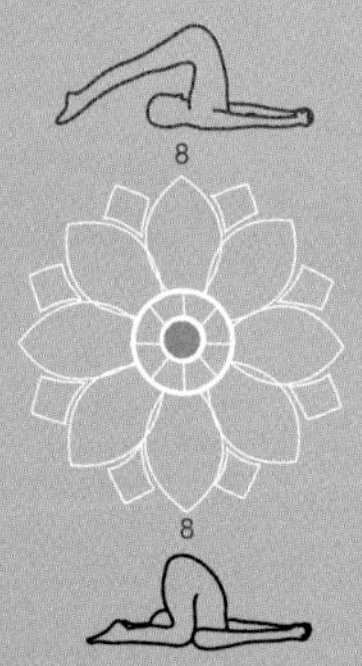

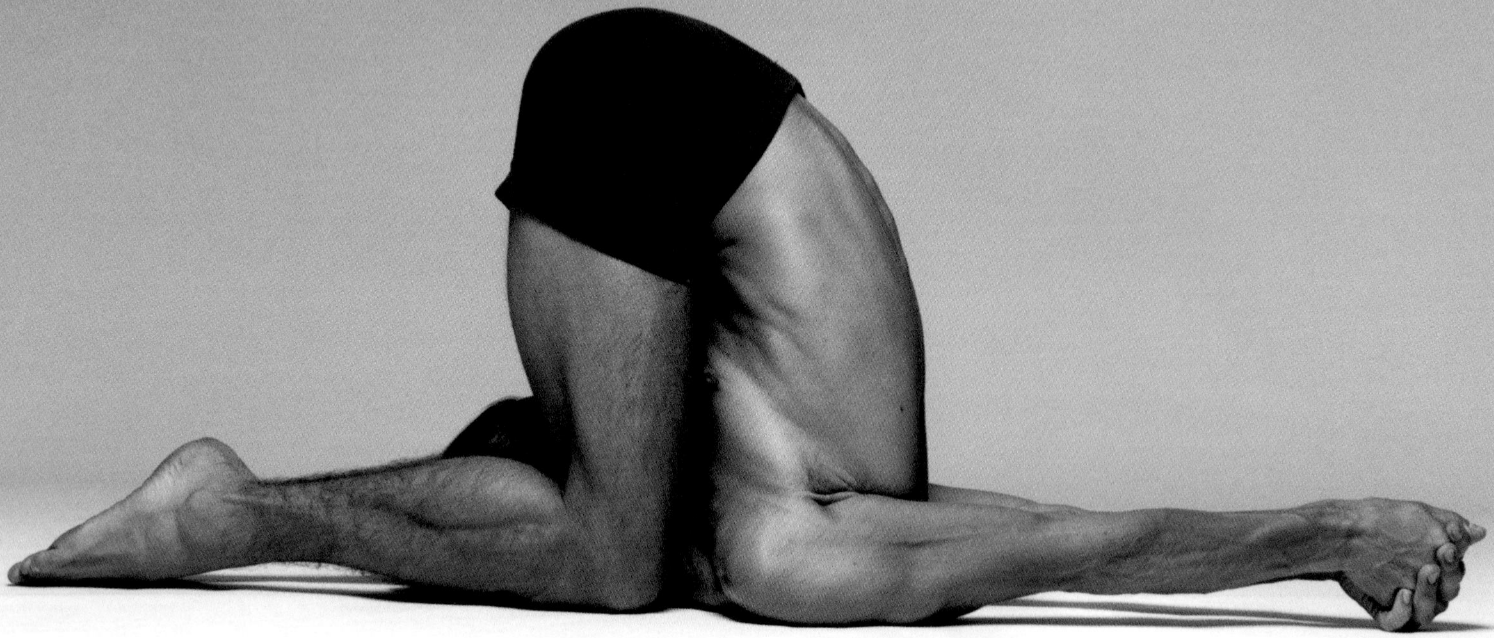

Vinyāsa	Prāṇa (breath)	Āsana (posture)	Dṛṣṭi (gazing point)	Bandha (muscle lock)
Samasthitiḥ		stand straight		
Vinyāsas 1–6 according to Sūrya-namaskāra A				
7 Sapta	in & out	jump through, lie down, hold the pose		
8 Aṣṭau	in & out	lift the legs up, bend knees to the ears		
state of the āsana; hold for 8–10 deep breaths				
9 Nava	in & out	chakrasana, backwards roll, chatvari pose		
10 Daśa	in	upward-facing dog		
11 Ekādaśa	out	downward-facing dog		
12 Dvādaśa	in	jump forwards, stretch the spine, head up		
13 Trayodaśa	out	bend forwards		
Samasthitiḥ	in	come up, stand straight		

Karṇa-pīḍāsana [ear pressure pose]

13 vinyāsas

Karṇa – ear; *pīḍā* – pressure, pressing; *āsana* – seat, posture

Karṇa-pīḍāsana comes directly after Halāsana's 8th vinyāsa.

8 Aṣṭau
Exhale, keep the feet and toes together with the feet pointed. The hands and arms stay behind the back, as they were in Halāsana. Lower the knees to the floor, and squeeze the inner knees into the ears. This is the state of the āsana. Breathe here eight to ten times and gaze at the tip of the nose.

After the last exhalation in Karṇa-pīḍāsana (8th vinyāsa) move to the next āsana, the 8th vinyāsa in Ūrdhva-padmāsana.

Beginners: Refer back to shoulderstanding.

- If your knees do not touch the floor, breathe deeply to open the spine up and slowly work the knees closer to the floor. Keep the feet together.
- Try to interlace the fingers behind the back and press the palms closer together; next, work on straightening the arms and pressing them into the floor.

Ūrdhva-padmāsana

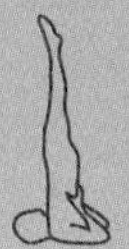

8

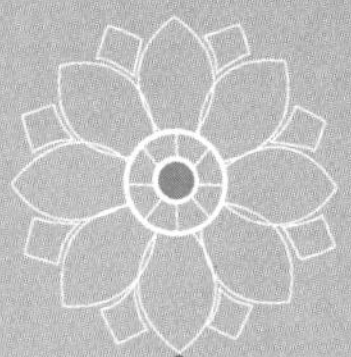

9

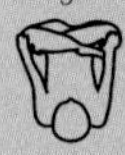

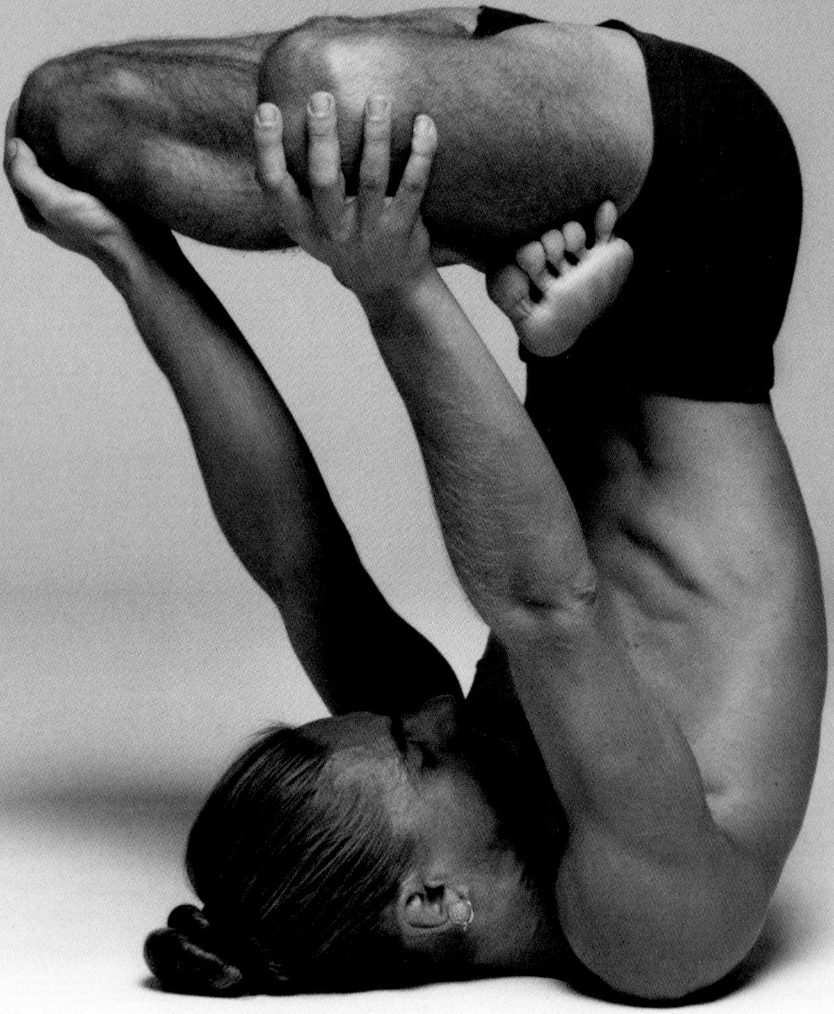

Ūrdhva-padmāsana *[upward lotus pose]*

14 vinyāsas

Ūrdhva – upwards; *padma* – lotus, lotus blossom; *āsana* – seat, posture

Ūrdhva-padmāsana comes after the 8th vinyāsa in Karṇa-pīḍāsana.

8 Aṣṭau
Inhale, raise the legs and move the hands back to support the spine, as in Salamba-sarvāṅgāsana. Gaze at the tip of the nose.

9 Nava
Exhale, balance the body on the shoulders with the back of the head and upper arms as a support. Lower the right foot into the left inner thigh and groin. Take hold of the foot with one hand and turn the sole of the foot out and place the back of the foot in the crease of the upper left thigh, with the heel pointing towards the left side of the navel. Then draw the left foot in, likewise, to the right inner thigh and groin, with the heel towards the right of the navel. This is an upside-down lotus (Padmāsana) position.

Note: Advanced students can work to bring the legs into lotus without using the hands to help. In this case, the hands would stay on the back and one would move into lotus using the strength of the muscles, the breath and the rhythm of the movement.

Continue with this āsana by straightening the spine, opening the chest and engaging the bandhas. Place the palms to the knees with the fingers on the kneecaps and straighten the arms. This is the state of the āsana. Breathe deeply eight to ten times. Gaze at the tip of the nose.

After the last inhalation in the 9th vinyāsa, go directly to the 9th vinyāsa in Piṇḍāsana.

Beginners: Refer back to shoulderstanding.

- If you are unable to come into full lotus at first, cross the legs, hold the knees and straighten the arms.

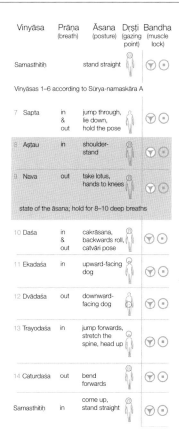

Vinyāsa	Prāṇa (breath)	Āsana (posture)	Dṛṣṭi (gazing point)	Bandha (muscle lock)
Samasthitiḥ		stand straight		
Vinyāsas 1–6 according to Sūrya-namaskāra A				
7 Sapta	in & out	jump through, lie down, hold the pose		
8 Aṣṭau	in	shoulder-stand		
9 Nava	out	take lotus, hands to knees		
state of the āsana; hold for 8–10 deep breaths				
10 Daśa	in & out	cakrāsana, backwards roll, catvāri pose		
11 Ekadaśa	in	upward-facing dog		
12 Dvādaśa	out	downward-facing dog		
13 Trayodaśa	in	jump forwards, stretch the spine, head up		
14 Caturdaśa	out	bend forwards		
Samasthitiḥ	in	come up, stand straight		

Vinyāsa	Prāṇa (breath)	Āsana (posture)	Dṛṣṭi (gazing point)	Bandha (muscle lock)
Samasthitiḥ		stand straight		
Vinyāsas 1–6 according to Sūrya-namaskāra A				
7 Sapta	in & out	jump through, lie down, hold the pose		
8 Aṣṭau	in	shoulder-stand		
9 Nava	out	take lotus pose, bring legs into the chest, bind the hands		
state of the āsana; hold for 8–10 deep breaths				
10 Daśa	in & out	cakrāsana, backwards roll, catvāri pose		
11 Ekadaśa	in	upward-facing dog		
12 Dvādaśa	out	downward-facing dog		
13 Trayodaśa	in	jump forwards, stretch the spine, head up		
14 Caturdaśa	out	bend forwards		
Samasthitiḥ	in	come up, stand straight		

Piṇḍāsana [embryo pose]

14 vinyāsas

Piṇḍa – embryo; *āsana* – seat, posture

Piṇḍāsana comes directly after the 9th vinyāsa in Ūrdhva-padmāsana.

9 Nava
Exhale and lower the legs (still in lotus) towards the chest, rounding the spine. The shins will come to either side of the face and the knees on either side of the head. Wrap the arms around the outsides of the thighs, bind one wrist and make a soft fist with the free hand. You can also take hold of the fingers instead of binding. Draw the lotus into the chest with the arms, but do not force the knees to the floor. Balance on the shoulders. This is the state of the āsana. Breathe deeply eight to ten times and gaze at the tip of the nose.

After the 9th vinyāsa, move into the next āsana, the 8th vinyāsa in Matsyāsana.

Beginners: Refer back to shoulderstanding and upward-facing lotus.

- If you are unable to come into full lotus at first, cross your legs and pull the legs into the chest.

Piṇḍāsana

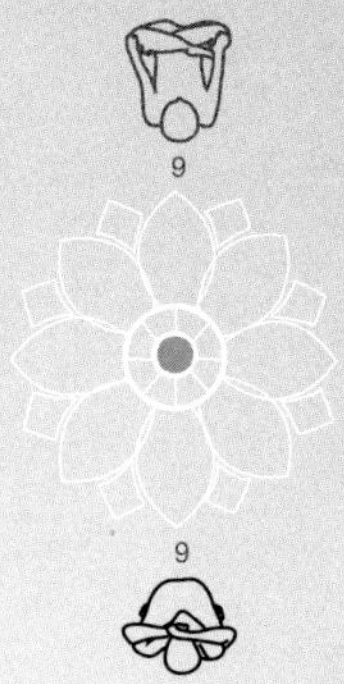

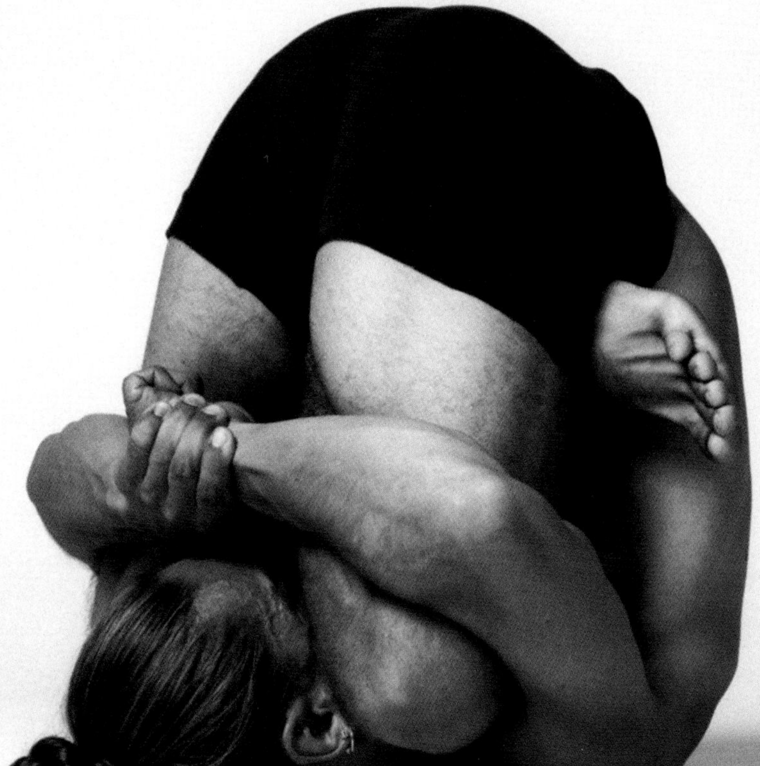

Matsyāsana

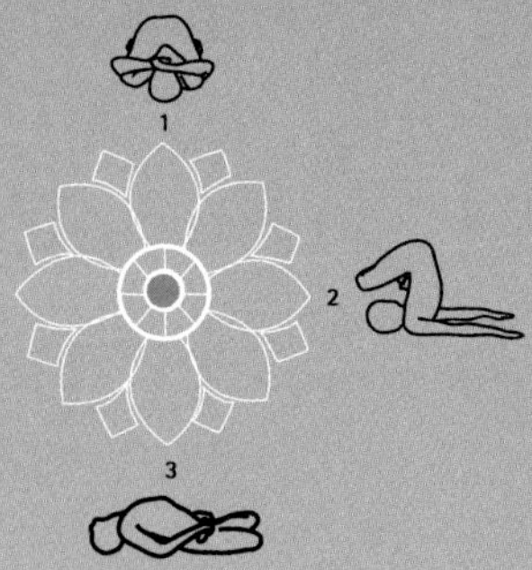

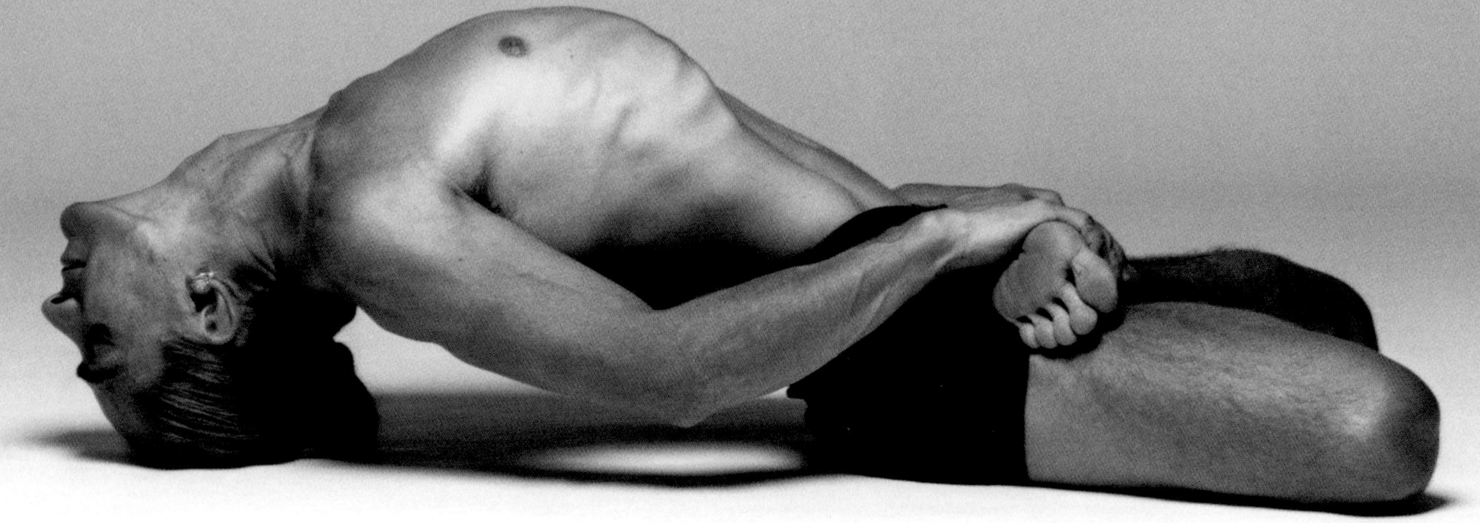

Vinyāsa	Prāṇa (breath)	Āsana (posture)	Dṛṣṭi (gazing point)	Bandha (muscle lock)
Samasthitiḥ		stand straight		
Vinyāsas 1–6 according to Sūrya-namaskāra A				
7 Sapta	in & out	jump through, lie down, hold the pose		
8 Aṣṭau	in & out	legs in lotus, (roll down) chest up, crown of head to floor		
state of the āsana; hold for 8–10 deep breaths				
9 Nava	in & out	cakrāsana, backwards roll catvāri pose		
10 Daśa	in	upward-facing dog		
11 Ekadaśa	out	downward-facing dog		
12 Dvādaśa	in	jump forwards, stretch the spine, head up		
13 Trayodaśa	out	bend forwards		
Samasthitiḥ	in	come up, stand straight		

Matsyāsana [fish pose]

13 vinyāsas

Matsya – fish; *āsana* – seat, posture

Matsyāsana is done after the 9th vinyāsa in Piṇḍāsana.

8 Aṣṭau
Exhale and straighten the arms back onto the mat with the palms down. Round the back and slowly lower the legs, keeping them in lotus, down to the floor. The back of the head stays on the floor as you roll down. Continue exhaling, engage uḍḍīyana-bandha and lift the upper back off the floor into an arch then place the crown of the head on the floor. Take hold of the middle part of the feet and pull back slightly, creating an opposing action to the upwards arch. Press the knees down into the floor and straighten the arms. This is the state of the āsana. Breathe deeply eight to ten times. Gaze at the tip of the nose.

Note: After the photographs in this book were taken, it was decided by Pattabhi Jois to straighten the arms in this āsana.

After the last inhalation in the 8th vinyāsa, go directly to the 8th vinyāsa in Uttāna-pādāsana.

Beginners: It can take some time to be practise Matsyāsana correctly.
- If you have neck problems, consult an experienced teacher.
- Lower down into Matsyāsana with a rounded back, keeping the legs in the same position (lotus).
- Press the elbows into the floor to help as you lift the chest and set the crown of the head on the floor.
- If the legs are not in lotus, support yourself in the pose by pressing the palms into the floor, or by placing them onto the thighs.

Note:
There are two breaths in the 9th vinyāsa.

Vinyāsa	Prāṇa (breath)	Āsana (posture)	Dṛṣṭi (gazing point)	Bandha (muscle lock)
Samasthitiḥ		stand straight		
Vinyāsas 1–6 according to Sūrya-namaskāra A				
7 Sapta	in & out	jump through, lie down, hold the pose		
8 Aṣṭau	in & out	crown of head to floor, lift arms and legs to angle		
state of the āsana; hold for 8–10 deep breaths				
9 Nava	in & out	cakrāsana, backwards roll, catvāri pose		
10 Daśa	in	upward-facing dog		
11 Ekadaśa	out	downward-facing dog		
12 Dvādaśa	in	jump forwards, head up		
13 Trayodaśa	out	bend forwards		
Samasthitiḥ	in	come up, stand straight		

Uttāna-pādāsana [extended foot pose]

13 vinyāsas

Uttana – strong, deep stretch, extended; *pāda* – foot; *āsana* – seat, posture

Uttāna-pādāsana is done after the 8th vinyāsa in Matsyāsana.

8 Aṣṭau
Leave the chest and head where they are as you exhale and open the lotus. Straighten out the legs and lift them into the same angle as in Navāsana. Lift the arms up, align them parallel to the legs and press the palms together. Point the feet and keep an extension in the arms by lengthening through the shoulders. This is the state of the āsana. Breathe deeply eight to ten times. Gaze at the tip of the nose.

9 Nava
Inhale and relax the head and back to the floor while the legs stay in the same position. Place the hands on the floor by the ears, fingers towards the shoulders. Engage the bandhas to support the body and raise the hips and back up off the floor. Keep the legs together and lift them straight overhead. Lower them onto the floor behind the head, about half a foot to a foot apart from each other. Exhale, round the spine and the back of the neck and, using the strength of the arms, lift the body off the floor, roll in a straight line over the head, through Cakrāsana and into Catvāri. Straighten the body and land in Catvāri position. Gaze at the tip of the nose.

Vinyāsas 10 and 11 are the same as the 5th and 6th vinyāsas in Sūrya-namaskāra A.

After vinyāsa 11, go directly to the next āsana, the 7th vinyāsa in Śīrṣāsana.

Beginners:
- If you have neck problems, speak with a teacher regarding this āsana and Cakrāsana.
- If you are at the beginning stages with Cakrāsana, as described in the 9th vinyāsa, refer to the instructions for the 24th vinyāsa in Supta-pādāṅguṣṭhāsana. Another option is to sit up, cross the legs and jump back as described in the 11th vinyāsa in Paścima-tānāsana.

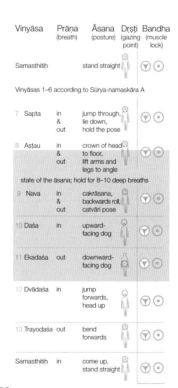

Uttāna-pādāsana

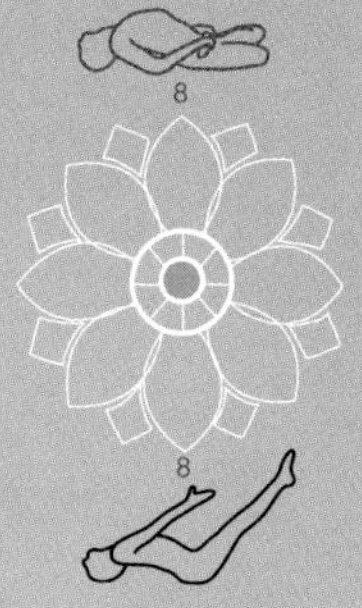

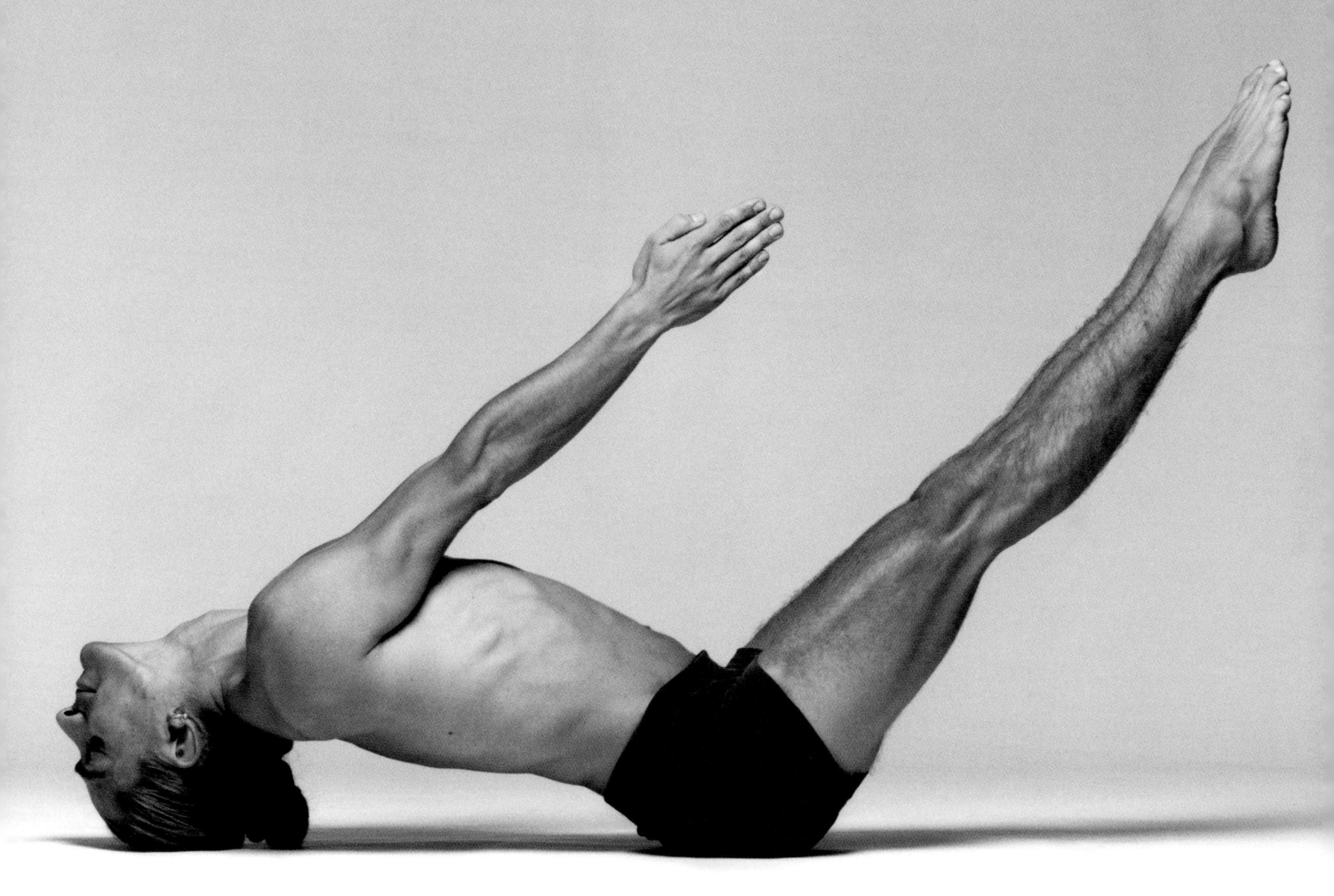

Śīrṣāsana

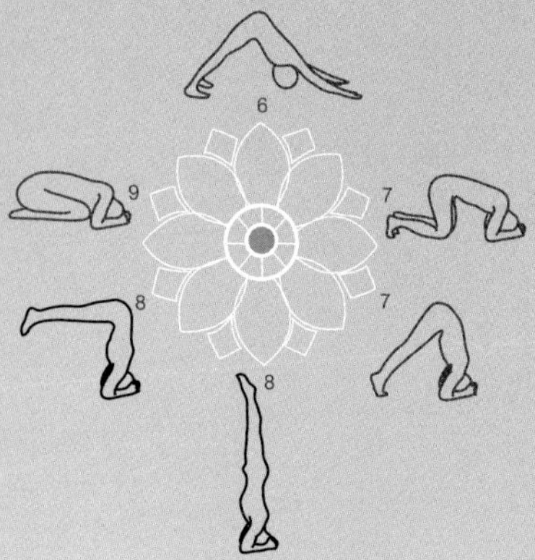

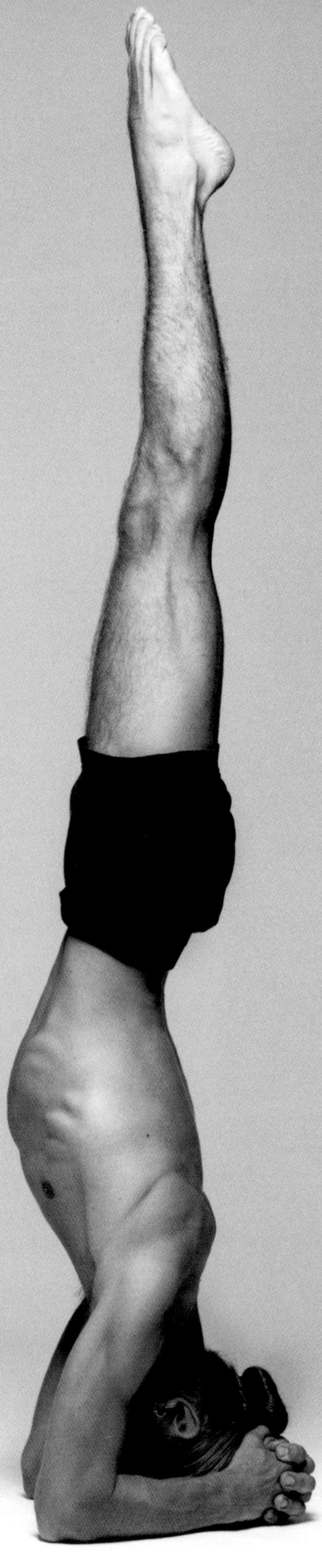

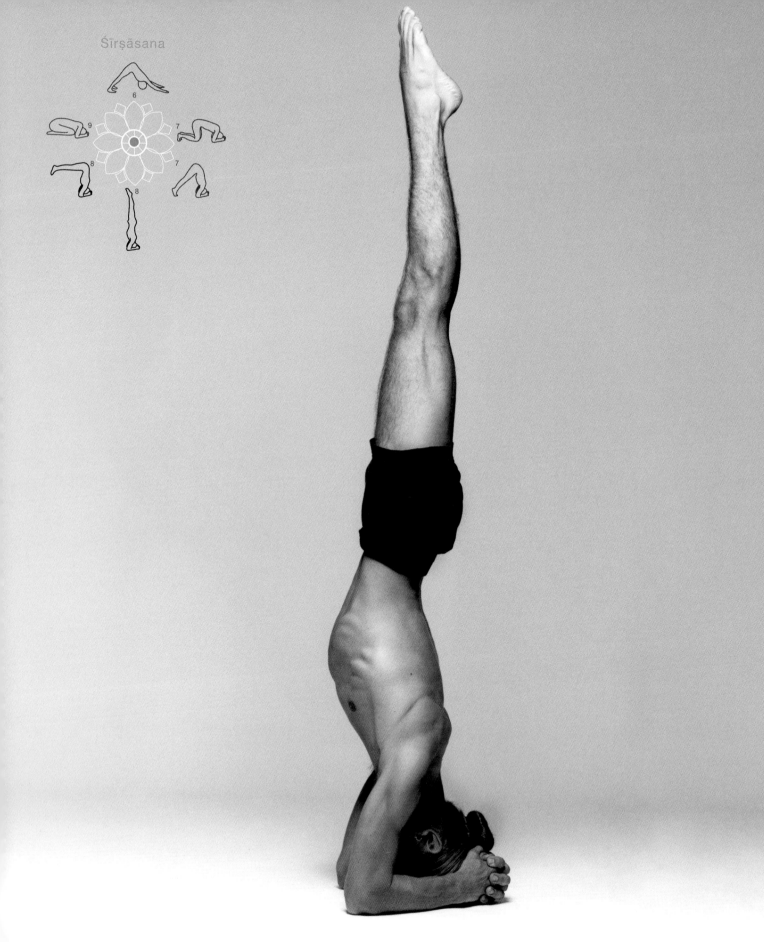

Śīrṣāsana [headstand pose]

13 vinyāsas

Śīrṣa – head; *āsana* – seat, posture

Śīrṣāsana is done after the 11th vinyāsa in Uttāna-pādāsana.

7 Sapta
Inhale, lower the knees to the floor behind the hands, and curl the toes under so that the balls of the feet are on the ground. Place the elbows on the floor in front of the knees, a forearm's length apart. You can measure this distance by placing both hands over the forearms, fingertips touching each elbow. Open the hands out and interlace the fingers. Place the outside edge of the hands into the mat, keeping the palms open, forming a rounded base. The hands and the elbows should make a triangle which serves as the foundation for the headstand. Place the front part of your head (the area between the forehead and the crown of the head) on the floor. Press the crown of the head onto the support you have made with your interlaced fingers and palms.
Exhale, straighten the legs, and walk the feet in until the spine is straight and approximately in line with the shoulders. The hips should point up towards the ceiling. Keeping the toes on the floor with the heels up and legs together, press the forearms and outer edges of the hands into the floor. Try to distribute the weight of the body more on the hands than on the head.

8 Aṣṭau
Inhale, engage the upper arms and mūla-bandha to lift the hips. Draw in uddīyana-bandha to straighten the spine and support the entire body. Straighten the legs and lift them up slowly and with control, keep the legs together and the feet pointed. This is the state of the āsana. The head can be slightly lifted up off the floor, supported by the forearms and shoulders. This position of the head is beneficial for blood circulation and it enables the release of energy from the more delicate sira nāḍīs, the nervous system in the crown of the head. Take 10–50 deep breathes here. Gaze at the tip of the nose.
Note: *Yoga Mala* states that one can practise Śīrṣāsana for a minimum of five minutes up to a maximum of three hours, and anywhere in between, in order to receive the full benefits of this āsana.
For a more challenging variation of headstand, stretch through the shoulders and strengthen the arms to lift the head up in between the shoulders. Draw the chin in towards the chest. Point the feet and gaze up at the toes. Balance here and breathe deeply. After holding Śīrṣāsana, exhale and lower the legs to a 90-degree angle, keeping the legs straight and the feet pointed. Gaze at the tip of the nose and stay here for ten deep breaths. On an inhalation, lift the legs back up once more to Śīrṣāsana.
Note: As soon as you can remain steady in Śīrṣāsana for an extended amount of time, you can begin to practise this variation as well. Since it is part of the 8th vinyāsa, it does not have its own vinyāsa number.

9 Nava
Exhale and slowly lower your straight legs down, gently touching the toes first to the mat. Without lifting the head, bend the knees and place the shins on the floor. Sit back on your heels and place your forehead on the floor in Balāsana (child's pose). The hands and arms are in front of you and remain in the same position as they were in headstand, but the elbows are released out to the sides. Breathe deeply here for a minute or two, balancing out the blood pressure and circulation. Gaze at the tip of the nose.
Note: After a long headstand (more than fifteen minutes), it is essential to rest in child's pose for a sufficient amount of time. Take rest for at least two minutes.
Continue by inhaling and lifting the head up. Place the hands on the floor, next to the shoulders and curl the toes under. Jump back on the exhalation, straightening the legs as you go, and land in Catvāri. Gaze at the tip of the nose.

Vinyāsas 10 and 11 are the same as the 5th and 6th vinyāsas in Sūrya-namaskāra A. After vinyāsa 11, move into the next āsana, the 7th vinyāsa in Baddha-padmāsana.

Beginners: Headstand is an āsana which can bring up mixed feelings and is often approached with apprehension. It is well worth it practising with a teacher first to receive individual instruction on how to balance the body, where to place the head, and how to fall out of the position without injuring yourself. It is also recommended that you begin practising headstand only once the shoulderstand is strong and stable. The shoulderstand prepares the back of the neck and the finer muscles along the spine for a safe headstand.
- If you have neck or back problems, speak with a teacher regarding this āsana.
- Begin the practice bit by bit. First, place your hands and head as described in the 7th vinyāsa, lift the hips, straighten the spine and walk your legs in towards the head.
- Next, try lifting one leg at a time, bending the knees in towards the chest. You can then try to slowly straighten both legs up to the ceiling. Do not hop or kick the legs up into headstand, as the movement has to be controlled from the beginning.
- Once the previous steps are in place, try to lift both legs up at the same time while keeping them bent. Find the balance first with bent legs, then slowly try to straighten them up. When this feels steady, continue with the description in the 8th vinyāsa.
- Always practise with plenty of space around your mat.
- If you should fall backwards, release the position of the hands and round through the back of the neck and spine, rolling down with as much control as possible.
- Engage and lengthen through the shoulders and upper arms, and try to lift the head, easing pressure on the crown of the head.
- Hold the āsana for as long as possible and come down slowly to rest. Try the 90-degree variation only when the headstand feels stable.
- Never do the headstand on its own or out of sequence. It is a finishing pose and the blood has to be warm before attempting the pose. It is to be followed only by the lotus pose and its variations and the relaxation pose.

Note 1:
There are two breaths in the 7th vinyāsa and three breaths in the 9th vinyāsa.

Note 2:
Child's pose is part of the 9th vinyāsa.

Note 3:
Vinyāsa 8 includes an extra variation: the 90-degree bend.

Vinyāsa	Prāṇa (breath)	Āsana (posture)	Dṛṣṭi (gazing point)	Bandha (muscle lock)
Samasthitiḥ		stand straight		
Vinyāsas 1–6 according to Sūrya-namaskāra A				
7 Sapta	in & out	hands and head to floor, straighten legs		
8 Aṣṭau	in	lift the legs to headstand		
state of the āsana; take 10–50 deep breaths here. Exhale down to 90 degrees; breathe 10 times; inhale back up				
9 Nava	iout & in & out	legs down, rest 1 minute, hand on floor, jump to catvāri position		
after coming down, rest 1–2 minutes				
10 Daśa	in	upward-facing dog		
11 Ekadaśa	out	downward-facing dog		
12 Dvādaśa	in	jump forwards, stretch the spine, head up		
13 Trayodaśa	out	bend forwards		
Samasthitiḥ	in	come up, stand straight		

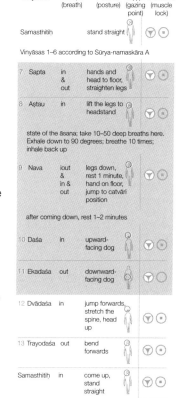

Baddha-padmāsana & Yoga-mudrā [bound lotus pose & sealed pose]

16 vinyāsas

Baddha – bound; *padma* – lotus; *āsana* – seat, posture; *yoga* – union, one-pointed focus; *mudrā* – close, set a seal on

Baddha-padmāsana is done right after the 11th vinyāsa in Śīrṣāsana.

7 Sapta
Inhale, jump through to sitting. Gaze at the tip of the nose.

8 Aṣṭau
Exhale and bring the right foot up into the crease of the left inner thigh. Turn the foot so the sole of the foot faces up; the back of the foot presses into the crease of the inner left thigh and groin, and the heel points towards the left side of the navel. Relax in the right hip joint to lower the right knee towards the floor, at a 45-degree angle. Lift the left foot over the right calf, and place it likewise into the crease of the upper right thigh and groin. This is lotus pose, Padmāsana.
Note: Advanced students can try to bring the legs into lotus without the help of the hands, using the bandhas, breath and momentum. Leave the palms on the floor by the hips as you fold the legs into lotus. Continuing with the exhalation, extend the left shoulder and wrap the left arm around the back to bind the left big toe with the first two fingers and thumb. The palm is turned down. Do the same with the right hand, binding the right big toe. Pull lightly on the toes, press the knees down towards the floor and flex the feet so the heels press in to the sides of the navel. Bow the head and lower the chin down. This is Baddha-padmāsana. Take a slow inhalation here, open the chest and lengthen the upper body. Gaze at the tip of the nose.

9 Nava
Exhale, keep the chest open while folding the body forwards and down onto the heels and shins, reaching the chin out towards the floor. Grip the big toes firmly while still pressing the heels into the navel area, massaging the intestines and stimulating the inner organs and energy channels. Draw in uddīyana-bandha to lengthen the body out and to create space for the heels and calves. Mūla-bandha presses the hips down, counter-balancing the forward-bending. This is Yoga-mudrā. Take ten deep breaths here. Gaze in between the eyebrows.

10 Daśa
Inhale, keep hold of the big toes and come back up to Baddha-padmāsana with a straight back and strong bandhas. Gaze at the tip of the nose.

After the 10th vinyāsa, on an exhalation, go directly to the next āsana, the 8th vinyāsa in Padmāsana.

Beginners: *Baddha-padmāsana* is one variation of the lotus postures. It can take some time before the hips, knees and ankles are flexible and strong enough to feel comfortable in this āsana.

- If you cannot bring the legs into lotus, bring the right leg into half-lotus and bend the left leg under the right. You can also sit in a cross-legged position.
- If you are still working towards lotus pose, bring the arms behind the back and take hold of the forearms or elbows.
- It can take many breaths to come into either half- or full lotus. Breathe slowly and deeply, trying to use as few breaths as possible when you take the pose.

Note 1:
In the 9th vinyāsa (Yoga-mudrā), you can also keep the gaze at the tip of the nose.

Note 2:
There are two breaths in the 8th and 10th vinyāsas.

Vinyāsa	Prāṇa (breath)	Āsana (posture)	Dṛṣṭi (gazing point)	Bandha (muscle lock)
Samasthitiḥ		stand straight		
Vinyāsas 1–6 according to Sūrya-namaskāra A				
7 Sapta	in	jump through		
8 Aṣṭau	out & in	lotus, bind toes, open chest		
this is Baddha-padmasana, hold for 1 deep inhalation				
9 Nava	out	bend forward, chin to floor		
this is Yoga-mudra; hold for 10 deep breaths				
10 Daśa	in & out	back to Baddha-padmasana, hold the pose		
11 Ekadaśa	in	hands on the floor, lift up		
12 Dvādaśa	out	catvāri position		
13 Trayodaśa	in	upward-facing dog		
14 Caturdaśa	out	downward-facing dog		
15 Pañcadaśa	in	jump forward, stretch the spine, head up		
16 Ṣoḍaśa	out	bend forward		
Samasthitihi	in	come up, stand straight		

Baddha-padmāsana
& Yoga-mudrā

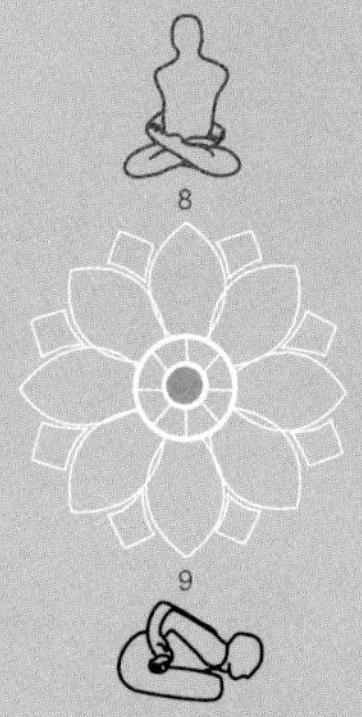

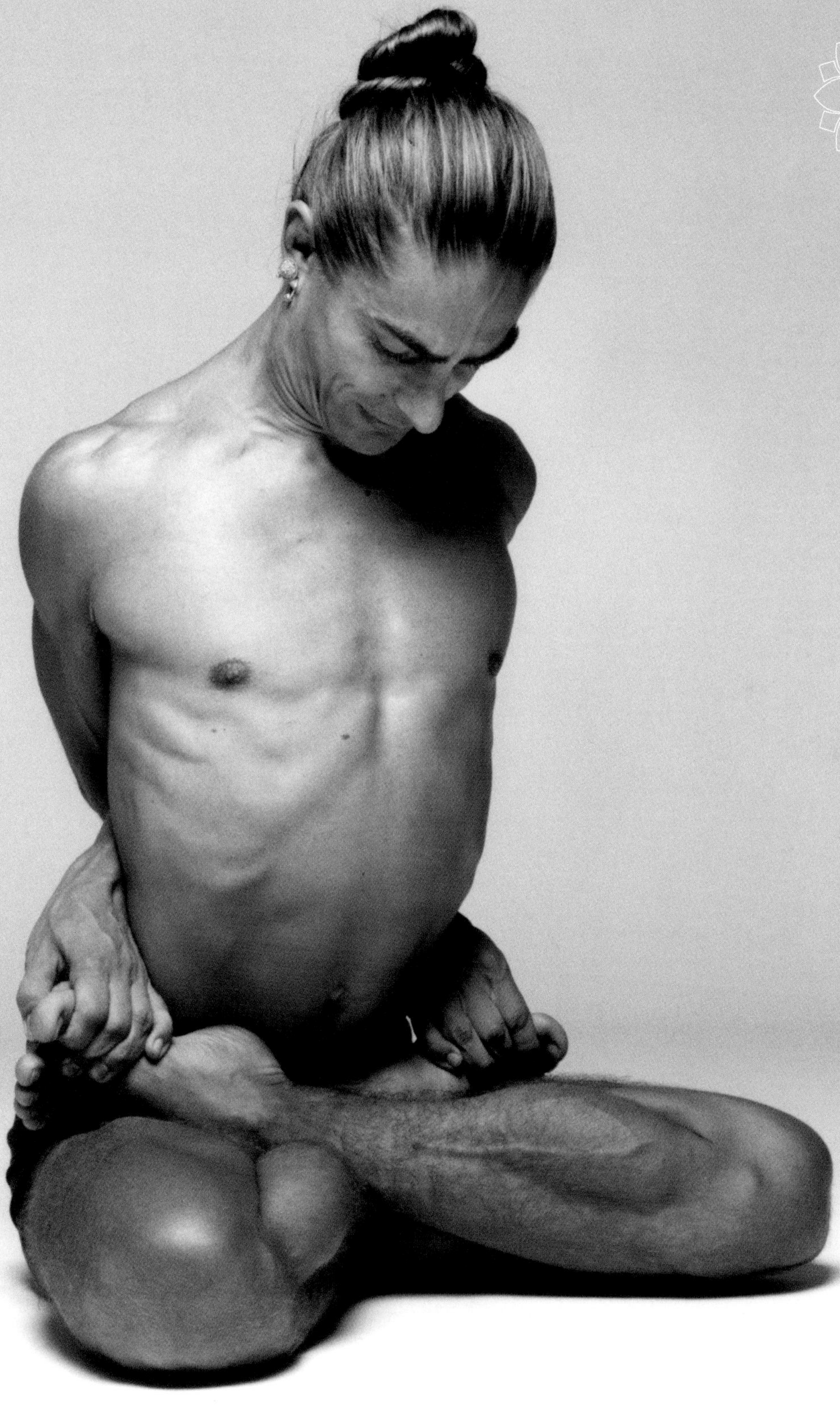

Padmāsana &
Utplutiḥ

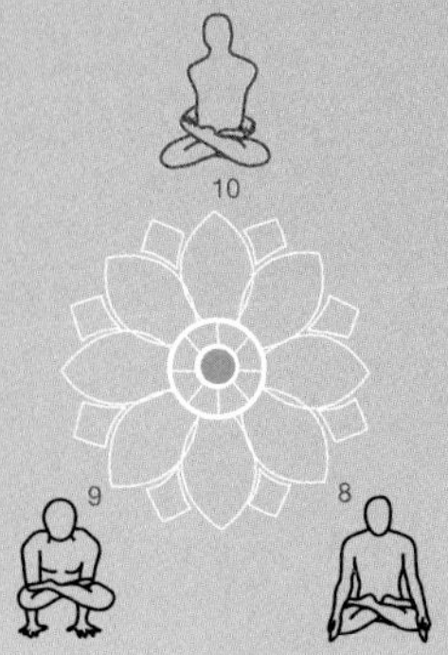

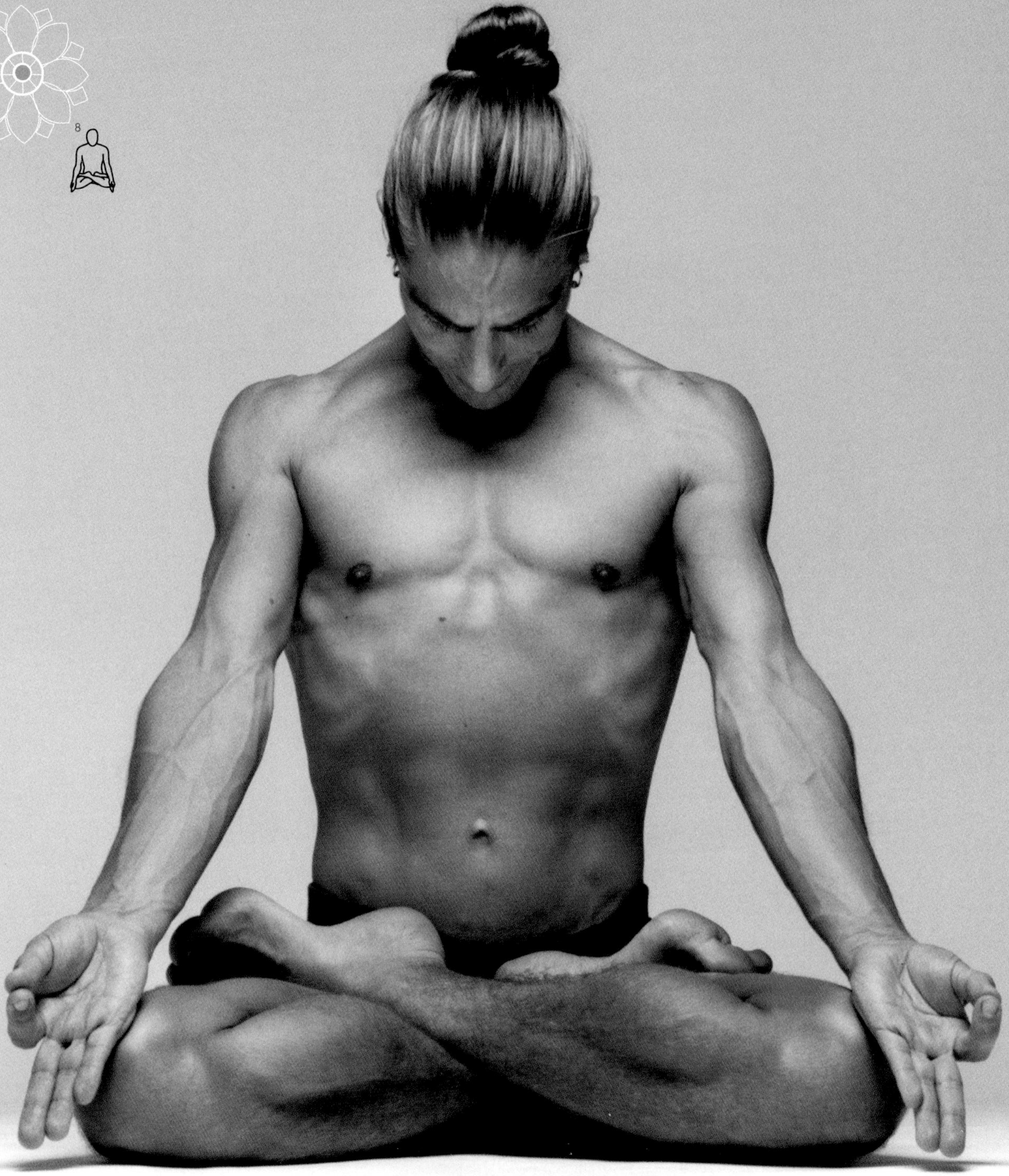

Padmāsana & Utplutiḥ [lotus pose & strong lift]

14 vinyāsas

Padma – lotus; *āsana* – seat, posture; *ut* – deep, strong; *pluti* – lift, take off, rise up

Padmāsana follows directly after the 10th vinyāsa in Baddha-padmāsana.

8 Aṣṭau
On an exhalation, straighten the arms and place the hands (palms out) on the tops of the knees. Touch the tips of the index finger and thumb and straighten the middle, ring and little fingers. Keep them together and pointed towards the floor. This position of the hands is jñāna-mudrā. Lift mūla-bandha to ground the body; engage uddīyana-bandha to elongate the spine and to expand and broaden the chest. Widen the shoulders and draw the chin down towards the collarbones. Lower the knees to the floor and flex the feet. Push the lower abdomen slightly forwards, so that the heels press in on either side of the navel. Separate the knees wider than in other lotus-based positions to open the hips, support the energy flow into the nāḍīs and to increase the lengthening of the spine. This is the state of the āsana. Hold for 10–25 deep breaths. Gaze at the tip of the nose. Note: According to *Yoga Mala*, advanced students can sit in this āsana and meditate for over three hours. This opens the āsana up on a profound level; the mind can reach new states of clarity while the body becomes light and free.

9 Nava
Inhale, press the palms into the floor by the hips. Stretch through the shoulders, engage the arms and lift the body up off the floor, still keeping the legs in lotus. The upper body and legs should create, more or less, a 90-degree angle at the hip crease. Using mūla- and uddīyana-bandha will increase the sense of lightness in this āsana, while building strength in both bandhas. Straighten the spine, keep the head up and open the chest. This is the state of Utplutiḥ. Hold for 10–25 deep breaths (see photo on p. 153). Gaze at the tip of the nose. With the last inhalation, lift the hips up higher and move the legs through the arms without touching the feet to the floor.

10 Daśa
Exhale, release the lotus pose and straighten the legs. When the feet touch the ground, bend the elbows and land in Catvāri. If the legs do not stay in the air during the entire jump-back, keep them lifted for as long as you can. Release the lotus, touch the feet to the floor, and jump back into catvāri. Gaze at the tip of the nose.

Vinyāsas 11–14 are the same as vinyāsas 5–8 in Sūrya-namaskāra A.

Samasthitiḥ
Inhale and come up to standing with a straight body, arms to the sides, and gaze at the tip of the nose. Traditionally, one chants the closing mantra/prayer here, with the head bowed and hands together in front of the heart (kara-mudrā or anjali-mudrā).

Beginners: During these āsanas, one stays in Padmāsana for many breaths. Open the legs to the cross-legged position if Padmāsana starts to feel too uncomfortable. If you cannot bring the legs into lotus, bring the right leg into half-lotus and bend the left leg under the right, or sit in a cross-legged position.

- It is also recommended that beginners practice lotus in the opposite way as well, bringing the left leg first to half lotus and placing the right leg on the top. This will balance the right and left sides.
- It can take many breaths to come into half- and full lotus. Bring the legs into lotus with the help of deep, slow breathing.

Note 1:
The breath is even longer and deeper now than in the earlier finishing poses.

Note 2:
After Padmāsana, take the vinyāsa up to Samasthitiḥ to chant the closing mantra, Śānti mantra (p. 67).

Vinyāsa	Prāṇa (breath)	Āsana (posture)	Dṛṣṭi (gazing point)	Bandha (muscle lock)
Samasthitiḥ		stand straight		
Vinyāsas 1–6 according to Sūrya-namaskāra A				
7 Sapta	in	jump through		
8 Aṣṭau	out	legs in lotus, hands on the knees in jñana mudrā		
state of Padmasana; hold for 10–25 deep breaths				
9 Nava	in	hands on the floor, lift up		
this is Utplutiḥ; hold for 10–25 deep breaths				
10 Daśa	out	jump-back to catvāri position		
11 Ekadaśa	in	upward-facing dog		
12 Dvādaśa	out	downward-facing dog		
13 Trayodaśa	in	jump forwards, stretch the spine, head up		
14 Caturdaśa	out	bend forwards		
Samasthitiḥ	in	come up, stand straight, closing mantra		

sukhāsana

Note:
Pattabhi Jois called this pose resting pose; Sharath Jois calls it Sukhāsana, easy pose. It is commonly known as Sāvāsana, corpse pose.

Sukhāsana, relaxation pose, is done after the āsana and prāṇāyama practice. Prepare yourself for comfortable relaxation by keeping the body warm and making sure you will not be disturbed. Put on warm, dry clothes or use a blanket that will protect you from any draft or chill. The final resting pose is of utmost importance as the body and mind need some time to recover after the practice. Muscles receive the chance to soften and the nervous system can settle, bringing a peaceful state to your mind and deserved release for your body.

Do vinyāsas 1–6 of Sūrya-namaskāra A after chanting the closing mantra.

7 Sapta

Inhale, jump through to sitting and come to lie down. Open the legs and arms so that the feet are about mat-width apart, with hands by the sides. The palms can either face up towards the ceiling or face down and touch the floor. Lengthen the back of the neck by drawing the chin down slightly. Close the eyes and relax the eyelids. Lengthen the hips by stretching the legs out. Relax and widen the shoulders and let the spine settle comfortably along the floor. Slow the breathing down even more, releasing all tension from the body and mind. Open the mouth slightly and release the body further, including more subtle areas, such as your facial muscles, scalp, tongue, corners of the mouth, fingers and toes. Relax the body effortlessly and breathe calmly. If other thoughts arise, simply return the focus peacefully to your breathing. Allow the feelings of light, freedom and happiness to be fully absorbed within. If you continue to feel tension arising in a specific area of the body, direct the breath to that place, release the tension using your breath and return to relaxing the entire body.

Stay here for 5 to 15 minutes.

In this resting pose, the mind can become conscious of the different phases and levels of relaxation. Avoid drifting off into sleep, as that will lessen the body's ability to create restorative energy, increasing the level of tamas guṇa instead (see p.49)

When you have finished resting, take a deep, energizing inhalation and exhalation. Wake the body up again with small movements and stretches (e.g. move the fingers and toes, circle the ankles and wrists, stretch the arms over the head, bring the knees into the chest, and roll slowly onto the back). Open your eyes and slowly come up to sitting. You should feel peaceful, clear-minded, renewed and fully energized.

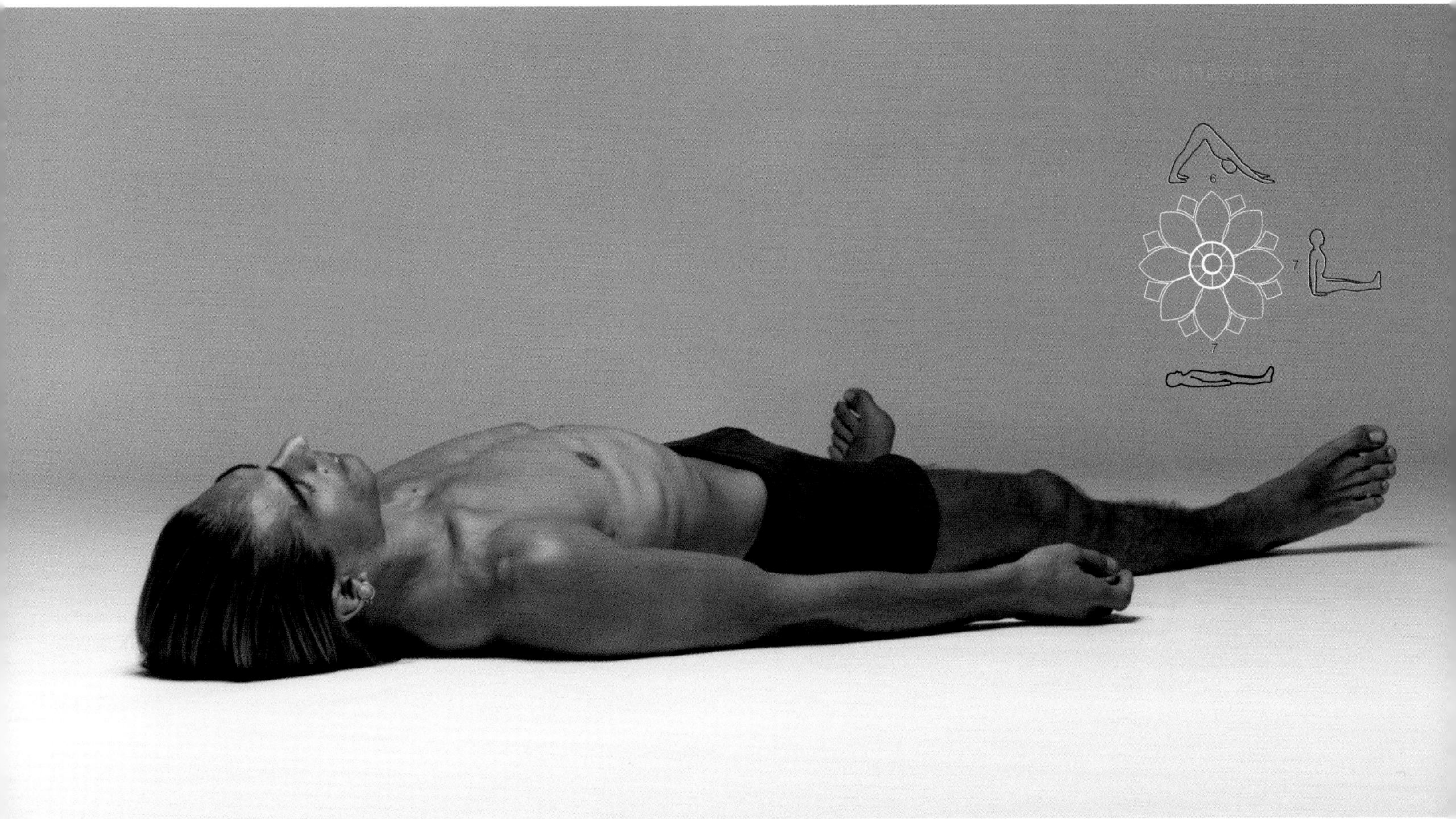
6
7
7

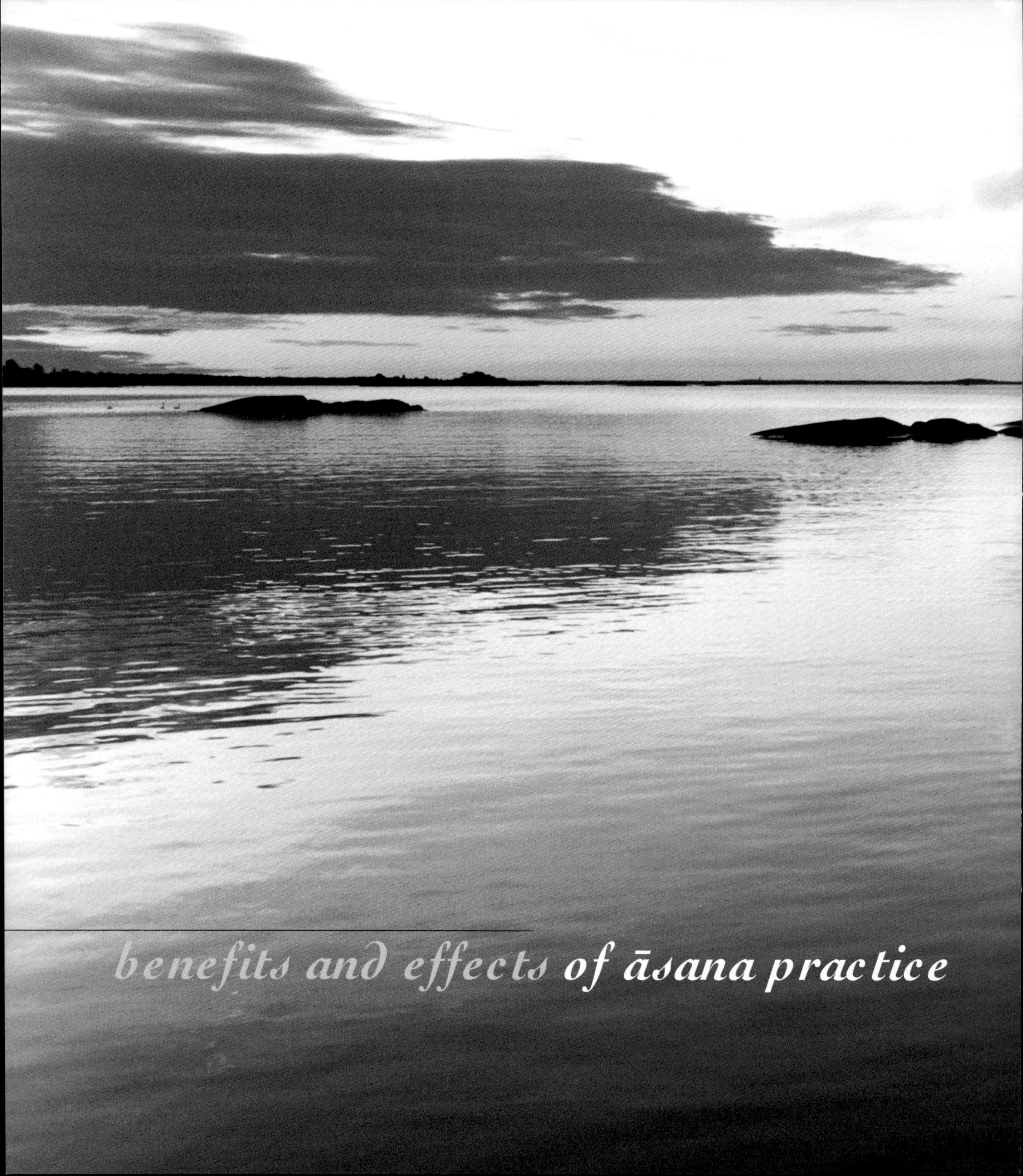

benefits and effects of āsana practice

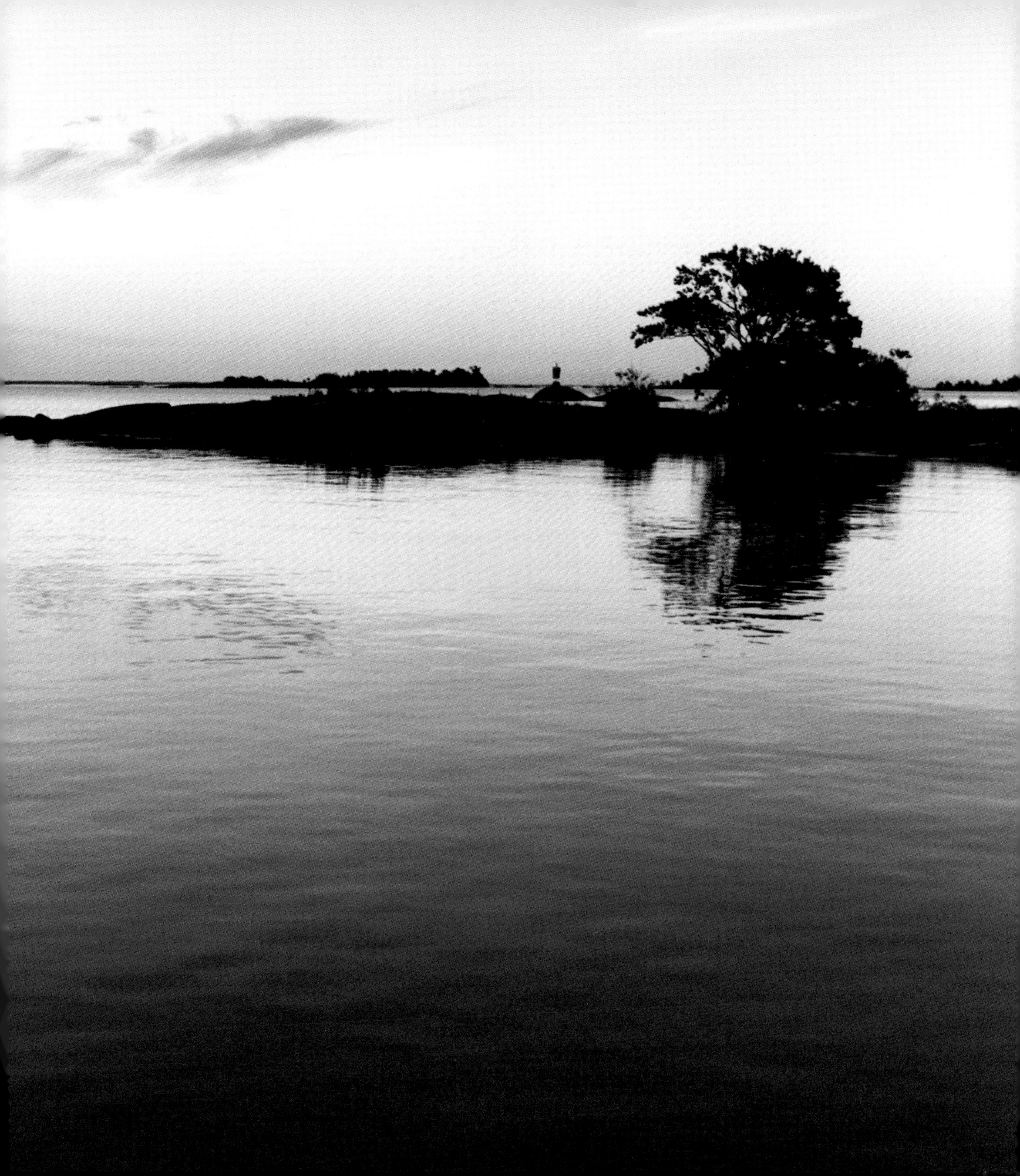

external effects

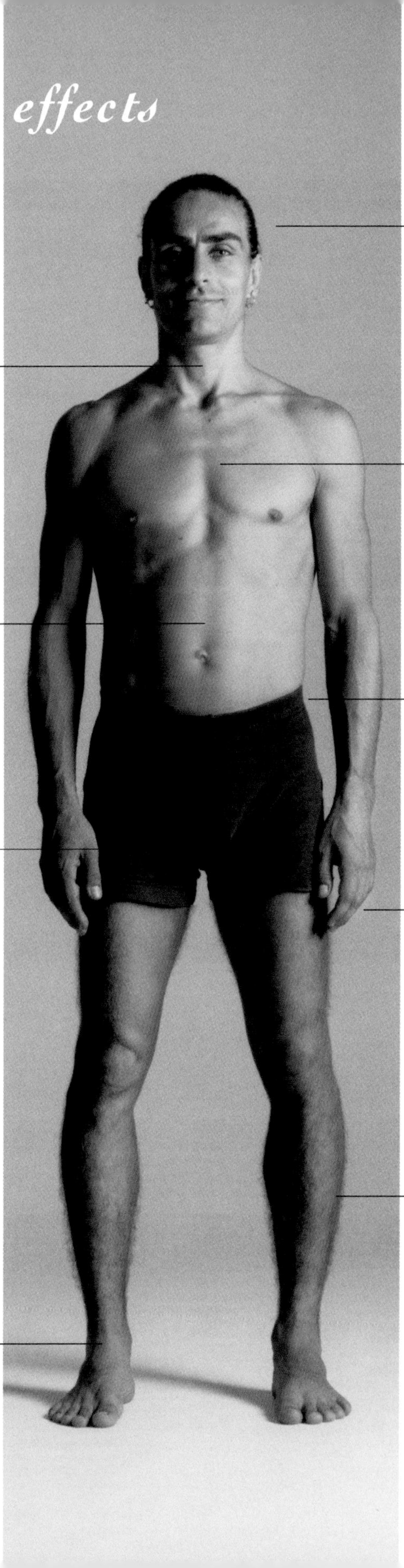

Throat and neck

Headstand and other inversions strengthen the finer muscles along the upper spine and neck, providing more range of motion to this area. These āsanas bring clarity to the voice and strengthen the respiratory system. Key āsanas: Setu-bandhāsana, Salamba-sarvāṅgāsana.

Stomach and lower back

When strong and elastic, the muscles in the stomach and lower back balance and support the entire body. They also protect inner organs, such as the liver, gall bladder, kidneys and spleen, from stress and injury. Organs such as these are both stimulated and cleansed by the practice. Key āsanas: Ardha-baddha-padmottānāsana, Navāsana, Kūrmāsana, Ūrdhva-mukha-paścimottānāsana, Ūrdhva-dhanur-āsana.

Tailbone and sexual organs

The tailbone, or base of the spine, is the origin of the body's strength. Mūla-bandha is rooted at the base of the spine, and when it is strong, the body feels light and mobile. Strengthening and gaining control of the muscles around the anus and recturm can help with such ailments as hemorrhoids and lazy bowel syndrome. When the muscles of the sexual organs are strong, the quality of sperm and ova improve and such ailments as incontinence and impotence may improve. Key āsanas: Jānu-śīrṣāsana B, Baddha-koṇāsana, Garbha-piṇḍāsana and Kukkuṭāsana.

Feet

The entire body is supported by the feet. Stretching them and releasing tension from the joints in the feet helps with balance, improves mobility through the spine, and brings a sense of lightness and ease when on the feet. Āsana practice can correct misalignment in the feet and toes and can prevent injury of the ligaments. Key āsanas: standing āsanas.

Head

Due to the reverse flow of blood, inversions are most beneficial for the head and brain, enriching these areas with fresh oxygen, vitamins and trace elements. The physical effects of inversions include hair growth and improved skin conditions. We also benefit mentally and emotionally from inversions, as they positively affect the quality of our thoughts and leave us feeling energized.
Key āsanas: Salamba-sarvāṅgāsana, Śīrṣāsana.

Chest and sternum

Stretching and relaxing deeply through the chest, sternum, shoulders and collarbones creates more space in the lungs and heart area. The muscles located around the shoulder blades, which support the back and improve posture, are strengthened, improving overall health and happiness. When the chest is free from blockages, ailments such as asthma and heart problems are alleviated. Key āsanas: Sūrya-namaskāra A & B, Setu-bandhāsana, Ūrdhva-dhanur-āsana.

Pelvis and hips

The hips and pelvis are the basis for the majority of the āsanas. Strong and open hips bring depth to the postures. When the hips are mobile, excess fat is dissolved and the intestines are purified, which improves digestion. The yoga āsanas which focus on the hip area strengthen the womb, diminishing the risk of a miscarriage and helping with delivery during childbirth. Key āsanas: Paścima-tānāsana, Marīcy-āsana C & D, Baddha-koṇāsana, Upaviṣṭa-koṇāsana.

The arms and hands

Most of the āsanas stretch and strengthen the arms and increase the flow of blood. The arms get stronger, the hands warmer and the sense of touch becomes refined. Key āsanas: Sūrya-namaskāra A and B, Prasārita-pādottānāsana C, Pārśvottānāsana.

Legs

The standing āsanas develop both strength and flexibility in the muscles and joints of the legs. Circulation throughout the body is improved as the blood pumps more efficiently through the thighs and hamstrings. Stiffness through major joints such as the knees, hips and ankles is alleviated, and flexibility in the muscles surrounding the knees supports and creates space in the knee joints. Stiffness in the knees or hyperextension will decrease. Strong legs protect against varicose veins as well as prevent a general sense of fatigue and pain in the body.
Key āsanas: Utthita-trikoṇāsana A & B, Utkaṭāsana, Vīrabhadrāsana A & B.

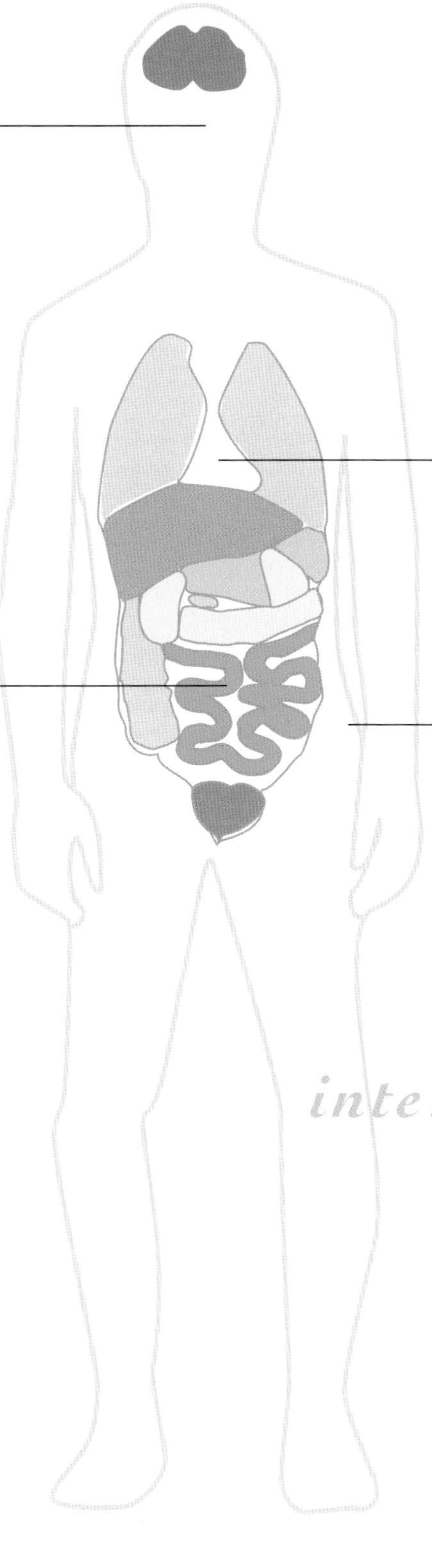

Head

Dṛṣṭi, or gazing points, and sound breathing provide the following benefits:
- Dṛṣṭi strengthens the eye muscles and sharpens the sense of sight.
- Sound breathing awakens the sense of smell and sense of hearing.
- Yoga āsanas, and inversions in particular, clarify and activate the senses.
- Inversions move amṛta-bindu (p. 46) and prāṇa towards the crown of the head, promoting overall health and longevity and awaken spirituality.

Key āsanas: Salamba-sarvāṅgāsana & Śīrṣāsana

Stomach and lower back

The body and senses are cleansed by agni, the fire of digestion that burns in the stomach energy center (vaishvanara). When this energy is activated, one might sense a warm or even burning sensation in the stomach. This energy is responsible for digestion. mūla-bandha, uddīyana-bandha and firm hip muscles all contribute to efficient digestion. Furthermore, the small and large intestines are cleansed, and ailments and energy blocks in this region of the body are removed. Key āsanas: Navāsana, Ūrdhva-mukha-paścimottānāsana, Ūrdhva-dhanur-āsana.

Chest and sternum

The chest and sternum surround the heart, both on the physical and energetic level. The heart cakra lies within the chest and is the body's fourth energy center. Opening the heart center cultivates trust in our intuition and a willingness to accept things as they are, and increases our capacity for compassion, self-acceptance and love. Key āsanas: all, when done with the right, meditative intention.

Hips and pelvis

The root of the energy centers, and the origin of the energy channels, lie within the hips and pelvis. The energy channels begin at the kāṇḍa or kāṇḍasthana (pp. 42), an egg-shaped energy center located deep within the pelvis. When both the hips and pelvis are strong and mobile, energy from the lower cakras can flow unrestricted to other parts of the body.

internal effects:

Āsana and prāṇāyama have an enormously positive effect on the muscles, circulation, nervous system and inner organs. They serve to activate the energy centers, cleanse the paths of the energy channels and distribute the flow of energy throughout the body. It usually takes more time to sense and trust the more quiet and subtle layers of the practice than it does to notice the tangible effects that occur on the physical level.

Every āsana will have various effects on the part of the body being activated in the particular pose. To access the āsanas on a more therapeutic level, it is recommended to hold poses that open up problematic or stiff areas longer than usual. These can be held for 10–80 breaths. It is not suggested, however, that you do only a few āsanas as therapy poses. It is essential to practice āsana in the proper sequence, as the order is an integral part of the yoga-cikitsā series, which was created as a systematic and holistic practice of therapy.

specific effects and benefits of the āsanas

Pādāṅguṣṭhāsana & Pāda-hastāsana

- strengthen the stomach, hips and leg muscles
- stimulate and purify the liver and spleen
- cleanse the urine and increase the quantity of digestive fluids
- heal the rectum and anus
- reduce gas
- dissolve excess fat from the stomach and hips

Utthita-trikoṇāsana A & B

- strengthen the feet, hip- and back muscles
- dissolve excess fat from the hips and waist
- improve digestion and increase digestive fluids
- relieve difficulties in breathing and expand the trachea and chest
- circulate the breath more freely in the throat and chest
- strengthen the spine and relax the nervous system (mainly in the rotation in Trikoṇāsana B)

Utthita-pārśvakoṇāsana A & B

- strengthen the back, hips and legs
- open the ankles and knees
- dissolve excess fat from the hips and waist
- stimulate the digestive organs
- relieve lower back pain
- alleviate breathing issues (mainly in the rotation in Pārśvakoṇāsana B)
- correct the alignment of the spine
- release the nerves around the spine

Prasārita-pādottānāsana A, B, C & D

- stretch and lengthen the hamstrings, feet, hips and back
- reverse the blood flow and bring nourishment to the brain (when the head is down)
- dissolve excess fat from the hips and stomach

C-variation:

- releases tension from the shoulders and shoulder blades
- stretches the wrists
- increases blood circulation in the upper body
- clears blockages in the air way

Pārśvottānāsana

- increases flexibility in the hips, feet and back
- releases tension through the shoulders and shoulder blades
- opens the chest and expands the breathing
- dissolves excess fat from the stomach and hips
- stabilizes the hips, feet, stomach and back

Utthita-hasta-pādāṅguṣṭhāsana

- strengthens the leg muscles
- increases flexibility in the hips and back
- develops balance and muscle control
- removes excess fat from the hips and waist
- strengthens and purifies the kidneys

Ardha-baddha-padmottānāsana

- increases mobility in the feet, ankles, knees and hips
- stimulates the intestines, spleen and the liver; right leg stimulates the spleen (on the left side of the navel) and left leg the liver (on the right side of the navel)
- activates digestion
- dissolves excess fat from the hips and waist
- relieves abdominal swelling and heals damaged stomach tissue (resulting from poor eating and drinking habits or illness)
- reverses complications caused by eating disorders

Utkaṭāsana

- engages the legs, hips, stomach and back
- stretches the Achilles tendon, ankles and shoulders
- removes excess fat from the hips and waist
- purifies the rectum
- heals slipped disks and relieves pain in the sacrum
- straightens out scoliosis
- relieves rheumatic pain of the back and pelvis

Vīrabhadrāsana A & B

- strengthen the legs, hips, and spine
- purify the lower abdomen, spine and sexual organs
- open the respiratory system (Vīrabhadrāsana A)
- expand the shoulders and back of the neck
- stimulate the throat cakra (viśuddha)
- relieve cramping and rheumatism in the legs, feet and joints

Paścima-tānāsana A, B & C

- enable proper digestion
- activate the digestive fire (agni) and stimulate a poor appetite
- remove excess fat from the waist and hips
- stimulate the liver
- cures dizziness and lethargy
- stretch the hamstrings, calves, hips and spine
- open the nāḍīs so that prāṇa can enter the body

Pūrvatanāsana

- increases flexibility in the feet, ankles and shoulders
- purifies the anus, rectum, waist and spine
- develops the muscles in the thighs, hips, stomach, back and arms
- rejuvenates, relaxes and strengthens the nervous system
- fortifies the heart and lungs

Ardha-baddha-padma-paścima-tānāsana

- stretches and strengthens the ligaments in the ankles and knees
- increases the range of motion in the legs, back and hips
- stimulates the intestines and the liver
- activates digestion
- dissolves excess fat from the hips and waist
- diminishes swelling of the abdomen
- improves damaged stomach tissue resulting from poor eating habits

Tiryaṅ-mukhaikapāda-paścima-tānāsana

- opens the ankles, knees, and hips
- softens joints made stiff from previous injury or surgery
- stimulates the lymph nodes
- reduces swelling of the feet
- cures sciatic pain and hemorrhoids
- purifies the small and large intestines

Jānu-śīrṣāsana A, B & C

- open the joints of the feet, back, ankles, knees and hips
- stimulate the spleen, liver, pancreas and kidneys
- rejuvenate sexual organs, increase the quality of the sperm and other fluids (shukra; vīrya (sperm) and śoṇita (female sexual fluids) via the vīrya- and śīvani-nāḍīs
- the śīvani-nāḍī purifies inner organs and strengthens the male and female sexual fluids
- support proper retention and elimination of urine from the bladder
- purify vīrya-nala-nāḍī (at the perineum in men and closer to the navel in women)
- reduce the effects of diabetes through the vīrya-nala-nāḍī (connected to the pancreas and responsible for insulin production)

Marīcy-āsana A

- dissolves excess fat from the stomach and hips
- reduces gas
- relieves menstrual cramps and strengthens the uterus
- lowers the risk of miscarriage
- purifies the large intestine and gall bladder
- activates the third cakra (maṇipura)

Marīcy-āsana B

- increases flexibility and heals injuries in the ankles, knees, hips and back
- purifies the kidneys, liver, spleen, intestines and rectum
- dissolves excess fat from the stomach and hips
- improves digestion and blood circulation
- alleviates gas
- relieves menstrual pain and strengthens the uterus
- lowers the risk of miscarriage
- purifies the large intestine and gall bladder
- invigorates the third cakra (maṇipura)

Marīcy-āsana C

- releases the nerves around the spine
- reduces mental stress
- extends range of motion along the spine
- reduces stiffness in the outer thigh and hip
- increases mobility in the shoulder joints
- increases flexibility and heals injuries in the ankles, knees, hips and back
- purifies the kidneys, liver, spleen, intestines and rectum
- dissolves excess fat from the stomach and hips
- improves digestion and blood circulation
- alleviates gas
- relieves menstrual cramps and strengthens the uterus
- lowers the risk of miscarriage
- purifies the large intestine and gall bladder
- invigorates the third cakra (maṇipura)

Marīcy-āsana D

- refer to Marīcy-āsana B & C

Navāsana

- strengthens the legs, hips, stomach muscles, lower back
- straightens the spine
- purifies the digestive system and alleviates gas
- dissolves excess fat from the abdomen

Bhuja-pīḍāsana

- strengthens the wrists, arms, shoulders and stomach muscles
- naturally develops mūla-bandha and uddīyana-bandha
- increases muscle control and balance
- purifies the throat (anna nala)

Kūrmāsana & supta-kūrmāsana

- open the chest and shoulders and improve posture
- straighten the spine and release tension in the back
- free the nerve channels (e.g. sciatic nerve) that travel along the spine and into the legs
- lighten the hips and legs
- expand the chest, lungs and back, and improve blood circulation
- deeply stretch the hamstrings and lower back, as well as the finer muscles among the ribs and collarbones
- balance the energy flows (prāṇa-vāyu and apāna-vāyu), deepen the breath and calm the mind
- stimulate the kidneys and release excess phlegm from the air passages (a kapha doṣa imbalance)
- activate kāṇḍa, the source of the nāḍīs

Garbha-piṇḍāsana

- purifies the intestines, liver, rectum and spleen
- activates the three cakras by the tailbone, lower abdomen and navel
- dissolves excess fat around the abdomen
- strengthens the uterus and lowers the risk of miscarriage
- massages, softens and releases the spine (rolling action) after Supta-kūrmāsana
- increases flexibility in the ankles, knees and hip joints
- releases tension in the calves

Kukkuṭāsana

- strengthens the wrists, arms, shoulders and stomach muscles
- activates the first three cakras, or energy centers, by the tailbone, lower abdomen and navel
- cleanses the liver and spleen
- dissolves excess fat
- releases excess phlegm from the air passages (a kapha doṣa imbalance)
- purifies the intestines, liver, rectum and spleen

Baddha-koṇāsana

This is the most effective āsana to cure ailments of the rectum and anus.

- heals hemorrhoids, constipation, digestive problems, bladder problems, irregularity in the menstrual cycle and sciatica
- alleviates problems with dhātus related to a decrease in the production of sexual fluids
- softens the joints in the ankles, knees and hips
- opens the chest and shoulders and improves posture
- aids in childbirth by softening and opening the hips

Upaviṣṭa-koṇāsana

- stretches the hamstrings and hip joints
- improves posture and opens the chest and shoulders
- releases tension in the back
- improves circulation through the hips
- strengthens the perineal muscles
- invigorates grdhasi-nāḍī (located at the perineum; serves as a link between all the other nāḍīs)
- keeps the hips and back strong and supple
- cures problems associated with sciatica
- improves the functioning of the intestines and dissolves excess fat from the hips and stomach

Supta-koṇāsana

This āsana has similar effects to the two preceding poses. Furthermore, as the first part of the āsana is an inversion, it has some of the effects of shoulderstand, Salamba-sarvāṅgāsana.

- opens the chest and shoulders and improves posture
- releases tension in the back
- stimulates agni, digestive fire
- heals illnesses related to the intestines and hips, such as hemorrhoids (mulavyadhista), constipation, bladder problems, irregularity in the menstrual cycle and sciatica
- improves control over the hips and stomach muscles, which helps in childbirth
- stimulates gridhasi-nāḍī
- purifies the throat and stimulates viśuddha-cakra, which encourages clarity in the voice
- fortifies the heart, purifies the lungs and alleviates asthma-related problems
- improves the functioning of the intestines and dissolves excess fat from the hips and stomach

Supta-pādāṅguṣṭhāsana

This āsana is the supine version of Utthita-hasta-pādāṅguṣṭhāsana. As you are now lying down, it may be easier to stretch the legs.

- develops control of the bandhas, and strengthens the stomach muscles and the upper body
- dissolves excess fat from the hips and stomach
- purifies and strengthens the kidneys
- purifies the urinary tract, rectum, blood vessels, cures hemorrhoids and strengthens the vas deferens (vīrya nala)
- massages the spine (Cakrāsana, backwards-roll)
- simultaneously strengthens and releases the back of the neck

Ubhaya-pādāṅguṣṭhāsana

- improves posture and opens the chest and shoulders
- releases tension in the back and massages the spine
- improves balance
- improves blood circulation through the spine
- purifies the stomach, anus, rectum, sexual organs and lumbar region (katti granthi)
- cures hemorrhoids as well as problems related to the urinary tract
- opens the three energy knots, granthi-traya, allowing prāṇa to flow to the suṣumnā-nāḍī

Ūrdhva-mukha-paścimottānāsana

- improves posture and opens the chest and shoulders
- releases tension in the back and massages the spine
- improves balance
- utilizes the back and stomach muscles
- stimulates svādhiṣṭhāna-cakra, located at the sacrum
- purifies the region around hips and stomach

Setu-bandhāsana

- develops the muscles in the back of the neck
- increases mobility in the neck and enhances use of the voice and throat
- activates the root cakra (mūlādhāra) and throat cakra (viśuddha)
- improves balance
- aids in the proper functioning of the esophagus, lungs and heart

Ūrdhva-dhanur-āsana

- releases muscle and nerve tension
- realigns the spine
- extends the front of the thighs, chest and shoulders
- stretches and strengthens the wrists
- simultaneously engages and releases the arms and shoulders
- strengthens the inner organs
- improves digestion
- expands the chest
- purifies the lungs, throat and esophagus

Salamba-sarvāṅgāsana

It is said that this āsana cures all ailments. The benefits of the āsana will increase the longer you hold the pose. Refer also to the benefits of the finishing āsanas (pp. 152–53).

- improves posture and opens the chest and shoulders
- releases tension in the back
- increases control of mūla-bandha, uddīyana-bandha, and jalandara bandha, the throat lock
- purifies the throat and stimulates viśuddha-cakra, which enhances the voice
- clarifies the voice and makes it melodious
- cures ailments of the throat, asthma and heart-related illnesses
- revives the lungs, heart and limbs
- balances the thyroid-gland hormones
- helps cure insomnia and mental illnesses (through long-term, sustained practice)

Halāsana

Refer to pp. 152–53

- aligns the hips
- purifies and strengthens the hips, intestines and stomach
- cures all ailments of the throat and chest, including respiratory problems such as asthma and chronic bronchitis; heart problems, sore throat, unclear speech and loss of speech

Karṇa-pīḍāsana

Refer to pp. 152–53

- alleviates ear infections, tinnitus and other ear-related problems
- purifies the ears and improves the sense of hearing

Ūrdhva-padmāsana

Refer to pp. 152–53

- purifies the rectum and urinary tract
- strengthens the stomach and back

Piṇḍāsana

Refer to pp. 152–53

- stimulates purification of the stomach, intestines, liver, spleen and spine

Matsyāsana

This āsana works as a counter-pose to the shoulderstanding āsanas.

- releases tension in the back of the neck
- increases mobility through the neck
- purifies the esophagus and lungs and strengthens the heart
- opens the throat and clarifies the voice
- purifies the anus, rectum, liver and spleen
- stimulates the root cakra, mūlādhāra-cakra (see above)

Uttāna-pādāsana

The effects of this āsana are similar to Matsyāsana.

- strengthens the legs, hips and stomach muscles

Śīrṣāsana

Headstand belongs to the (inverted) finishing poses (viparīta-karaṇi) and many of its benefits are listed on pp. 152–53. It is considered to be the "king of the yoga āsanas."

- improves balance and increases confidence
- engages the muscles needed for balance, and familiarizes one with being upside-down
- rejuvenates the nāḍīs and carries blood to the head
- replenishes the crown of the head and the sense organs
- improves and increases sensitivity in the senses of sight, smell and hearing
- releases tension in the muscles and nerves throughout the body
- encourages feelings of lightness, relaxation and peace of mind
- purifies the sahasrāra-cakra, the crown cakra, and helps contain amṛta-bindu within the head

Baddha-padmāsana & Yoga-mudrā

- simultaneously strengthen and increase flexibility in the ankles, knees, hips and lower back
- open the chest, shoulders and upper back
- purify the intestines, liver, lower back, spleen, anus and rectum
- remove excess fat from the waist and hips

Padmāsana & Utpluti

Refer to pp. 152–53

- bring flexibility to the ankles, knees, and hip joints
- expand the lower back
- facilitate the flow of energy through the nāḍīs
- calm the mind and focus the concentration
- unlock the three energy knots, granthi-traya, allowing pranic energy to flow to the suṣumnā-nāḍī
- burn off old karma and heal all ailments (according to ancient texts)
- develop the strength and awareness of the bandhas (Utpluti)

aṣṭāṅga yoga and natural rhythms

Pattabhi Jois can be quoted as having said that aṣṭāṅga yoga is not meant for lazy people. All those who follow the traditional vinyāsa method will certainly agree. The practice consists of six āsana series (Primary, Intermediate, Advanced A, B, C and D) which require increasing levels of proficiency. The week traditionally begins on Sunday, when one would do the Intermediate series; on Monday, Advanced A; Tuesday, Advanced B; Wednesday, Advanced C; Thursday, Advanced D; and on Friday, the Primary series. Saturday is meant for resting, when one refrains from strenuous physical and mental activity. The necessity of this day of rest must not be underestimated, as it is crucial for the body and mind to recover.

If you are currently working on the Primary series, this will be your weekly practice. When a teacher starts to add poses from the Intermediate series, continue with the Primary series from Sunday to Thursday, adding on the new Intermediate poses after Setu-bandhāsana. When you have come more or less halfway along the Intermediate series, the teacher may split the two series. At this point, from Sunday to Thursday, you would stop doing Primary and practice the Intermediate series as far as it has been taught. Fridays are always reserved for the Primary series only.

When one progresses through to the end of the Intermediate series and starts to work on the Advanced A series, the weekly schedule is as follows: Sunday, Intermediate series; from Monday to Thursday, Intermediate series and individually-taught poses from Advanced A. Similarly, when one has come more or less half-way through Advanced A, the teacher can split the practice. At which point, one reserves Sunday for the Intermediate series, Monday through Thursday for Advanced A and Friday for the Primary series. One moves through the six series with the same pattern. However, the Primary series is always consistently practised on Fridays. Note that moon days are not considered to be rest days in this weekly practice pattern. Therefore, the regular routine is maintained up to the day before, and carried on after, the moon day. This weekly rhythm follows the traditional way, as taught by Pattabhi Jois, and is still carried out in this manner by Sharath and Saraswati Jois in Mysore. However, various circumstances in our daily lives can often prevent us from following this exact rhythm and chances are, you might have to adjust according to what suits you best. For example, if your schedule doesn't permit Saturday to be your rest day, do the Primary series the day before your allocated rest day.

In addition to Saturdays, rest days are taken on the holidays that are observed in your own religion, culture and country. It is also advisable to take rest after a long journey or after particularly exhausting work, simply allowing the body to recover. If you feel up to practising, go through only part of the series, keeping it light and gentle.

Beginners

In spite of the recommended traditional six-day-a-week practice schedule, develop a rhythm that supports your situation in life. Finding the time to practice six days a week requires some reorganization of time, work, family, hobbies and relationships. Incorporate the practice into your daily life gradually. Stay calm and tolerant of people who may seem skeptical or sarcastic regarding the efficacy of yoga. Often their disbelief in, and resistence to, the practice will diminish as they see you grow stronger, healthier and happier.

Moon days

As human beings are an integral part of nature and the surrounding environment, people are affected by the movements and activity of the solar system. For example, farmers, hunters and fishermen became aware, over the ages, of the influence of the solar system on the cyclical rhythm of nature. They gave careful consideration in determining the exact days and times most beneficial for setting traps, casting nets, or planting seeds and cultivating the harvest. In India, an astrological chart is always consulted regarding the important events that mark daily life. People will check an astrological chart and consult an astrologer to determine the most auspicious and appropriate day(s) for such events as weddings and important rituals. Astrologers and astrological charts are also used for determining a person's compatibility when choosing a spouse.

Many of us are unconscious of the effects the full and new moon have on us and our surroundings. Some people may feel it physically, in the quality and quantity of their sleep, or in how much or how little energy they have. In this tradition of aṣṭāṅga yoga, moon days are not considered favorable for yoga practice. The Jyotishas, Vedic astrologers, check the exact time of the moon day and its energetic effects, based on the position of the moon and stars. Pattabhi Jois mentioned that it is not an easy calculation to make and has to be done by a skilled Jyotisha. The moon day is generally considered to be the 23-hour period before the exact moment of either a full or new moon, and is thought to be an unstable time for both the body and mind. On these days, the risk of injury increases as the concentration and energy required for the practice is disturbed.

Menstruation

Menstruation is a natural cleansing process, which follows the moon cycle. An average menstrual cycle lasts, more or less, for about 28 days or four weeks. After which, if an ovum has not been fertilized by sperm, hormones are secreted that initiate the shedding of the uterine walls, which typically lasts about three to five days. This process cleanses the inner organs, and creates helpful bacteria which keep the uterus clean. In a healthy body, the menses, the fluid that comes out that contains blood and endometrial tissue, is generally red in color and should have a neutral smell.

"Acid purifies bronze, a river is purified by its own stream, and a woman is purified during menstruation."
– Vinod Verma: The Kāma Sūtra for Women

Women go through several physical and mental changes during menstruation. It is especially important to allow for the menses to flow out freely, without disturbing this natural cleansing cycle by practising intense āsana, or engaging in other extreme physical or mental practices and activity.

Pattabhi Jois recommended that women take rest for the first three days of menstruation. On the morning of the fourth day, a hot bath is recommended to relieve the symptoms that can arise at this time. After this, she can return to her normal practice. If somehow menstruation has stopped and there is no sign of pregnancy, at every full moon (until her period starts again), the woman should take three days off from practicing, as she would if she was having her period. This may help to bring the natural rhythm back to her cycle.

"Woman should understand the process of menstruation and its cause, perceive herself better, and get a firm grip on her femininity and life."
– Vinod Verma: The Kāma Sūtra for Women

Some women feel stronger during their period, and others find that the āsanas relieve the cramps that can accompany menstruation. For these reasons, many continue practising during this time. According to Pattabhi Jois, this can perhaps provide a feeling of relief, but he claimed it was not that advantageous for the inner cleansing process. This is an important point to understand, as this internal process of cleansing has longer-lasting effects on both body and mind. Furthermore, the downwards flow of blood utilizes apana energy, making it much more difficult to control the bandhas or to use them effectively. Nor is it particularly helpful to engage the bandhas during menstruation, which naturally causes energy to flow down and out. Disturbing this natural downwards-moving flow can create an imbalance in the body as things, quite literally, go against the stream. If women continue to practise during menstruation, it can lead to cycle irregularity, amenorrhea or, in worst-case scenarios, a damaged uterus. Giving the body time to rest from āsana regulates the cycle, strengthens the female reproductive organs, and restores balance in the body and mind.

Pregnancy

The process of creating a new life brings us into contact with the same creation that brought about the entire universe. Before, during and after pregnancy, it behooves the mother and father to assure that this new life gets the best start possible.

A yogic lifestyle supports activity which strengthens and revives both the mother and child during all phases of pregnancy, delivery and postpartum.

One of yoga's most important tasks is to encourage the creation of healthy offspring with the possibility for spiritual development. A sound body and mind in both parents can bring about a healthy child. Āsanas strengthen the uterus, improve control of the muscles in the groin in particular, and the whole body in general, and lower the risk of miscarriage. Sound breathing can help alleviate pain, cleanse the inner organs and nervous system as well as calm and strengthen the mind, teaching patience and gratitude for life.

"During pregnancy, it is necessary to follow a healthy lifestyle, practice yoga and use rejuvenating products. With their help, the womb will become healthy, the joints mobile and the mind stable."
– Vinod Verma: The Kāma Sūtra for Women

Special care should be taken when approaching the Marīcy-āsana series, Garbha-piṇḍāsana and other postures which require the body to twist or in which the core is squeezed deeply. One should move slowly and calmly through the āsanas, breathing deeply and listening carefully to the body.

After childbirth, a woman's body needs time to recover and heal. This is important not only for her and the new-born child, but for the family as well, having gone through a large transformation. The child and the family is now the most important thing in life, and that is reason enough to give plenty of time, care and love to the new arrival.

The earliest one should return to āsana is three months after delivery. First begin with the sun salutations, then add on part of the standing poses. Let this process take time, as returning too quickly to the full series can lower the production of milk and can be too demanding on the stomach muscles and lower back. By accepting the change that pregnancy, childbirth, and, now, child-rearing, has brought to your body, you can find an inner calm and enjoy the gradual process of returning to your āsana practice.

simple sanskrit pronunciation guide

Since the Sanskrit alphabet is made up of more letters than the Roman alphabet, one has to understand the use of special dots and lines known as diacritical marks, which indicate the correct sounds. This book follows the standard system for this and is explained briefly below. While this may seem complicated at first glance, Sanskrit is in fact a logical language and the letters are consistently pronounced in the same way.

Sanskrit has thirteen vowels, classified as long and short. For correct pronunciation, it is essential to differentiate between the two. The short vowels are as follows:

a – pronounced as the "u" in "but"
i – as the "i" in "pin"
u – as the "u" in "push"
ṛ – rolling r; in North India today, often pronounced as "ri", in South India as "ru"
ḷ – Rolling l; sometimes pronounced as "li"

Some of the long vowels are doubled-up versions of short vowels. They are pronounced as follows:

ā – as "a" in "far"
ī – as the "ee" in "beet"
ū – as the "u" in "rule"
ṝ – as ṛ above but twice as long

There are two vowels that have only long versions:

e – as the "e" in "met" but twice as long
o – as the "o" in "bored"

Finally, there are two diphthongs that are counted as long vowels:

ai – as the "uy" in "buy"
au – as the "ow" in "how"

Between vowels and consonants, there are two special letters:

ṁ – nasal m, often pronounced like m (found in bilabial section opposite)
ḥ – final h, nowadays usually pronounced so that the preceding vowel is slightly echoed after it; aḥ thus "aha", iḥ "ihi". Within verses, pronounced as a slight aspiration.

The consonants are divided into groups depending on which part of the mouth is used for pronunciation.

The gutturals are pronounced at the back of the mouth:

k – as "k" in "kite"
kh – as the "ckh" in "Eckhart". This is a separate letter from "k" above.
The "h" in Sanskrit letters is always a clearly heard aspiration.
g – as "g" in "give"
gh – as "gh" in "dig hard"
ṅ – as "ng" in "sing"

In the palatals, your tongue will be up against the palate at the front of the mouth.

c – as in "ch" in "chair"
ch – the same, but with added aspiration, as "chh" in "staunch-heart"
j – as "j" in "joy"
jh – the same, but with added aspiration, as "dgeh" in "hedgehog"
ñ – as "ny" in "canyon"

In the cerebrals, your tongue will touch the top of the mouth, kind of curving backwards, making a sharp sound. The following are approximate values:

ṭ – as "t" in "tub"
ṭh – as "th" in "light-heart"
ḍ – as "d" in "dove"
ḍh – as "dh" in "red-hot"
ṇ – as "n" but with the tongue in the same place as for the other cerebrals. As in "rna", preparing to say the "r"and say "na", as in renown.

In the dentals, the tongue should touch your teeth. This is important, since it differentiates them from the cerebrals above.

The bilabials are sounded by bringing the lips together:

p – as "p" in "pine"
ph – as "ph" in "uphill". Not as "ph" in "philosophy"! There is no "f" in Sanskrit.
b – as "b" in "bird"
bh – as "bh" in "rub hard"
m – as "m" in "mother"

There are four semi-vowels in Sanskrit. These letters are counted as consonants:

y – as "y" in "yes"
r – as "r" in "run"
l – as "l" in "light"
v – as "v" in "vine"

There are three sibilants:

ś – this is a palatal letter (see opposite), as "sh" in shame
ṣ – this is a cerebral (see opposite), as "sh" in "shine". This sibilant and the preceding one are often quite similar in their pronunciation.
s – as "s" in "sun"

There is also a separate aspirate:

h – as "h" in "home"

bibliography

www.kpjayi.org
www.ashtanga.com
www.astanga.fi
www.petriraisanen.com
www.ashtangabook.com
petri@ashtangabook.com
www.namarupa.org

Broo, Måns. *Joogan Filosofia Patanjalin Yoga-sutra*. Helsinki: Gaudeamus, 2010.

Desikachar, Kausthub. *The Yoga of the Yogi*. Chennai: Krishnamacharya Yoga Mandiram, 2005.

Desikachar, T.K.V. *The Heart of Yoga*. Chennai: Inner Traditions,1995.

Desikachar, T.K.V. and R.H. Cravens. *Yoga and the Living Tradition of Krishnamacharya*. Chennai: Aperture Foundation Inc., 1998.

Devananda, Swami Viṣṇu. *Haṭha-yoga-pradīpikā*. Canada: Motilal Banarsidass Publishers and Om Lotus Publications, 1987. As written down in the 17th century from ancient sources by Yogi Swatmarama.

Frawley, David. *Yoga & Ayurveda*. USA: Lotus Press, 1999.

Gheranda-saṁhitā. Munshiram Manoharlal Publishers, 1999. Translated by Rai Bahadur Shrisha Candra Vasu from the first edition. Delhi: 1914.

Iyengar, B.K.S. *Light on Yoga*. Pune: Harper Collins, India, 1966.

Javanainen, Juha. *Bockin Perheen Saaga, Väinämöisen Mytologia*. Ior Bock, Finland: Synchronicity Publications, 1996.

Krishnamacharya, Tirumalai. *Yoga-makaranda* (1934). Revised ed. Chennai: Media Garuda, 2011.

Krishnamacharya, T. and T.K.V Desikachar. *Yoga-rahasya*. Chennai: Krishnamacharya Yoga Mandiram, 1998.

van Lysebeth, Andre. *Tantra: The Cult of the Feminine*. Boston: Samuel Weiser, 1995.

van Lysebeth, Andre. *Prāṇāyama: The Yoga of Breathing*. London: Unwin Paperbacks, 1979.

Miele, Lino. *Ashtanga Yoga under the guidance of Śrī K. Pattabhi Jois.* Mysore: self-published by author, 1994.

Mohan, A.G. *Krishnamacharya: His Life and Teachings*. Shambhala Publications: USA, 2010.

Namapura, periodical. 2004–2008 and on-line issues 2009–2013

Pattabhi Jois, Śrī K. *Yoga-mala*. Mysore: self-published by author, 1962. 1st English ed. New York: Eddie Stern/Patanjali Yoga Shala, 1999, 2002.

Pattanaik, Dr. Devdutt. *Mith = Mithya, A Handbook of Hindu Mythology*. New Delhi: Penguin Books, 2006.

Prasad, Ramananda. *The Bhagavad-Gītā*. 2nd ed. Delhi: Motilal Banarsidass Publishers, 1996.

Ramaswami, Srivatsa. *The Complete Book of Vinyāsa Yoga*. New York: Marlowe & Company, 2005.

Ramaswami, Srivatsa & David Hurwitz. *Yoga Beneath the Surface.* New York: Marlowe & Company, 2006

Scott, John. *Ashtanga Yoga*. London: Gaia Books Ltd., 2000

Śaṅkarācārya, Ādī. *Yoga Tārāvalī.* Chennai: Krishnamacharya Yoga Mandiram, 2003. Written in the 7th century. Translated by and with commentary from T.K.V. Desikachar and Kausthub Desikachar.

Stern, Eddie and Deirdre Summerbell. *A Tribute*. Mysore & New York: published by Eddie Stern and Gwyneth Paltrow, 2002.

Śiva Samhita. Munshiram Manoharlal Publishers, 1999. Translated by Rai Bahadur Shrisha Candra Vasu from 1st ed. Delhi, 1914.

Svoboda, Robert E. *Prakṛti. Your Ayurvedic Constitution.* Albuquerque: Lotus Press, 1989.

Verma, Vinod. *Kāma Sutra for Women*. Kodansha America Inc, 1997, and Penguin Books India, 2000.

Zimmer, Heinrich. *Philosophies of India*. USA: Princeton University Press, 1951. (Heinrich Zimmer 1890–1943. A posthumous book completed by Joseph Campbell).

The World's Best Anatomical Charts. USA: Anatomical Chart Company, 1993.

acknowledgements

Warm thanks goes to my family, friends and students, and to all those who read this book and help spread the teachings of yoga.

I would like to sincerely thank the following people who have contributed to the making of this book, and who have supported my passion for yoga.

My guru
Śrī K. Pattabhi Jois

My teachers
R. Sharath Jois, Tove Palmgren, Derek Ireland, Lino Miele, Eddie Stern

Contributors
Sanskrit Devanagaris, Mantra transliteration and pronunciation chart – **Måns Broo**
English Editor – **Wambui Njuguna**
Photograph of "Gurujī and Sharath" – **Jenni Banerjee**
Photograph of "Gurujī and Petri" – **Ilaria Perra**
Assistant Photo Editor – **Erica Fae**

Thank you to Ammaji (Savitramma Jois), Saraswati Jois, my first haṭha-yoga teacher Alexander Takis, Radha Warrell, Tina Pizzimenti, Gwendoline Hunt, Manju Jois, John Campbell, Juha Javanainen, Joseph Dunham, Ior Bock, Richard Freeman, Noah Williams, Nancy Gilgoff, Alex Medin, Govinda Kai, Guy Donahaye, Jeff Lewis, Janne Kontala, Timo Kiiskinen, and folk-healers, Raimo Holtti and Heikki Nurminen for their beneficial teachings, encouragement and kind-heartedness.

I am especially grateful for my lovely Wambui, for editing the book and for her endurance and support.

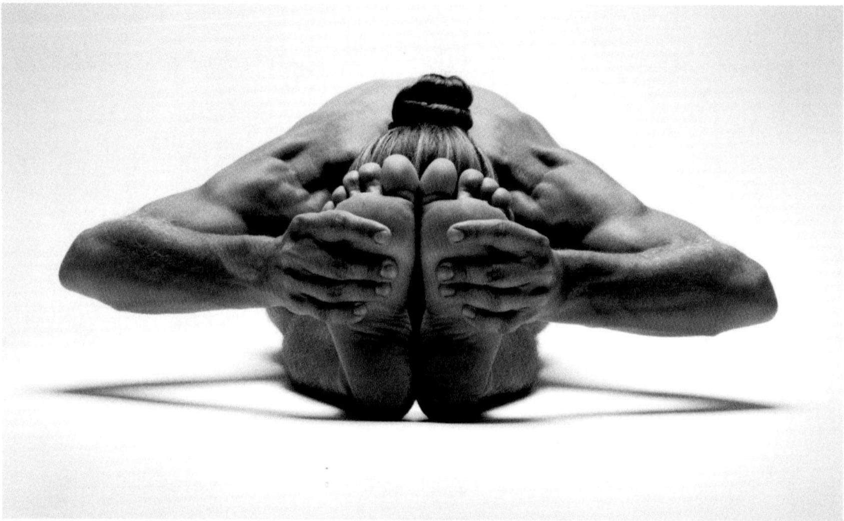

Photographs by Alexander Berg